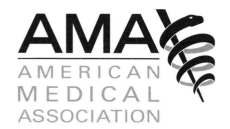

BASIC DISASTER LIFE SUPPORT™

v.3.0

Course Manual

Editors-in-Chief

Raymond E. Swienton, MD

Italo Subbarao, DO, MBA

Deputy Editor

David S. Markenson, MD, MBA

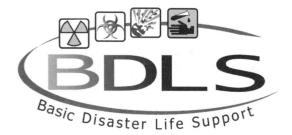

Executive Vice President, Chief Executive Officer: James L. Madara, MD
Chief Operating Officer: Bernard L. Hengesbaugh
Senior Vice President, Publishing and Business Services: Robert A. Musacchio, PhD
Vice President, Business Operations: Vanessa Hayden
Vice President, Publications and Clinical Solutions: Mary Lou White
Senior Acquisitions Editor: Janet Thron
Manager, Book and Product Development and Production: Nancy Baker
Senior Developmental Editor: Michael Ryder
Production Specialist: Meghan Anderson
Director, Sales, Marketing and Strategic Relationships: Joann Skiba
Director, Sales Business Products: Mark Daniels
Director, Marketing: Erin Kalitowsk
Marketing Manager: Lori Hollacher

© 2012 by the American Medical Association
All rights reserved.
Printed in the United States of America

No part of this publication may be reproduced, stored in a retrieval system, or transmitted, in any form or by any means electronic, mechanical, photocopying, recording, or otherwise, without the prior written permission of the publisher.

Internet address: www.ama-assn.org

The American Medical Association ("AMA") and its authors and editors have consulted sources believed to be knowledgeable in their fields. However, neither the AMA nor its authors or editors warrant that the information is in every respect accurate and/or complete. The AMA, its authors, and editors assume no responsibility for use of the information contained in this publication. Neither the AMA, its authors, or editors shall be responsible for, and expressly disclaims liability for, damages of any kind arising out of the use of, reference to, or reliance on the content of this publication. This publication is for informational purposes only. The AMA does not provide medical, legal, financial, or other professional advice and readers are encouraged to consult a professional advisor for such advice.

The contents of this publication represent the views of the author(s) and should not be construed to be the views or policy of the AMA, or of the institution with which the author(s) may be affiliated, unless this is clearly specified.

Additional copies of this book may be ordered by calling 800 621-8335 or from the secure AMA Web site at www.amabookstore.com. Refer to product number OP426610.

Core Disaster Life Support®, CDLS®, and PRE-DISASTER Paradigm™ are trademarks of the American Medical Association.
Advanced Disaster Life Support™, ADLS®, Basic Disaster Life Support™, BDLS®, DISASTER Paradigm™, National Disaster Life Support™, and NDLSF™ are trademarks of the National Disaster Life Support Foundation, Inc.

BP09:11-P-038:03/12
ISBN 978-1-60359-207-9

CONTENTS

Preface   xiii

Acknowledgments   xv

About the Editors   xvii

About the Contributing Editor and Contributors   xix

Reviewers   xxv

Course Objectives   xxvii

CHAPTER | **ONE**

All-Hazards Disaster Casualty Management

1.1   Purpose   1-1

1.2   Learning Objectives   1-2

1.3   Background   1-2

1.4   Definitions and Taxonomy   1-4

　　1.4.1 The PRE-DISASTER Paradigm™   1-5

　　1.4.2 The DISASTER Paradigm™   1-6

1.5   Health-Related Considerations in Disaster Planning   1-8

　　1.5.1 Risk Analysis   1-10

　　1.5.2 Population Vulnerability Assessment   1-10

　　1.5.3 Health System Surge Planning   1-12

　　1.5.4 Legal and Ethical Planning Considerations   1-13

　　1.5.5 Exercises and Drills   1-13

1.6   Health-Related Considerations in Disaster Response   1-14

　　1.6.1 Situational Awareness and Detection   1-14

　　1.6.2 Hazard Assessment   1-16

　　1.6.3 Incident Management   1-17

　　　　1.6.3.1 Emergency Operations Center   1-18

　　　　1.6.3.2 Disaster Communications   1-18

　　　　1.6.3.3 Logistical Support Services   1-19

　　　　1.6.3.4 Disaster Forensics   1-20

　　1.6.4 Health Care Facility Surge Management   1-20

　　　　1.6.4.1 Space, Staff, and Supplies   1-21

　　　　1.6.4.2 Surge-Based Health Care Facilities   1-23

1.7   Recovery and Beyond   1-25

　　1.7.1 Continuity of Operations in Health Care Facilities   1-25

　　1.7.2 After-Action Review   1-26

　　1.7.3 Preparation and Planning for Future Events   1-27

　　1.7.4 Building Community Readiness and Resilience for Future Events   1-28

1.8   Summary   1-29

1.9   Discussion Points   1-30

　　References   1-32

CHAPTER | **TWO**

Public Health Response to Disasters

2.1   Purpose   2-1

2.2   Learning Objectives   2-1

2.3   Background   2-2

2.4   The Public Health System   2-2

2.5 Public Health Agencies and Organizations   2-4

2.5.1 Local Health Agencies   2-4

2.5.2 State Health Agencies   2-5

2.5.3 Federal Health Agencies   2-5

2.5.4 Nongovernmental Organizations (NGOs) and Private Governmental Organizations (PGOs)   2-6

2.5.5 Global Health Agencies and Organizations   2-7

2.6 Public Health Role in Disaster Response   2-8

2.6.1 Emergency Public Health Powers   2-9

2.6.2 Epidemiologic Surveillance and Investigation   2-11

2.6.3 Enhanced Public Health Reporting   2-14

2.6.4 Incident Management   2-15

2.6.4.1 Health System Integration   2-15

2.6.4.2 Multiagency Coordination   2-16

2.6.5 Crisis and Emergency Risk Communication   2-17

2.6.6 Community Evacuation Considerations   2-18

2.6.7 Population-Based Surge Management   2-19

2.6.8 Communicable Disease Prevention and Control   2-22

2.6.9 Laboratory Services   2-23

2.6.10 Mass Care Services   2-24

2.6.11 Environmental Health Services   2-24

2.7 Recovery and Beyond   2-25

2.8 Summary   2-26

2.9 Discussion Points   2-27

References   2-29

CHAPTER | **THREE**

Population Health and Mental Health in Disasters

3.1 Purpose   3-1

3.2 Learning Objectives   3-1

3.3 Background   3-2

3.4 Children and Disasters   3-2

3.4.1 Pediatric Vulnerabilities in Disasters   3-3

3.4.1.1 Anatomic Considerations   3-3

3.4.1.2 Physiologic Considerations   3-5

3.4.1.3 Immunologic Considerations   3-5

3.4.1.4 Developmental Considerations   3-6

3.4.1.5 Mental and Behavioral Health Considerations   3-6

3.4.2 Pediatric Casualty Care   3-6

3.4.2.1 Communicating with Children   3-7

3.4.2.2 Communicating with Parents   3-8

3.4.2.3 Decontamination   3-8

3.4.2.4 Pediatric Medications, Equipment, and Supplies   3-9

3.4.3 Family Identification and Reunification   3-9

3.4.4 Pediatric Health Challenges   3-10

3.4.4.1 Lodging and Shelter   3-11

3.4.4.2 Environmental Health, Nutrition, and Communicable Disease Control   3-11

3.4.4.3 Children with Chronic Illness and Injury   3-12

3.4.4.4 Pediatric Health Care Access in Disasters   3-12

3.4.4.5 Child Maltreatment   3-13

3.4.5 Pediatrics, First Responders, and First Receivers   3-13

3.5 Women's Health in Disasters   3-13

3.6 People with Chronic Illness in Disasters   3-16

3.6.1 Medical and Health Record Access   3-16

3.6.2 Medical Care Access   3-17

3.6.3 Planning Considerations   3-17

3.7 People with Functional and Access Needs in Disasters   3-18

3.7.1 Definitions   3-19

3.7.2 Communication Challenges   3-20

3.7.3 Evacuation Challenges   3-21

3.7.4 Sheltering Considerations   3-22

3.7.5 Health Care Considerations   3-23

3.8 Mental and Behavioral Health in Disasters   3-25

3.8.1 Planning Goals and Priorities   3-26

3.8.2 Stress and Psychological Trauma   3-27

3.8.3 Mental Health Disorders and Syndromes Associated with Disasters   3-28

3.8.4 Mental Health Considerations for Adults   3-31

3.8.4.1 Psychological Triage   3-31

3.8.4.2 Psychological First Aid (PFA)   3-32

3.8.4.3 Outreach and Information Dissemination   3-33

3.8.4.4 Technical Assistance, Consultation, and Training   3-33

3.8.4.5 Treatment   3-34

3.8.4.6 Implications for the Emergency Response Workforce   3-34

3.8.5 Mental Health Considerations for Children and Adolescents   3-35

3.9 Summary   3-36

References   3-36

CHAPTER | **FOUR**

Workforce Readiness and Disaster Deployment

4.1 Purpose   4-1

4.2 Learning Objectives   4-2

4.3 Background   4-2

4.4 Predeployment Preparation and Planning   4-3

4.4.1 Volunteerism and Team Membership   4-4

4.4.2 Maintaining Deployment Readiness Status   4-4

4.4.3 Personal Health and Wellness   4-7

4.4.4 Personal Equipment and Packing   4-8

4.4.5 Professional Credentials and Equipment   4-9

4.4.6 Predeployment Education and Training   4-9

4.4.7 Legal Issues for Volunteer Health Responders   4-11

4.4.7.1 Professional Liability   4-11

4.4.7.2 Scope of Practice   4-12

4.5 Personal Risk Awareness and Mitigation   4-13

4.6 Workforce Activation and Mobilization   4-15

4.7 Workforce Protection   4-16

4.7.1 Disaster Scene Exclusion Zones   4-17

4.7.2 Selection and Use of PPE   4-18

4.7.2.1 PPE Levels   4-20

4.7.2.2 PPE Challenges   4-21

4.8 Casualty Decontamination   4-22

4.8.1 Types of Decontamination   4-22

4.8.2 Special Decontamination Considerations   4-23

4.9 Workforce Demobilization and Deployment-Related Stress   4-25

4.10 Summary   4-26

References   4-27

CHAPTER | **FIVE**

Mass Casualty and Fatality Management

5.1 Purpose   5-1

5.2 Learning Objectives   5-2

5.3 Background   5-2

5.4 General Principles of Mass Casualty Triage   5-3

5.4.1 Mass Casualty Triage Systems   5-5

5.4.2 Limitations of Triage Systems   5-7

5.4.3 Triage Categories   5-7

    5.4.3.1 Immediate (Red) Triage Category   5-8

    5.4.3.2 Delayed (Yellow) Triage Category   5-8

    5.4.3.3 Minimal (Green) Triage Category   5-8

    5.4.3.4 Expectant (Gray) Triage Category   5-8

    5.4.3.5 Dead (Black) Triage Category   5-9

5.4.4 Triage Tags and Casualty Care Documentation   5-11

5.5 SALT Mass Casualty Triage Methodology   5-12

5.5.1 SALT Step 1: Global Sorting   5-13

5.5.2 SALT Step 2: Individual Assessment   5-13

5.6 Casualty Assessment   5-15

5.6.1 Primary Assessment   5-15

5.6.2 Secondary Assessment   5-18

    5.6.2.1 Casualty History   5-18

    5.6.2.2 Casualty Physical Examination   5-19

5.6.3 Implications of PPE for Casualty Management   5-19

5.7 Casualty Transport and Evacuation   5-19

5.8 Mass Fatality Management   5-20

5.8.1 Mass Fatality Event Definition   5-22

5.8.2 Field Fatality Management   5-22

5.8.3 Morgue Operations   5-22

5.8.4 Provider and Survivor Management   5-23

5.9 Casualty Reporting, Identification, and Tracking   5-24

5.9.1 Casualty Reporting   5-24

5.9.2 Casualty Identification and Tracking   5-24

5.10 Professionalism and Ethics in Mass Casualty Care   5-25

5.11 Summary   5-27

References   5-28

CHAPTER | SIX

Explosions and Traumatic Disasters

6.1 Purpose   6-1

6.2 Learning Objectives   6-2

6.3 Background   6-2

6.4 Types of Explosions   6-3

6.4.1 Nuclear Explosion   6-3

6.4.2 Mechanical Explosion   6-3

6.4.3 Chemical Explosion   6-4

6.5 Mechanisms of Blast Injury   6-6

6.5.1 Primary Blast Injury   6-6

6.5.2 Secondary Blast Injury   6-7

6.5.3 Tertiary Blast Injury   6-8

6.5.4 Quaternary Blast Injury   6-8

6.6 Situational Awareness and Detection   6-9

6.7 Clinical Decision Making   6-10

6.7.1 Lifesaving Skills   6-11

6.7.2 Pulmonary Blast Injury   6-11

6.7.3 Arterial Gas Embolism   6-12

6.7.4 Traumatic Asphyxiation   6-13

6.7.5 Traumatic Amputation   6-14

6.7.6 Crush Injury   6-15

6.7.7 Compartment Syndrome   6-16

6.7.8 Gastrointestinal Blast Injury   6-17

6.7.9 Auditory Blast Injury   6-17

6.7.10 Ocular Blast Injury   6-17

6.7.11 Flash Burns   6-18

6.7.12 Blunt Ballistic Injury   6-18

6.7.13 Penetrating Ballistic Injury   6-19

6.7.14 Penetrating Stab or Impaling Injury   6-20

6.8 Public Health Considerations   6-20

6.9 Mental Health Considerations   6-20

6.10 Pediatric Considerations   6-21

6.11 Summary 6-21

6.12 Discussion Points 6-22

References 6-24

CHAPTER | **SEVEN**
Nuclear and Radiologic Disasters

7.1 Purpose 7-1

7.2 Learning Objectives 7-2

7.3 Background 7-2

7.4 Radiation Basics 7-3

7.4.1 Radiation Measurement Terms and Units 7-4

7.4.2 Radiation Exposure and Contamination 7-5

7.4.3 Biologic Consequences of Radiation Exposure 7-5

7.5 Characteristic Injuries After Nuclear and Radiologic Disasters 7-6

7.5.1 Trauma Injuries 7-6

7.5.2 Thermal Burns 7-6

7.5.3 Radiation Toxicity 7-7

7.5.4 Electromagnetic Pulse 7-8

7.6 Situational Awareness and Detection 7-8

7.6.1 Scene Assessment 7-8

7.6.2 Radiation Detection Technology 7-9

7.7 Hazard Assessment 7-9

7.8 Incident Management Challenges 7-11

7.8.1 Radiation Field Determination 7-11

7.8.2 Logistical Support Services 7-12

7.8.3 Personnel Shortages 7-13

7.8.4 Information Sharing 7-13

7.8.5 Media Cooperation 7-14

7.9 Workforce Protection 7-14

7.9.1 Scene Safety and Security 7-15

7.9.2 Personal Protective Equipment (PPE) 7-16

7.9.3 Radiation Exposure Monitoring 7-17

7.9.4 Casualty Decontamination 7-18

7.10 Casualty Management 7-19

7.10.1 Mass Casualty Triage 7-19

7.10.2 Casualty Transport to Receiving Facilities 7-20

7.11 Clinical Management of Radiation Casualties: Basic Concepts and Principles 7-21

7.11.1 Clinical Clues to Radiation Exposure 7-22

7.11.2 Patient Assessment and Clinical Decision Making 7-23

7.11.3 Trauma Care 7-25

7.11.4 Diagnostic Testing 7-26

7.11.5 Therapeutic Interventions 7-27

7.11.6 Altered Care Environment 7-27

7.12 Management of Acute Radiation Syndrome (ARS) 7-28

7.12.1 Treatment of Emesis and Diarrhea 7-30

7.12.2 Infection Control 7-31

7.12.3 Cytokine Therapy 7-31

7.12.4 Stem Cell Transplants 7-32

7.13 Cutaneous Radiation Syndrome (CRS) 7-32

7.14 Management of Internal Radioisotope Contamination 7-33

7.14.1 Isotope Determination 7-33

7.14.2 Decorporation Techniques and Countermeasures 7-34

7.15 Public Health Implications of Nuclear and Radiologic Disasters 7-37

7.15.1 Crisis and Emergency Risk Communication 7-37

7.15.2 Mental and Behavioral Health Considerations 7-38

7.15.3 People with Functional, Access, or Other Special Needs 7-38

7.15.4 Age-Related Vulnerabilities 7-39

7.15.5 Risk to Pregnant Women and Fetuses 7-39

7.15.6 Population Monitoring 7-40

7.16 Summary   7-41

7.17 Discussion Points   7-43

References   7-45

CHAPTER | **EIGHT**
Chemical Disasters

8.1 Purpose   8-1

8.2 Learning Objectives   8-1

8.3 Background   8-2

8.3.1 Chemical Emergencies   8-2

8.3.2 Chemical Disasters   8-3

8.4 Situational Awareness and Detection   8-3

8.4.1 Chemical Exposure Clues   8-4

8.4.2 Chemical Detection Devices   8-6

8.5 Incident Management and Workforce Protection   8-7

8.6 General Casualty Management Considerations   8-8

8.6.1 Triage Considerations   8-9

8.6.2 Casualty Assessment   8-10

8.6.3 Treatment Principles for Chemical Casualties   8-12

8.7 Clinical Management of Selected Chemical Agents   8-12

8.7.1 Blister Agents (Vesicants)   8-13

8.7.1.1 Blister Agent (Vesicant) Pathophysiology   8-13

8.7.1.2 Diagnosis of Blister Agent (Vesicant) Exposure   8-14

8.7.1.3 Blister Agent (Vesicant) Treatment Considerations   8-14

8.7.2 Choking/Pulmonary Agents   8-17

8.7.2.1 Pathophysiology of Choking or Pulmonary Agents   8-17

8.7.2.2 Diagnosis of Exposure to Choking or Pulmonary Agents   8-18

8.7.2.3 Treatment Considerations for Choking or Pulmonary Agents   8-19

8.7.3 Cyanide Agents   8-19

8.7.3.1 Cyanide Pathophysiology   8-20

8.7.3.2 Diagnosis of Cyanide Exposure   8-23

8.7.3.3 Cyanide Treatment Considerations   8-24

8.7.4 Nerve Agents   8-26

8.7.4.1 Nerve Agent Pathophysiology   8-27

8.7.4.2 Diagnosis of Nerve Agent Exposure   8-27

8.7.4.3 Nerve Agent Treatment Considerations   8-28

8.8 Pediatric Treatment Considerations   8-33

8.9 Selected Large-Scale Chemical Disasters: Learning From Experience   8-35

8.9.1 Bhopal, India (1984)   8-35

8.9.2 Tokyo Sarin Subway Attack (1995)   8-35

8.9.3 British Petroleum Oil Spill, Gulf of Mexico (2010)   8-36

8.10 Summary   8-37

8.11 Discussion Points   8-38

References   8-40

CHAPTER | **NINE**
Biologic Disasters

9.1 Purpose   9-1

9.2 Learning Objectives   9-2

9.3 Background   9-2

9.4 Basics of Infectious Disease Exposure and Transmission   9-2

9.5 Types of Biologic Disasters   9-5

9.5.1 Epidemics and Pandemics   9-6

9.5.2 Bioterrorism   9-6

9.6 Characteristics of Biologic Agents   9-7

9.7 Situational Awareness and Detection   9-9

9.8 Clinical Decision Making   9-10

9.8.1 Public Health Notification   9-11

9.8.2 Transmission-Based Infection Control   9-12

9.8.3 Triage   9-13

9.8.4 Clinical Assessment and Diagnosis   9-13

9.8.5 Therapeutic Interventions   9-14

9.9 Biologic Agent–Specific Issues   9-14

9.9.1 Anthrax *(Bacillus anthracis)*   9-15

9.9.1.1 General   9-15

9.9.1.2 Clinical Features   9-15

9.9.1.3 Diagnosis   9-16

9.9.1.4 Treatment   9-17

9.9.1.5 Prophylaxis   9-17

9.9.1.6 Infection Control   9-18

9.9.2 Botulism *(Clostridium botulinum* Toxin)   9-18

9.9.2.1 General   9-18

9.9.2.2 Clinical Features   9-18

9.9.2.3 Diagnosis   9-19

9.9.2.4 Treatment   9-19

9.9.2.5 Prophylaxis   9-19

9.9.2.6 Infection Control   9-20

9.9.3 Pneumonic Plague *(Yersina pestis)*   9-20

9.9.3.1 General   9-20

9.9.3.2 Clinical Features After a BT Attack   9-20

9.9.3.3 Diagnosis   9-20

9.9.3.4 Treatment   9-21

9.9.3.5 Prophylaxis   9-21

9.9.3.6 Infection Control   9-21

9.9.4 Severe Acute Respiratory Syndrome (SARS)   9-22

9.9.4.1 General   9-22

9.9.4.2 Clinical Features   9-22

9.9.4.3 Diagnosis   9-22

9.9.4.4 Treatment   9-23

9.9.4.5 Prophylaxis   9-23

9.9.4.6 Infection Control   9-23

9.9.5 Smallpox *(Variola major)*   9-23

9.9.5.1 General   9-23

9.9.5.2 Clinical Features   9-24

9.9.5.3 Diagnosis   9-25

9.9.5.4 Treatment   9-25

9.9.5.5 Prophylaxis   9-26

9.9.5.6 Infection Control   9-26

9.9.6 Tularemia *(Francisella tularensis)*   9-26

9.9.6.1 General   9-26

9.9.6.2 Clinical Features   9-26

9.9.6.3 Diagnosis   9-26

9.9.6.4 Treatment   9-27

9.9.6.5 Prophylaxis   9-27

9.9.6.6 Infection Control   9-27

9.9.7 Viral Hemorrhagic Fevers (VHFs)   9-28

9.9.7.1 General   9-28

9.9.7.2 Clinical Features   9-28

9.9.7.3 Diagnosis   9-28

9.9.7.4 Treatment   9-29

9.9.7.5 Prophylaxis   9-29

9.9.7.6 Isolation   9-29

9.9.8 Clinical Considerations for Pediatric Casualties   9-30

9.10 Public Health Actions in a BT Attack   9-32

9.10.1 Threat Assessment   9-33

9.10.2 Medical Countermeasures and Point-of-Distribution Access   9-33

9.11 Summary   9-34

9.12 Discussion Points   9-35

References   9-37

CHAPTER | TEN

Natural Disasters

10.1 Purpose   10-1

10.2 Learning Objectives   10-2

10.3 Background   10-2

10.4 Natural Disaster–Specific Considerations   10-3

   10.4.1 Situational Awareness   10-4

   10.4.2 Health Facility Expansion of Surge Capability   10-5

10.5 Casualty Management   10-5

10.6 Earthquakes and Tsunamis   10-8

   10.6.1 Causes and Characteristics   10-9

   10.6.2 Early Detection and Warning Systems   10-10

   10.6.3 Acute Hazards and Effects   10-11

   10.6.4 Clinical Implications: Immediate and Long Term   10-11

   10.6.5 Public Health Considerations   10-12

   10.6.6 Prevention and Mitigation of Future Events   10-14

10.7 Floods   10-14

   10.7.1 Causes and Characteristics   10-14

   10.7.2 Early Detection and Warning Systems   10-15

   10.7.3 Acute Hazards and Effects   10-16

   10.7.4 Clinical Implications: Immediate and Long Term   10-16

   10.7.5 Public Health Considerations   10-17

   10.7.6 Prevention and Mitigation of Future Events   10-17

10.8 Heat Emergencies   10-18

   10.8.1 Causes and Characteristics   10-18

   10.8.2 Early Detection and Warning Systems   10-18

   10.8.3 Acute Hazards and Effects   10-19

   10.8.4 Clinical Implications: Immediate and Long Term   10-19

   10.8.5 Public Health Considerations   10-20

   10.8.6 Prevention and Mitigation of Future Events   10-20

10.9 Hurricanes, Cyclones, and Typhoons   10-21

   10.9.1 Causes and Characteristics   10-21

   10.9.2 Early Detection and Warning Systems   10-22

   10.9.3 Acute Hazards and Effects   10-22

   10.9.4 Clinical Implications: Immediate and Long Term   10-23

   10.9.5 Public Health Considerations   10-25

   10.9.6 Prevention and Mitigation of Future Events   10-26

10.10 Tornadoes   10-26

   10.10.1 Causes and Characteristics   10-27

   10.10.2 Early Detection and Warning Systems   10-28

   10.10.3 Acute Hazards and Effects   10-29

   10.10.4 Clinical Implications: Immediate and Long Term   10-29

   10.10.5 Public Health Considerations   10-29

   10.10.6 Prevention and Mitigation of Future Events   10-30

10.11 Volcanic Eruptions   10-30

   10.11.1 Causes and Characteristics   10-31

   10.11.2 Early Detection and Warning Systems   10-32

   10.11.3 Acute Hazards and Effects   10-32

   10.11.4 Clinical Implications: Immediate and Long Term   10-33

   10.11.5 Public Health Considerations   10-35

   10.11.6 Prevention and Mitigation of Future Events   10-35

10.12 Wildfires   10-35

   10.12.1 Causes and Characteristics   10-35

   10.12.2 Early Detection and Warning Systems   10-36

   10.12.3 Acute Hazards and Effects   10-36

   10.12.4 Clinical Implications: Immediate and Long Term   10-37

10.12.5 Public Health Considerations   10-37

10.12.6 Prevention and Mitigation of Future Events   10-38

10.13 Winter Storms   10-38

10.13.1 Causes and Characteristics   10-39

10.13.2 Early Detection and Warning Systems   10-39

10.13.3 Acute Hazards and Effects   10-40

10.13.4 Clinical Implications: Immediate and Long Term   10-40

10.13.5 Public Health Considerations   10-41

10.13.6 Prevention and Mitigation of Future Events   10-41

10.14 Summary   10-41

10.15 Discussion Points   10-42

References   10-44

Appendices

Appendix A: PRE-DISASTER Paradigm™ and DISASTER Paradigm™   A-A1

Appendix B: Competencies for Health Professionals in Disaster Medicine and Public Health Preparedness Addressed in the BDLS® v.3.0 Course Manual and Course Objective Linkage   A-B1

Appendix C: List of Acronyms and Abbreviations   A-C1

Glossary   G-1

Index   I-1

PREFACE

The potential for tremendous numbers of casualties from disasters and public health emergencies demand that we have a health and medical workforce that is well prepared, ready to serve, and willing to engage when needed. The Basic Disaster Life Support™ (BDLS®) course (v.3.0) and supporting course manual are competency-based and designed to teach "basic" concepts and "all-hazards" principles to help learners manage disaster-related injuries and illnesses, as well as mass casualty and population-based care, across a broad range of disasters. The overarching theme that captures the essence of BDLS® (v.3.0) is disaster casualty management.

BDLS® is an awareness-level course, which is aimed at the broad range of audiences that share a common likelihood of providing health care and assistance in a disaster or public health emergency. This includes health care, public health, and allied health professionals; emergency medical services personnel; and all medical first responders and receivers. It builds upon information presented in the Core Disaster Life Support® course (v.3.0) and prepares the learner for the Advanced Disaster Life Support™ course (v.3.0), thus integrating a standardized curriculum throughout the National Disaster Life Support™ family of courses.

The BDLS® course manual is refreshing and exciting, containing timely and comprehensive updates of the previous edition, as well as new content areas. This includes updated and redesigned chapters on public health, population health, and mental health. New and expanded topics include situational awareness, workforce safety and readiness, disaster deployment, surge capacity management, mass casualty triage and management, crisis standards of care, and mass fatality management. It is both a resource that supports the course, as well as a reference, containing expanded subject matter, summary tables, and comprehensive citation listings.

The BDLS® course and supporting course manual have been developed by—and for—members of our health and medical workforce, in whom the casualties of the future will entrust their lives. We invite you to take the course, read this manual, and trust that you will agree that BDLS® is a valuable resource in preparing for disaster casualty management.

Raymond E. Swienton, MD
Co-Editor-in-Chief, Basic Disaster Life Support™ Version 3.0

Italo Subbarao, DO, MBA
Co-Editor-in-Chief, Basic Disaster Life Support™ Version 3.0

ACKNOWLEDGMENTS

The editors acknowledge the contributions toward the development of BDLS® v.3.0 made by the other NDLS™ course editors:

Phillip L. Coule, MD
John A. Mitas II, MD
John H. Armstrong, MD
Richard B. Schwartz, MD

CONTRIBUTING EDITOR
Jim Lyznicki, MS, MPH

The American Medical Association and the National Disaster Life Support Foundation, Inc., extend sincere appreciation to the founding authors and editors of the NDLS™ course curricula for their continued vision and leadership in advancing and promoting excellence in education and training of all health care professionals in disaster medicine and public health preparedness:

Phillip L. Coule, MD
Cham E. Dallas, PhD
James J. James, MD, DrPH, MHA
Scott Lillibridge, MD
Paul E. Pepe, MD, MPH
Richard B. Schwartz, MD
Raymond E. Swienton, MD

Developed in collaboration with:

The National Disaster Life Support Education Consortium™
Medical College of Georgia
University of Texas Southwestern Medical Center at Dallas
University of Texas School of Public Health at Houston
University of Georgia

ABOUT THE EDITORS

About the Editors-in-Chief

Raymond E. Swienton, MD, is is associate professor of emergency medicine and director of the Section of Emergency Medical Services, Homeland Security and Disaster Medicine at the University of Texas Southwestern Medical Center at Dallas. Dr Swienton is one of the original creators of the National Disaster Life Support™ (NDLS™) series of courses. He is one of the founding and current board members of the National Disaster Life Support Foundation, Inc., and the Executive Committee of the National Disaster Life Support Educational Consortium™.

Dr Swienton began his career in emergency medicine and disaster medicine as an EMT-paramedic, and as a physician board certified in emergency medicine has continued his dedication to these disciplines through clinical practice, operational deployments, publications, and educational training program development world-wide. His commitment to medical education and passion for teaching is conveyed in the phrase "See one, do one, teach…many."

Italo Subbarao, DO, MBA, is the director of the Public Health Readiness Office at the American Medical Association Center for Public Health Preparedness and Disaster Response; the deputy editor of the journal *Disaster Medicine and Public Health Preparedness*, an official AMA publication; and the medical director for the NDLS™ Program Office. Dr Subbarao is a leader in domestic and international disaster response, including terrorism. He has provided field and technical support to the Haiti earthquake; the Mumbai shootings; Hurricanes Gustave, Ike, and Katrina; the Pakistan earthquake; the Virginia Tech mass casualty incident; the F-5 tornado that impacted Greensborough, Kansas; the San Diego wildfires; and the Iowa floods. He has published and edited more than 40 books and articles and has been an invited speaker to many domestic and international conferences and symposiums, including HHS-, CDC-, and NATO-sponsored events.

Dr Subbarao is a board-eligible emergency medicine physician and has completed additional fellowship training in disaster medicine at Johns Hopkins University. Dr Subbarao completed his emergency medicine residency training at Lehigh Valley Hospital-Muhlenberg, in Bethlehem, Pennsylvania, where he won three national resident research awards. He is a graduate of the Philadelphia College of Osteopathic Medical School joint DO/MBA program in health care administration.

About the Deputy Editor

David S. Markenson, MD, MBA, is the medical director for Disaster Medicine and Regional Emergency Services at Westchester Medical Center and director of the Center for Disaster Medicine at the School of Health Sciences and Practice at New York Medical College School of Public Health. Dr Markenson is the national chair of the American Red Cross Scientific Advisory Council. In additional to his hospital appointments, Dr Markenson is a professor of public health at the School of Public Health and professor of pediatrics at New York Medical College.

His career has been dedicated to improving the approach to pediatric care, disaster medicine, emergency medical services, and emergency medicine. He is the principal investigator on multiple federal grants related to pediatric disaster medicine, pediatric prehospital care, and pediatric emergency medicine. He recently created national emergency preparedness guidelines for pediatrics and persons with disabilities. Dr Markenson is a graduate of the Albert Einstein College of Medicine, Bronx, New York.

ABOUT THE CONTRIBUTING EDITOR AND CONTRIBUTORS

Contributing Editor

Jim Lyznicki, MS, MPH, is the associate director of the Center for Public Health Preparedness and Disaster Response at the American Medical Association. He holds master's degrees in medical microbiology and in environmental and occupational health. Prior to joining the AMA, he spent 10 years as a clinical microbiology laboratory supervisor at the University of Chicago Medical Center and the Rush Medical Center, and 2 years as an environmental health scientist at the University of Illinois School of Public Health.

Contributors

William Bell, PhD, is senior research scientist at the Institute for Health Management and Mass Destruction Defense at the University of Georgia. His work in weapons of mass destruction modeling has encompassed the detailed predictions of health effects from potential terrorist nuclear events for more than 40 cities in the United States and in the Middle East.

John Broach, MD, MPH, is assistant professor of emergency medicine and member of the Division of Disaster Medicine and Emergency Preparedness at the University of Massachusetts Medical School and UMass Memorial Medical Center in Worcester, Massachusetts. Dr Broach has experience as a disaster responder and teaches extensively about disaster preparedness and response strategies. John is also a member of the Massachusetts DMAT MA-2 and the Mobile Acute Care Strike Team program through the National Disaster Medical System.

Apryl R. Brown, MD, MPH, oversees the operations of the Detroit Medical Reserve Corps, which is headquartered out of the Office of the Surgeon General. At Wayne County Community College District, she is an adjunct biology professor. In the American Public Health Association, she serves on the education board and governing council, and she is a board of director for the Michigan Public Health Association Board.

Frederick M. Burkle, Jr, MD, MPH, DTM, is senior fellow and scientist, the Harvard Humanitarian Initiative, Harvard School of Public Health and senior associate faculty and research scientist at the Center for Refugee and Disaster Response, Johns Hopkins University Medical Institutes. He also served as a senior public policy scholar, Woodrow Wilson Center for International Scholars, Washington, DC.

Allen Cherson, DO, is assistant director of emergency medicine at Brookdale University Hospital and Medical Center in Brooklyn, New York. Prior to this he was deputy medical director for the Fire Department of New York. During his time with FDNY, Dr Cherson helped manage numerous major incidents, was responsible for training and field response and was one of the medical team managers for NYC USAR Task Force 1. He is residency trained in emergency medicine and fellowship trained in prehospital care. Dr Cherson is also an active participant in emergency medical services in both New York City and Nassau County, New York.

COL Ted Cieslak, MD, received his medical doctorate at Ohio State University and completed training in pediatrics at Baylor and in infectious diseases at Walter Reed. Following 9 years of clinical practice, Dr Cieslak went on to hold leadership roles at USAMRIID, the San Antonio Military Pediatric Center, the CDC, and the Army's Medical Command. He remains active in the area of bioterrorism defense and served as biodefense consultant to the Surgeon General.

Michael Colvard, DDS, is a periodontal surgeon and associate professor of oral medicine and diagnostics sciences, Department of Oral Medicine and Diagnostic Sciences, College of Dentistry, at the University of Illinois in Chicago (UIC). He is director of the Illinois Department of Public Health and UIC Dental, Dental Emergency Medicine Readiness Team (DEMRT) Office. Dr Colvard is a consultant for disaster response, Council on Dental Practice, American Dental Association.

Arthur Cooper, MD, MS, is professor of surgery at the Columbia University College of Physicians and Surgeons; director of trauma and pediatric surgical services at the Harlem Hospital Center; and affiliate faculty at the National Center for Disaster Preparedness of the Columbia University Mailman School of Public Health. He is a member of the Central Leadership Council of the New York City Pediatric Disaster Coalition and a founding member of the American Board of Disaster Medicine, with expertise in the fields of pediatric trauma, disaster medicine, and emergency preparedness.

Cham Dallas, PhD, is professor and director, Institute for Health Management and Mass Destruction Defense, at the College of Public Health, University of Georgia. Dr Dallas has more than 30 years of experience in weapons of mass destruction issues, including a decade of research on-site in Chernobyl, has published extensively, and served as principal investigator over the past decade for emergency response research and training.

Alexander Eastman, MD, MPH, is an assistant professor and trauma surgeon in the Division of Burns, Trauma and Critical Care at UT Southwestern Medical Center/Parkland Memorial Hospital. He is board certified in both general surgery and surgical critical care and has a Master's Degree in Public Health from the University of Texas Health Science Center–Houston. In addition, he is the deputy medical director of the Dallas Police Department (DPD), the lead medical officer for DPD SWAT, and a Dallas police officer.

Daniel B. Fagbuyi, MD, is the medical director of disaster preparedness and emergency management at Children's National Medical Center in Washington, DC. He is assistant professor of pediatrics and emergency medicine at the George Washington University School of Medicine and was recently appointed by the US Secretary of Health and Human Services, Kathleen Sebelius, to the National Biodefense Science Board. He is an advisor and subject matter expert instrumental in numerous national and local initiatives and committees.

George Gentile, RN, BSN, MPH, serves as the director of Emergency Preparedness and Continuity of Operations for HHS, Health Resources and Services Administration. Mr Gentile has expertise in public health system response and recovery planning and in emergency nursing.

Elin A. Gursky, ScD, MSc, is a corporate fellow in the Division of National Strategy Support of ANSER/Analytic Services, Inc, a not-for-profit research institute in Arlington, Virginia. Dr Gursky is an infectious disease epidemiologist with expertise in biodefense, health security, and public health systems and strategy for disease detection and outbreak control.

Alison Hayward, MD, has completed a fellowship in disaster medicine and emergency preparedness at the University of Massachusetts Memorial Medical Center and is currently an associate consultant in emergency medicine at the Mayo Clinic in Rochester, Minnesota. Dr Hayward also serves as the executive director of the Uganda Village Project. Her main interests include complex humanitarian disasters and global public health.

James J. James, MD, DrPH, MHA, is director of the American Medical Association (AMA) Center for Public Health Preparedness; editor-in-chief, *Disaster Medicine and Public Health Preparedness*; and reviewer on the HHS National Biodefense Science Board. Prior to joining the AMA, he served as the director of the Miami Dade County Health Department and served 26 years with the US Army Medical Department, his last assignment being commanding general of William Beaumont Army Medical Center in El Paso, Texas.

Seth C. Jones, NR-Paramedic, BS, is a paramedic field trainer with the Denver Health Paramedic Division. During his time at Denver Health, he brought the NDLS™ Regional Training Center to Denver; he has also developed and delivered curricula in disaster training, planning, and preparedness for providers within Denver Health and around the Rocky Mountain region.

Daniel Kirkpatrick, RN, MSN, is the associate director for workforce development at the National Center for Medical Readiness, Boonshoft School of Medicine, Wright State University. A retired Air Force colonel and nurse, Dan has extensive experience in medical readiness and disaster preparedness in both military and civilian environments.

Kelly R. Klein, MD, is the medical director for hospital emergency preparedness at the Eastern Maine Medical Center in Bangor, Maine. She is also a physician with Michigan-1 DMAT and has participated in many national disaster responses. She reviews for multiple journals, has been widely published, and has lectured extensively in the US and internationally on topics of disaster preparedness, response, and the psychosocial aspects of disasters.

J. Marc Liu, MD, MPH, is associate professor of emergency medicine at the Medical College of Wisconsin and serves as associate director of medical services for Milwaukee County Emergency Medical Services. Dr Liu has provided field medical support and technical advising for a number of local, state, and federal agencies, where he works to promote coordinated efforts in medical incident planning and response.

William Maliha, MD, served for seven years as medical director of the New York State Department of Health, Health Emergency Preparedness Program. He is board certified in both emergency medicine and family medicine and serves as affiliate faculty at the Columbia University, Mailman School of Public Health, National Center for Disaster Preparedness. Dr Maliha currently serves on the Expert Advisory Board for Global Emergency Resources, Inc. Previously, Dr Maliha served as full-time faculty for the Albany Medical Center Department of Emergency Medicine and has directed multiple emergency departments and psychiatric emergency departments over the span of his career. He is a member of the Alpha Omega Alpha Medical Honor Society.

Mary-Elise Manuell, MD, MA, is the director of the Division of Disaster Medicine and assistant professor of emergency medicine at the University of Massachusetts Medical School. She serves as director of the CEEPET (Center of Excellence in Emergency Preparedness Education and Training) at the medical school, chair of the Hospitals and Clinics Committee for the Worcester MMRS (Medical Metropolitan Response System), and cochair of the hospital disaster committee at UMass Memorial Medical Center.

Andrew Milsten, MD, MS, is with the Disaster Medicine Division at the University of Massachusetts Medical School, where he serves as the director of the Disaster Medicine Fellowship. Dr Milsten is an emergency medicine physician at UMass Memorial Medical Center and also the associate director of CEEPET (The Center of Excellence for Emergency Preparedness Education and Training). Dr Milsten has expertise in mass gathering medical care.

Steven J. Parrillo, DO, is the chair of the Albert Einstein Healthcare Network's Emergency Management Committee. He serves as medical director and faculty for the Philadelphia University Disaster Medicine and Management Masters Program, where he is an adjunct professor in the School of Science and Health. His publications include articles in emergency medicine journals, disaster journals, and textbooks. Dr Parrillo is also an associate professor of emergency medicine at both Jefferson Medical College and Philadelphia College of Osteopathic Medicine.

Glen I. Reeves, MD, MPH, is a principal scientist at Applied Research Associates, Inc., in Arlington, Virginia. He is board certified in therapeutic radiology and aerospace medicine. His expertise is in the medical effects of ionizing radiation from radiologic dispersal and exposure devices and nuclear weapons. He also provides input on the medical effects of chemical and biologic weapons.

Michael J. Reilly, DrPH, MPH, NREMT-P, CEM, is the director of planning and response at the National Center for Disaster Preparedness at Columbia University, Mailman School of Public Health. Dr Reilly was formerly assistant director of the Center for Disaster Medicine and assistant professor and director of the Graduate Program in Emergency Preparedness at New York Medical College. Dr Reilly has 15 years of experience in public safety, public health, and emergency planning and response, with a focus in worker safety and health system preparedness for disasters, terrorism, and public health emergencies.

Alessandra Rossodivita, MD, PhD, specialist in disaster medicine, is head of Semi-Intensive Cardiac Surgery Unit—San Raffaele Hospital Scientific Foundation—University of Medicine "Vita-Salute," Department of Cardiothoracic and Vascular Diseases. She has been a member of World Association of Disaster and Emergency Medicine (WADEM) since 2007 and of the public organization International Information Academy of Moscow (IIA), a public organization with general consultative status with the United Nations since 1995.

Charles Stewart, MD, MSc(DM), MPH, is a graduate of the European Master in Disaster Medicine program and is the director of the Oklahoma Disaster Institute and a professor of emergency medicine at the University of Oklahoma. He is the medical director for Oklahoma Task Force 1 (OKTF-1) Urban Search and Rescue unit. He is the author of numerous articles and books on disaster and emergency medicine.

Sandra Vyhlidal, MSN, RN, is emergency preparedness coordinator for Methodist and Methodist Women's Hospitals in Omaha, Nebraska. She is an active volunteer nurse for the Eastern Nebraska–Western Iowa Medical Reserve Corps (MRC) and deployed during the Katrina-Rita hurricane disaster. Sandra is a member of the Nebraska-1 Disaster Medical Assistance Team and Omaha Metropolitan Medical Response System. Sandra's nursing background includes medical-surgical, critical care, and infection prevention.

Michael Wainscott, MD, is the director for the Emergency Medicine Residency Program and a professor at the University of Texas Southwestern Medical Center at Dallas. Dr Wainscott has expertise in disaster management with a focus on disaster education and has helped establish emergency medicine residency programs and disaster medicine educational programs worldwide.

Lauren Walsh, MPH, is a research associate for the Center for Public Health Preparedness and Disaster Response (CPHPDR) at the American Medical Association. She earned her Master of Public Health degree in epidemiology from Columbia University and is currently pursuing her doctorate at the University of Illinois at Chicago. Prior to joining the AMA, she worked at Columbia University's National Center for Disaster Preparedness.

John C. White, CNMT, is the radiation safety officer for the VA North Texas Health Care System. He has been a certified nuclear medicine technologist since 1978 and is past president of the South Texas Chapter–Health Physics Society. Mr White is the founder and current chair of the North Texas Radiation Response Group. His professional experience includes work in the areas of radiologic emergency response, nuclear medicine, nuclear weapons effects engineering, reactor health physics, radioactive materials research, and radiation safety.

REVIEWERS

Chad Anspach, BS, AS, EMT-P
Indiana University Health

John H. Armstrong, MD
University of South Florida

Christine Bartholomew, BSN, RN
Columbus Community Hospital

Jamil Bayram, MD
Johns Hopkins University

Thomas Benzoni, DO, ABOEM
Mercy Air Care and *Iowa DMAT*

Edward Bottei, MD
Iowa Statewide Poison Control Center

Mona Bomgaars, MD, MPH
National Disaster Life Support Education Consortium™ Executive Committee

Apryl Brown, MD, MPH
Detroit Medical Reserve Corps

David Burich, MSN, APRN
Yale New Haven Health System

W. Thomas Burnett, MD
Virginia Tech Carilion School of Medicine and *The Carilion Clinic*

Stephen V. Cantrill, MD
Denver Health Medical Center

Ataf Chaudry, MD, EMT-P
Retired

Allen Cherson, DO
Brookdale University Hospital and Medical Center

Chester C. Clarke, MD, MPH, MA
American College of Preventive Medicine and *Exponent, Inc.*

Arthur Cooper, MD, MS
Columbia University

Robert L. Ditch, Colonel, USAF, Ret, EdD, CEM, NREMT-P
Synaptic Emergency Educational Services and
the George Washington University

Benjamin Godder, DMD
New York University College of Dentistry

Karen Hussey, RN
University of Missouri

Seth Jones, BS, NR-Paramedic
Denver Health

Howard Klausner, MD
Henry Ford Health System

AJ Kluthe, BS, EMS-I, NR-Paramedic
Center for Preparedness Education

George Kolo, DO
Kansas City University of Medicine and Biosciences

Corry Kucik, MD
US Navy

Thomas Lehman
University of Texas Southwestern Medical Center

Craig Llewellyn, MD, MDTM & H
Uniformed Services University of Health Sciences School of Medicine

John A. Mitas, II, MD
American College of Physicians

Paul E. Moore, MS, NREMT, CEM
University of Texas Southwestern Medical Center

Brandi Pond, MPH
Oologah-Talala EMS

John F. Ryan, CEM
Department of Defense, Fire and *Emergency Services*

Ann Sakaguchi, PhD, MPH
University of Hawaii

Paul N. Severin, MD
Rush Medical College and
John H. Stroger, Jr., Hospital of Cook County

Robin E. Stutman, MD, MSc
Cooper University Hospital

Gretchen Tighe, MPAS, PA-C
Des Moines University

David Welsh, MD
Surgical Associates of Southeastern Indiana

COURSE OBJECTIVES

Upon completion of the Basic Disaster Life Support™ (BDLS®) course (v.3.0), participants will be able to:

➤ Describe an all-hazards, standardized, scalable casualty management approach for use in disasters and public health emergencies, including life saving interventions and medical decision making in an altered care environment.

➤ Describe information sharing, resource access, communication, and reporting methods useful for health professionals during disasters and public health emergencies.

➤ Describe the purpose and importance of the incident management system for providing health and medical support services in a disaster or public health emergency.

➤ Describe field, facility, community, and regional surge capacity assets for the management and support of mass casualties in a disaster or public health emergency.

➤ Describe considerations and solutions to ensure continuity of and access to health-related information and services to meet the medical and mental health needs of all ages, populations, and communities affected by a disaster or public health emergency.

➤ Describe public health interventions appropriate for all ages, populations, and communities affected by a disaster or public health emergency.

➤ Identify the potential casualty population in a disaster or public health emergency, including persons with acute injuries or illnesses; those with pre-existing disease, injuries, or disabilities; those with age-related vulnerabilities or other functional and access needs; and their family/caregiver support network.

➤ Describe the deployment readiness components for health professionals in a disaster or public health emergency.

➤ Describe an all-hazards standardized, scalable workforce protection approach for use in disasters and public health emergencies, including detection, safety, security, hazard assessment, support, and evacuation or sheltering in place.

➤ Describe actions that facilitate mass casualty field triage utilizing a standard-ized step-wise approach and uniform triage categories.

➤ Describe the concepts and principles of mass fatality management for health professionals in a disaster or public health emergency.

➤ Describe the clinical assessment and management of injuries, illnesses, and mental health conditions manifested by all ages and populations in a disaster or public health emergency.

➤ Describe moral, ethical, legal, and regulatory issues relevant to the health-related management of individuals of all ages, populations, and communities affected by a disaster or public health emergency.

The BDLS® course and course objectives support a consensus-based competency framework,* which was endorsed by the National Disaster Life Support Education Consortium in 2009. A chart depicting the specific competencies and subcompeten-cies that are relevant to each chapter in this manual is presented as Appendix B.

*Source document: Subbarao I, Lyznicki J, Hsu E, et al. A consensus-based educa-tional framework and competency set for the discipline of disaster medicine and public health preparedness. *Disaster Med Public Health Preparedness*. 2008;2:57-68.

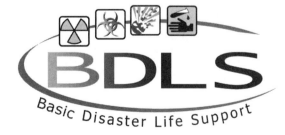

CHAPTER | ONE

All-Hazards Disaster Casualty Management

CHAPTER CHAIR

James J. James, MD, DrPH, MHA

CONTRIBUTING AUTHORS

Jim Lyznicki, MS, MPH

Sandra Vyhlidal, MSN, RN

Allen Cherson, DO

Daniel B. Fagbuyi, MD

Michael Colvard, DDS

Italo Subbarao, DO, MBA

1.1 PURPOSE

This chapter reviews concepts and principles in all-hazards disaster casualty management as delineated in the PRE-DISASTER Paradigm™ and DISASTER Paradigm™. An all-hazards approach is utilized to underscore that the basic tenets of disaster casualty management are the same, regardless of the cause of the event. The DISASTER Paradigm™ components "safety and security" and "triage and treatment" are introduced in this chapter, but more detailed discussion of these topics is contained in Chapter 4, "Workforce Readiness and Disaster Deployment," and Chapter 5, "Mass Casualty and Fatality Management," respectively.

1.2   LEARNING OBJECTIVES

After completing this chapter, readers should be able to:

➤ Discuss each component of the PRE-DISASTER Paradigm™ as it pertains to all-hazards disaster preparedness.

➤ Discuss each component of the DISASTER Paradigm™ as it pertains to all-hazards disaster response and recovery.

➤ Discuss health-related aspects of all-hazards disaster preparedness, including risk analysis, population vulnerability assessment, health system surge planning, and legal and ethical considerations.

➤ Describe principles for all-hazards disaster response and recovery with particular attention to situational awareness, incident management, health facility surge management, continuity of operations, and after-action review.

Learning objectives for this chapter are competency-based, as delineated in Appendix B.

1.3   BACKGROUND

According to the World Health Organization Center for Research on the Epidemiology of Disasters (WHO/CRED), the frequency of disasters worldwide has doubled since 1995. Global trends indicate that the frequency and magnitude (and thus the risk) of disaster hazards is on the rise. Part of the increase is attributed to better reporting due to improved surveillance and communication technologies such as the Internet and cellular telephones. Population vulnerability (eg, due to urbanization and overpopulation) is also a factor. Globalization, which connects countries through economic interdependencies, has led to increased international travel and commerce. Such activity also has led to overpopulation in cities around the world and increased movement of people to coastal areas and other disaster-prone regions. Increases in international travel may speed the rate at which an emerging infectious disease or bioterrorism agent spreads across the globe.

According to the WHO/CRED, in the previous century, about 3.5 million people were killed worldwide as a result of natural disasters; about 200 million were killed as a result of human-caused disasters (eg, war, terrorism, genocide). Each year in the United States, disasters cause hundreds of deaths and thousands of injuries and cost billions of dollars due to disruption of commerce and destruction of homes and critical infrastructure. Although the number of lives lost to disasters each year generally has declined, the economic cost of major disaster response and recovery continues to rise. In 2005, Hurricane Katrina brought an unprecedented level of attention to the impact of disasters on public health and health care delivery systems. Hospitals, medical facilities, and medical practices in the region, as well as the lives of many children and adults, were changed forever or completely lost. More than 5 years after this disaster, southern Louisiana and other states along the Gulf Coast continue recovery efforts, including the restoration of health care systems and infrastructures.

Response to a disaster is not the responsibility of any single agency or group. The sheer size of these events and the number of people involved requires cooperation among numerous agencies and individuals. This includes all levels of government and private sector responders. Organizations and individuals must be "interoperable" or able to work together to decrease duplication of effort, increase efficiency, and protect the safety of the community as well as that of responders. In 2009, the US Department of Health and Human Services (HHS) released the National Health Security Strategy (NHSS) as the first comprehensive approach for galvanizing national efforts to minimize the health consequences associated with large-scale incidents, including natural disasters, disease outbreaks, hazardous materials spills, nuclear accidents, and biologic and other terrorist attacks.[1] The NHSS is designed to achieve two goals: (1) build community resilience; and (2) strengthen and sustain health and emergency response systems.

In an all-hazards approach to disaster casualty management, health professionals must be cognizant of various potential risks and must prioritize preparedness efforts on the basis of the likelihood of risk occurrence. The public health implications of disasters can be widespread and variable, depending on many factors, including the nature, scale, and time of the event; level of preparedness; and response capacity. When making preparations for mass casualty incidents, it is essential that disaster planners recognize local health systems as part of the community's critical infrastructure and ensure continuity of operations to protect public health.

Objectives of the National Health Security Strategy[1]

The goals of the NHSS are supported by 10 strategic objectives, which describe what must be accomplished to address current gaps in national health security and to maintain improvements in health security over the longer term.

➤ Foster informed, empowered individuals and communities

➤ Develop and maintain the workforce needed for national health security

➤ Ensure situational awareness

➤ Foster integrated, scalable health care delivery systems

➤ Ensure timely and effective communications

➤ Promote an effective countermeasures enterprise

➤ Ensure prevention or mitigation of environmental and other emerging threats to health

➤ Incorporate postincident health recovery into planning and response

➤ Work with cross-border and global partners to enhance national, continental, and global health security

➤ Ensure that all systems that support national health security are based on the best available science, evaluation, and quality-improvement methods

1.4 DEFINITIONS AND TAXONOMY

Consensus definitions and terminology are extremely important to help ensure consistency in disaster education, training, and research. If events and data are identified with common definitions and taxonomies, they can be more easily studied and compared. In accordance with the all-hazards framework for disaster casualty management, the National Disaster Life Support™ (NDLS™) Program promotes the following definition of disaster: "An event and its consequences that result in a serious disruption of the functioning of a community and cause widespread human, material, economic, or environmental losses that exceed the capacity of the affected area to respond without external assistance to save lives, preserve property, and maintain the stability and integrity of the affected area."

DISASTER = NEEDS > RESOURCES

For operational purposes, a disaster can be defined as an event in which the needs exceed immediately available resources.

While various disaster classifications exist, the most inclusive taxonomy defines three distinct categories: natural disasters, human systems failure, and war and conflict as one dimension of classification; and time as another dimension (time-limited vs prolonged disasters).[2] The distinctions among these categories can become blurred, as in the case of industrial catastrophes, structural collapse of buildings, transportation-related emergencies, release of hazardous materials by fires or explosions, and infectious disease outbreaks. For example, Hurricane Katrina was a natural disaster, but the levee breaches and delayed response could be considered human systems failures. The radiation leakage from damaged nuclear power reactors at Fukushima following the 2011 Japan earthquake and tsunami is another example. Generally, a disaster is classified according to its primary categorization, and so Hurricane Katrina would be considered a natural disaster. Identical disasters may have differing consequences depending on the location of the event and the availability of resources.

Disasters are referred to as local "incidents" or "events" in that their impact is immediate and direct, while the time course, population, and geography are generally limited. Most natural disasters are limited in scale and time and are managed locally with subsequent infusion of regional or national resources as needed. In the developed world, localized disasters rarely result in a public health emergency unless they affect the public health infrastructure and system.

Public health emergencies can be defined as events that adversely affect the public health system and/or its protective infrastructure (ie, water, sanitation, shelter, food, fuel, and health), resulting in both direct and indirect consequences to the health of a population.[2,3] Direct consequences include the immediate injuries, illnesses, and deaths that are attributed directly to exposure to the hazard. Indirect consequences are measured as the excess injuries, illnesses, and deaths that are caused by the inability to access medical care. These are due to a variety of factors, including: significantly damaged medical and public health infrastructure, population displacement to areas without adequate medical care, lack of medical and public health providers for the vast numbers of injured or ill, and lack of security or governance to allow for medical and public health care. Deaths due to indirect consequences are often preventable and may supersede direct deaths.

Dealing with disasters and public health emergencies requires an all-hazards approach to better coordinate planning and response efforts. All-hazards preparedness refers to considering all potential hazards to a community and taking steps to mitigate and prepare for any potential hazard that may affect the community. Essential to the implementation of an all-hazards approach is the identification of actions that can be initiated immediately when an incident has occurred. This allows for an operational response to begin during the early phases of situational awareness acquisition. An analogy would be the initiation of cardiopulmonary resuscitation for a victim of cardiac arrest. Cardiopulmonary resuscitation is learned as part of an all-hazards approach to the management of cardiac arrest and should not be delayed until the exact cause of the cardiac arrest is determined. By considering and preparing the community for all hazards, planning gaps can be reduced, potentially resulting in a more effective response to the event. From the moment a disaster is recognized, the acute medical care and public health systems need to be engaged as part of an integrated response. Timely and accurate recognition of the public health impact is critical for disaster mitigation, preparedness, response, and recovery.

1.4.1 The PRE-DISASTER Paradigm™

For the NDLS program, the PRE-DISASTER Paradigm™ was introduced in the Core Disaster Life Support™ (CDLS®) course (v 3.0) and supporting course manual. It was developed to reinforce key elements for enhancing personal, organizational, and community preparedness. The "PRE" mnemonic encompasses:

➤ Planning and practice

➤ Resilience

➤ Education and training

Planning and practice: The strength of preparedness depends on careful and ongoing planning, as well as continual practicing of those plans. Planning includes the design, implementation, and ongoing evaluation of efforts to help communities, institutions, and individuals prepare for, respond to, and recover from disasters and public health emergencies. Effective planning requires integrated collaboration from the entire disaster response system to include emergency management and public safety agencies, local public health agencies, hospitals (both private and public), local clinics, emergency medical services (both private and public), businesses, and community groups. Contingencies must be considered to address scarcity of resources and ensure continuity of operations.

Resilience: Being prepared (through planning, education, and training) can reduce fear, anxiety, and losses associated with a disaster and build resilience. Resilience is the ability of individuals and communities to rebound to a reasonable state of normalcy after exposure to disasters, serious emergencies, and other traumatic, tragic, and stressful events (such as family and relationship problems, serious health problems, or workplace and financial stressors). In advance of a disaster, resilience can be built into a community by educating the population about local disaster planning and response efforts and assisting residents with the development of personal and family preparedness plans. Given that resources may be limited during a disaster, it is increasingly recognized that communities may need to be on their own for at least 96 hours before outside help arrives and thus need to build resilience before an incident occurs.

Education and training: Effective education programs can help minimize the impact of a disaster as well as build resiliency. The development and dissemination of comprehensive curricula to train health system responders for disasters and public health emergencies (such as through the NDLS™ program) is a challenge. This is because disasters, terrorism, and public health emergencies can occur in multiple scenarios with diverse clinical and public health outcomes. Many of these issues are not addressed in current health professional schools or continuing education programs. Certainly, the topic areas that need to be learned by all potential health system responders must be relevant to the roles they will play and be reasonably attainable, considering time and financial resources.

The elements of the PRE-DISASTER Paradigm™ are discussed and reinforced further in this chapter and other chapters of this manual.

1.4.2   The DISASTER Paradigm™

The DISASTER Paradigm™, also introduced in the CDLS® course (v3.0), is a practical learning tool to enhance communication consistency among disaster response personnel and agencies. Use of the DISASTER Paradigm™ can benefit all responders by helping them answer the question: "Do my needs exceed my resources?" It is a useful mnemonic device for identifying the following key elements of disaster response and recovery:

➤ *D*etection

➤ *I*ncident management

➤ *S*afety and security

➤ *A*ssess hazards

➤ *S*upport

➤ *T*riage and treatment

➤ *E*vacuation

➤ *R*ecovery

Detection: Detection is the first step for effective disaster response. Every time a crew or unit responds to an emergency call or event, they should immediately determine whether there is a disaster or mass casualty situation present. Do current needs exceed available capabilities and resources? Is there a suspected threat or hazardous material present?

Incident management: All disaster responders should understand core elements of the National Incident Management System (NIMS). Effective incident management requires command, coordination, and communication ("the three Cs"). In any disaster, effective incident management starts with communication. Does each responder know about the incident command system (ICS) and respective roles within that system? Is there a practiced plan for event notification and reporting? Are there simplified external and internal communication systems in place? How are messages with public health and emergency management agencies initiated and sustained? In a disaster, regular communication systems are immediately challenged, and the usual systems, such as paging or cell phones, may be down or overloaded. The basic principles of ICS and emergency management should be well known by all disaster responders. The tenets of incident command (ie, operations, logistics, planning, and finance) are important and serve as the building blocks for a functional ICS system.

Safety and security: The nature of emergency response is to save lives, which may involve responders putting their own safety at risk. If the precise cause of an incident is not immediately apparent, or if there is a suspicion that something is unusual, emergency responders should take necessary precautions to minimize risk to themselves and others. Even if real-time identification of the precise cause is not possible, responder safety remains paramount. Triage, treatment, and evacuation of casualties become secondary considerations if scene conditions do not permit intervention without endangering rescuers. The immediate scene may be too dangerous to allow any responders in to provide care. A well-meaning responder who becomes injured or acutely ill while attempting to help ends up becoming part of the problem and is now a new casualty, thus increasing the demands on the response rather than being part of the solution.

Assess hazards: A challenging feature of many disasters is the risk of structural collapse, fire, ruptured gas lines, downed power lines, and numerous other factors that may trigger additional casualties. Other concerns include the potential release of toxic chemicals and radiation, as well as respiratory hazards from byproducts of combustion (eg, smoke, carbon monoxide, cyanide, or dust). Emergency responders must remain vigilant for these hazards and take appropriate precautions to protect themselves and others. If they do not, detection of these situations may come too late to prevent further harm and destruction.

Support: Referring to logistics, *support* is a comprehensive term that means getting what is needed to get the job done. By its very nature, a disaster or serious mass casualty incident requires the coordination of resources and assets from myriad public- and private-sector agencies and organizations. Effective response, recovery, and mitigation require support planning by agencies, institutions, and communities well in advance of any emergency. This includes acquisition and deployment of essential personnel, supplies, facilities, vehicles, and other resources. It also means being prepared for surge: an influx of mass casualties exceeding daily abilities for care.

Triage and treatment: In a serious disaster, involving multiple casualties, the goal of triage is to do the greatest good for the greatest number of possible survivors. The initial objective is to prevent expansion of the casualty population by facilitating the movement of ambulatory casualties and uninjured bystanders away from the scene. Focusing on a severely injured casualty, before promoting the safety of the larger casualty population, would not achieve the goal of the greatest good for the greatest number. The next objective of disaster triage is to sort casualties and identify those with life-threatening injuries to initiate emergency treatment immediately. Once this is accomplished, casualties with less-serious injuries can be assessed further and triaged for removal from the scene on the basis of their level of injury and available resources. Effective triage "regulates" surge demands for staff, supplies, and space by finding the most critically injured or ill people and prioritizing them for transport from the scene to receiving facilities for more definitive medical and surgical care. Treatment continues until all casualties have been transported to hospitals or other treatment centers or all available resources have been exhausted.

Evacuation: Effective community preparedness requires planning for individual and community evacuation needs; understanding the target population, their concerns and nuances; and knowing where they can be safely relocated during a disaster. The number of people to be evacuated, the modes of transportation, and the rapidity with which the evacuation occurs vary with the situation at hand. Evacuation plans must account for complex scenarios, such as the evacuation of schools, high-rises, hospitals, and long-term care facilities (eg, nursing homes and rehabilitation facilities). In a disaster, usual transport may be nonfunctional because of the direct effect of the disaster on transport infrastructure or the indirect effect of overwhelming casualty transport needs. Evacuation with specified resources must be built into community and facility disaster response plans and, more importantly, practiced. Evacuation begins and ends with a self-determined evacuation plan and operational assessment.

Recovery: Recovery is the longest phase of any disaster and begins when the event occurs. It is best subdivided into "relief, rehabilitation, and restoration" to focus on recovery of the public health in its fullest. In terms of physical, economic, and community recovery, this phase may take months or years. The imprint disasters leave on medical and mental health can last a lifetime. Government agencies, businesses, and various organizations (eg, the American Red Cross, the Salvation Army) work together to provide community support during this period. The goal of recovery is to ensure the economic sustainability of a community and the long-term physical and mental well-being of its citizens, to rebuild and repair the physical infrastructure, and to implement mitigation activities to reduce the effect of future disasters. Recovery efforts seek to restore normalcy as soon as possible. This outcome reflects the resilience of the community in general, and its affected individuals in particular.

The elements of the DISASTER Paradigm™ are discussed and reinforced further in this chapter and other chapters of this manual.

1.5 HEALTH-RELATED CONSIDERATIONS IN DISASTER PLANNING

Disasters strike locally, and communities must bear the ultimate responsibility for planning for and mobilizing emergency and health care resources to ensure adequate disaster response capability and capacity. The goal of disaster planning is to achieve a satisfactory level of readiness to respond to any disaster situation through measures that strengthen the technical and managerial capacity of governments, organizations, and communities. During the planning process, government officials, business leaders, and other individuals develop policies and procedures to save lives, minimize damage, and enhance emergency response operations. The effectiveness of preparedness depends on knowledge of potential hazards and appropriate countermeasures, as well as the extent to which government agencies, nongovernmental organizations, and the general public are able to make use of this information in an emergency. Effective planning requires integrated collaboration from the entire disaster response system to include emergency management and public safety agencies, local public health agencies, hospitals (both private and public), local clinics, emergency medical services (both private and public), businesses, and community groups. Contingencies also must be considered (eg, to address scarcity of resources).

Disaster plans (also called *emergency operations plans* or EOPs) differ among jurisdictions because local hazards, laws, and resources vary. Plans must address short- and long-term objectives of preparedness, response, and recovery activities to include resources to protect public health and safety; restoration of essential government services; and provision of emergency relief to government, businesses, and affected populations. Disaster plans must be well coordinated to ensure efficient mobilization of assets from local, regional, and national sources in a predetermined manner. Any disaster preparedness and response plan needs to consider the physical, behavioral, and emotional factors underlying human responses to trauma, being cognizant of the unique vulnerabilities and responses of various populations, as well as mechanisms for coping with these factors. Community members should be encouraged to participate in disaster planning so they are informed about local response procedures.

Planning must involve a collaborative approach among local, state, and federal authorities, as well as a host of private agencies and organizations that provide support and counseling services under normal circumstances. It is recommended that these entities work together in advance to develop scripted public messaging that is informative, educational, calming, and supportive. Waiting to develop these until the actual occurrence of an event is a prescription for failure. Local authorities should develop contact lists with information for all locally available clinical and mental health professionals. Additionally, local authorities should work with state health officials in developing a mass mental health crisis response plan. All available partners should be included in the planning and response phases of this plan. These should include, but not be limited to, the American Red Cross, the Salvation Army, faith-based counseling services, and private mental health providers.

Community and health facility EOPs should outline how they will respond to hazards that are most likely to be encountered, identify response roles and responsibilities, and serve as road maps for incident preparation, response, and recovery. Various disaster casualty scenarios need to be planned for and practiced in advance to avoid comprising an effective community health system. Facility plans should address situations in which equipment and facilities suffer damage, which can affect patient and employee safety. Plans should be in place to provide for security resources as well as monitoring systems to create as safe an environment as possible for responders, rescue personnel, and health care facility personnel.

Extensive discussion of personal and community preparedness planning is provided in the CDLS® course (v 3.0) and supporting course manual. More information on community and health care facility disaster response operations is provided in the Advanced Disaster Life Support™ (ADLS®) course (v3.0) and supporting course manual.

1.5.1   Risk Analysis

Effective disaster planning begins with an assessment of the hazards that may be encountered and recognition of what could happen in specified scenarios. This requires consideration of numerous hazards and the potential affect that they have on different populations, facilities, human resources, and services. Risk analysis can be complicated by the high degree of uncertainty for various disaster events, both in predicting the occurrence of the events and in estimating their consequences. It requires thorough evaluation of potential hazards and vulnerabilities along with quantitative estimates of the probability and consequences of different possible disaster scenarios. Assessments can be conducted on a variety of spatial scales, from the exact city block where a health care facility is located to a global scale covering broad populations. Risk analysis involves four interrelated components:

➤ *Risk perception:* understanding how different people perceive and measure risk

➤ *Hazard analysis:* assessment of various hazards for a particular geographic area and the magnitude of impact given local resources, allowing for prioritization of response and mitigation options

➤ *Vulnerability assessment:* identifying particular infrastructures and populations at increased risk for damage or harm

➤ *Capacity assessment:* identifying available resources that can be used to reduce risk, enhance survival, and help affected individuals and populations cope with severe trauma

The first step in disaster planning is the development of a hazard vulnerability analysis (HVA). The HVA is a disaster needs assessment for an organization or community. It should address the types of emergencies most relevant to the community or facility, its geographic location, and the needs of the populations served.

While it is important that an EOP be broad enough to address all possible hazards, planners should determine the most likely risks for the region and give particular attention to these in the plan. Is the community or facility in a flood zone or hurricane-prone area? Does the plan include procedures for power outages during extreme temperatures? When deliberating such questions, it is important to understand the difference between the terms *risk* and *hazard*. A *hazard* is anything that has the potential to do harm to property, the environment, people, or animals. *Risk* is the probability of the potential hazard actually occurring.

1.5.2   Population Vulnerability Assessment

The public health implications of disasters can be widespread and variable, depending on many factors, including the nature, scale, and time of the event; level of preparedness; and response capacity. Lessons from past disasters continually demonstrate the disproportionate impact that these events can have on the most vulnerable members of society, including those with chronic diseases, children, the elderly, and minority populations. The need to address the great diversity of special health concerns, language and cultural barriers, and other life circumstances presents multiple challenges for disaster response and recovery systems. Minimizing adverse health outcomes requires cooperative efforts that cross traditional boundaries of health specialties, professions, and nationalities.

The affect of disasters varies greatly as a reflection of both the physical hazards and the vulnerabilities of the population being affected. Disasters result when vulnerable populations and infrastructure are exposed to physical hazards. It is this exposure that results in injuries, illnesses, deaths, and destruction. These outcomes reflect both the magnitude of the hazards and the level of vulnerability of the population and infrastructure. While disaster plans seek to prevent and control injuries and disease in all populations, people with access and functional needs must be identified and have valid emergency care plans in place. These should include plans for managing day-to-day problems related to their specific illness or disability, as well as plans for managing health-related needs in the event of a disaster or public health emergency.[4] In a large-scale emergency, medical supplies, equipment, and availability of medications may be limited and can pose a serious challenge for those with chronic diseases. During a prolonged lockdown or shelter-in-place situation, lack of availability of medications can pose a serious challenge for individuals with chronic diseases.

Disasters disproportionately affect at-risk or vulnerable populations. These populations tend to be ethnic minorities and possess a low socioeconomic status; reside in denser, more hazard-prone neighborhoods; possess a higher prevalence of chronic disease (both physical, mental, and chemically dependent); have low health literacy; and have greater barriers to access to medical care. Infants, children, the elderly,

Geospatial Technologies and Disaster Planning

Recognizing that disasters are inherently geographic processes, it makes sense that geospatial technologies are important tools in preparing for, responding to, and recovering from disasters. *Geospatial technology* is a general term used to describe a broad set of software and instruments for gathering, compiling, storing, analyzing, modeling, and visualizing geographic data. A geographic information system (GIS) is one type of geospatial technology that is used extensively in hazard assessment. Simply put, GIS is software for making maps. More specifically, a GIS user has the ability to store, manipulate, and represent spatial data. Therefore, one can look at the spatial extent of possible hazards overlaid on data that shows vulnerable populations and infrastructure.

Other geospatial technologies include global positioning systems (GPSs) and remote sensing (RS). A GPS provides precise measurements of an individual position. It utilizes a handheld receiver and a system of satellites. RS refers to instrumentation and data analysis techniques that provide data on location without visiting that location. Using RS, hazard scientists can map and quantify flood, seismic, and environmental hazards; detect biological and chemical signatures; and determine sources of water.

Every component of the health care community should identify potential disasters that may affect its area and should utilize applicable hazards tools to ensure effective preparedness, response, and recovery planning.

pregnant women, and the mentally and physically disabled are included in this definition. Children are particularly at risk because they have many distinct anatomic, physiologic, immunologic, developmental, and psychosocial characteristics; in addition, they have not yet developed adult coping strategies and are deficient of life experiences to help them understand what has happened. Population health issues and vulnerabilities are discussed in greater detail in Chapter 3, "Population Health and Mental Health in Disasters."

1.5.3   Health System Surge Planning

Most communities cannot realistically be expected to stockpile every possible durable medical item, pharmaceutical, or foodstuff in adequate supplies to have a significant impact on the repercussions suffered from all types of disasters. However, there are many actions that communities can take that will have a significant positive impact should such an event ever occur. Communities can organize themselves to assess and inventory various available resources. Hotel beds, auditoriums, schools, and places of worship can be inventoried.

Delays in the arrival of logistical support, limited personnel, transportation limitations, and disruption in public works (eg, electrical power, potable water) may be contributing factors that impact the ability to deliver normal or near-normal levels of health services. During these times, it is important to take all necessary steps to return to a desired standard of care as soon as possible. Communities and health care facilities must plan and prepare for this reality by increasing public and staff awareness about this issue, as well as by ensuring an adequate ethical and legal framework to provide care during mass casualty events. The goal is to keep the health system functioning to deliver the highest level of care possible to save as many lives as possible.[5-7]

Effective health system preparedness and response requires consideration of various "surge" strategies that address ways to reduce the demand for care and the need to augment inpatient and ambulatory care capacities and capabilities. The success of these strategies is dependent on personnel, space, bed availability, access to medical technology, medication reserves, and the extent of damage sustained by the health care infrastructure.[8-11] To successfully manage a large influx of casualties, there must be a surge capacity plan for the health system and individual health care facilities. Ideally, each facility will have its own plan, coordinated with a regional plan.

Surge-based planning includes community teamwork. Community planning allows facilities to develop mutual aid agreements, identify and use standardized equipment, train personnel collectively, test preparedness processes and procedures

Surge Capacity and Capability

Surge capacity is the ability of a health system to rapidly expand beyond normal services to meet the increased demand for care of patients. This surge occurs in physical space/hospital beds, qualified personnel, medical care, and public health services in the event of a large-scale disaster or public health emergency.

Surge capability combines capacity with what can be done for the casualties. Surge capability is measured in terms of the numbers of staff and resources truly available to provide the services for which these facilities and equipment are required (ie, the number of specialists and ventilators to navigate a mass casualty event). Surge capability must account not only for the care of affected populations, but for the care of those with regular emergencies unrelated to disaster, such as heart attack, stroke, labor, and acute illness.

through community-wide exercises, and provide opportunities to address identified gaps. Four key components are necessary in surge-based planning: (1) increasing health care facility capacity; (2) planning for supporting acute care sites/alternate care facilities; (3) developing electronic registries of volunteer health care providers; and (4) planning for altered care delivery (ie, crisis standards of care). To assist hospitals and responding organizations with these components, the federal government has provided funding, guidance, and other assistance at the state level.[11] State governments have been given the responsibility to develop plans that coordinate regional and local entities. Many hospitals have made efforts toward the first three key components, but the fourth one, establishing crisis standards of care, continues to be difficult. States have recommended different approaches to altering patient care in a serious disaster, but no agreement or standardization has occurred.[11] Surge capacity issues are discussed further in Section 1.6.4 of this chapter and in the ADLS® course (v 3.0) and supporting course manual.

1.5.4   Legal and Ethical Planning Considerations

In a crisis, state and local emergency management and public health leaders need a clearly defined set of legal and ethical principles to help them make sound, real-time decisions for managing the situation and allocating potentially scarce resources. The all-hazards approach to disaster casualty management requires that these principles be adaptable to a variety of emergencies, ranging from disease pandemics to terrorism to weather-related events. A sound ethical and legal framework is essential to assess and justify public health actions and interventions. Decisions made in a disaster situation will affect the health and lives of individuals and populations and are thus fundamentally moral in nature. In a disaster, ethics is closely intertwined with the legal framework that will be used to guide policy decisions. During the disaster planning process, it will become clear that serious moral and ethical issues must be confronted before, during, and after an event.

Policies, such as those that guide the allocation of scarce resources or limit individual liberty, may adversely affect segments of the population, thereby reducing public confidence and trust in decision makers. A lack of public trust may ultimately hinder compliance or cooperation with advice or orders, which is necessary for an effective response to a disaster situation. Ensuring that these difficult decisions are based on sound scientific and ethical principles and that health professionals and other responders act in accord with these standards will help to build and maintain public confidence and trust in a disaster. The application of ethical principles to public health policy necessitates that responders provide for the health needs of all affected persons without regard to age, race, ethnicity, nationality, religious beliefs, sexual orientation, residency status, or socioeconomic status. Legal and ethical issues confronting disaster responders are addressed in more detail in Chapter 4, "Workforce Readiness and Disaster Deployment," as well as in the CDLS® (v 3.0) and ADLS® (v3.0) courses and supporting course manuals.

1.5.5   Exercises and Drills

Once response plans have been developed, they must be tested rigorously through realistic exercises and drills, conducted to reflect actual conditions that would likely be encountered and the resources and personnel that would be available. Staff need to know when and why the plan is used and what roles they will play when the plan is activated. The ongoing testing of plans, policies, and procedures during exercises and drills is an important part of disaster preparedness. This allows participants to apply knowledge and skills and, at the same time, allows them to identify opportunities for improvement and develop action plans to fix identified gaps. All exercises should be followed by a detailed evaluation and action plan for improvement. Exercises include seminars, workshops, tabletop scenarios, functional drills, and full-scale drills.

Disaster exercises should be designed to test incident command and control, communications, logistics, laboratory coordination, and clinical capabilities, among others. These exercises may involve only the leadership of an organization and focus on planning and decision making (the command post exercise), they may involve notional play using a tabletop exercise, or they may involve actual hands-on training and evaluation in a disaster drill or field-training exercise. The JCAHO requires hospitals to conduct a hazard vulnerability analysis, develop an emergency management plan, and evaluate this plan twice yearly; one of these evaluations must include a community-wide drill.[12] Moreover, the Joint Commission specifically mandates that hospitals provide facilities (and training in the use of such facilities) for radioactive, biologic, and chemical isolation and decontamination.

1.6 HEALTH-RELATED CONSIDERATIONS IN DISASTER RESPONSE

Once a disaster occurs, the response phase involves implementation of personal, community, and facility disaster plans. Community response plans will be implemented through a local incident management structure, which may be scaled according to the disaster situation. The aim of disaster response is to provide immediate assistance to protect lives, preserve health, and support the morale of affected populations. The focus will be on meeting the basic needs of affected people until more permanent and sustainable solutions can be found.

During a disaster, myriad public- and private-sector agencies may be called on to deal with immediate response and recovery. To be able to respond effectively, their efforts must be rapid, flexible, sustainable, integrated, and coordinated at all levels, which requires experienced leaders, trained personnel, adequate transport and logistic support, appropriate communications, and standard operating procedures for working in disaster situations. Federal, state, and local government agencies have unmatched resources and legal authority to address disaster-related needs. Government authorities will coordinate extensive logistical efforts, such as moving large amounts of relief supplies.

1.6.1 Situational Awareness and Detection

In an all-hazards approach to disaster casualty management, response personnel must be aware of the environment they are operating in at all times. *Situational awareness* refers to the capability to maintain a constant vigil over important information, understand the relationship among various pieces of information being monitored, and project this understanding to make critical decisions.[13] This includes, but is not limited to, the arrival of additional casualties, changes in environmental conditions, time of day, personnel, and modes of communications in their area of operation. All of these have the potential to affect decisions regarding personal safety, security, triage, and therapeutic interventions, as well as the safety of individuals receiving care.

Situational awareness requires the ability to objectively quantify the magnitude of a disaster event and resources consumed and needed through multiple mechanisms, including radio and television networks, the Internet and social media, eyewitness accounts, disease and injury surveillance systems, clinic and hospital bed census and inpatient reporting, laboratory reporting, and death notices. Timely, credible, and reliable information is essential before, during, and after a disaster strikes. This includes up-to-date guidelines, recommendations, health alerts, and up-to-date, standards-based information systems that monitor data on injuries and diseases and enable efficient communication among public and private health organizations, the media, and the public.

A key initial step in mobilizing an emergency response for an affected population is to obtain information about the extent of the population's immediate needs and the status of the supporting health infrastructure. Situational awareness and disease and injury surveillance are often limited in accuracy in the early period following a disaster. Early on, information sharing is limited. Verification of information is difficult. Media coverage may be delayed because of challenges in accessing the local area.

Detection is the initial recognition that a threatening situation is imminent or exists. The key to detection of a disaster is ongoing vigilance and situational awareness of abnormal changes in the immediate environment, as well as awareness of unusual disease patterns and occurrences in the vicinity. Detection is not just about major emergencies—it may be simply identifying something outside the norm. The detection process involves recognizing that a situation exists that could overwhelm the resources available. Health professionals are on the front lines when dealing with injury and disease, every day and in emergencies, caused by microbes, environmental hazards, natural disasters, highway collisions, terrorism, or other calamities. Early detection and reporting are critical to minimize casualties through astute individuals and teamwork by public- and private-sector health and emergency response personnel.

Detection requires awareness of the environment, recognition of unusual circumstances, and, in some cases, a high index of suspicion. Knowing that something has occurred is not always as intuitive as it may seem. For natural disasters, nuclear detonations, and explosive events, prediction can be difficult or impossible, but detection after the event is very straightforward. For chemical emergencies, detection hinges on environmental clues and on familiarity with the characteristic presentations (toxidromes) of the major chemical classes. For biologic agents, environmental clues, patient

Situational Awareness

When it is evident that immediate response needs outweigh the available resources, a disaster exists. Actions taken in the ensuing minutes and hours will become extremely important to protect the health, safety, and security of all affected populations. In such situations, it will be critical to communicate effectively with the emergency management and response organizations, hospitals, and the public health system.

symptoms, disease syndromes, and careful surveillance are critical. For radiologic disasters, early detection may be difficult, especially for a covert release. As remote sensing and standoff detection technologies increase in capability and allow the development of miniaturized hand-held tools, emergency responders can expect to use these tools to assist in the detection and quantification of threats.

Detection may be complicated when the event is insidious or escalates over time. In 1999, the West Nile virus outbreak in New York City was discovered after "an unusual cluster of cases of meningoencephalitis associated with muscle weakness was reported to the New York City Department of Health."[14] Although this situation was not a disaster (by definition), the potential for a serious health emergency was certainly present had this been a more infectious agent. In July 1995, Chicago experienced a heat wave that took the lives of approximately 700 people over a 5-day period.[15] Initially, this was not perceived to be a major health crisis. But as the weather remained unseasonably hot and humid, and as the electrical grid began to succumb to additional stress, emergency department visits and emergency medical services (EMS) responses increased, and the situation escalated to become a very significant health emergency.

1.6.2   Hazard Assessment

Actual and potential hazards related to a disaster must be assessed continually. Hazards will vary according to the situation encountered and assignment given to the health responder. All disasters, regardless of the primary cause, create the possibility of secondary hazards capable of injuring anyone present at the scene, including responders. The detonation of a car bomb, for example, can be more than just a simple explosion. The bomb may be associated with the release of a chemical or radioactive agent. Another explosive device may be placed at the scene to explode when the device is moved or touched by response personnel. The explosion can cause additional damage to surrounding buildings and infrastructure. A challenging feature of many disasters is the risk of structural collapse, fire, ruptured gas lines, downed power lines, and numerous other factors, which may cause additional casualties. Other concerns include the potential release of toxic chemicals and radiation, as well as respiratory hazards from byproducts of combustion (eg, smoke, carbon monoxide, cyanide, or dust). Emergency responders must take appropriate precautions to protect themselves and others. If they do not, detection of these situations may come too late to prevent further harm and destruction.

In any emergency response environment, it is essential to understand that there are multiple hazards present. The approach to any scene should include an evaluation of the presence of hazardous materials in particular, but it also should include electrical and fire hazards, secondary explosive devices, or explosive hazards innate to heated objects or destabilized containment (eg, fuel storage or gas cylinders). Incident response can be complicated further by communications disruption; weather threats; loss of routes of ingress and egress; damage to emergency vehicles, equipment, and supplies; and even darkness. The all-hazards approach to disaster casualty management requires awareness of the possibility of such dangers and continual assessment at the scene to detect and protect against recognized and perceived threats.

1.6.3 Incident Management

Most emergency response planning scenarios involve the establishment of an incident command post at a substantial distance from the disaster scene. In any disaster, general principles of containment, decontamination, prehospital care, and field triage should be fully employed. Protective actions should be implemented to reduce or eliminate exposure of the public to actual and potential hazardous situations. The principal protective action decisions for consideration in the early and intermediate phases of an emergency are whether to shelter in place, evacuate, or relocate affected or potentially affected populations. Secondary actions include administration of medical countermeasures, decontamination (including decontamination of persons evacuated from the affected area), use of access restrictions, and use of restrictions on food and water. In some situations, only one protective action needs to be implemented, while in others, numerous protective actions will be necessary.

In 2003, Homeland Security Presidential Directive 5 called on federal departments and agencies to make adoption of NIMS a requirement, to the extent permitted by law, for providing federal preparedness assistance through grants, contracts, or other activities.[16] NIMS is designed to standardize disaster response across the United States to provide consistent incident management.[17] NIMS provides a nationwide template enabling government and nongovernmental responders to functionally operate in domestic incidents. Compliance with NIMS is now a prerequisite for receiving federal funding for disaster preparedness activities.

Under NIMS, the ICS has become the model for disaster management needs throughout the nation.[18,19] The current challenge is to maximize the use of ICSs across geographic and disciplinary borders so that this proven approach can be applied to incident management needs nationwide. Incident command typically involves a single agency as the primary responder. If there are multiple agencies involved, the situation requires use of unified command or area command structures. For most emergencies, the ICS will be composed of a network of professionals, working on common goals, under the leadership of one ultimately responsible commander. Response to a large-scale disaster or public health emergency will require an area command structure, involving multiple jurisdictions and agencies, to determine responsibilities and coordinate the allocation of potentially scarce health resources.

The ICS provides the operational structure to address the challenges and issues that disasters create in an efficient manner through the use of the concepts of unity of command and the utilization of the command staff and general staff structures to manage a disaster. At any disaster scene, there is a single designated supervisor, referred to as the *incident commander*, who is ultimately responsible for the overall management of the situation. Other key command staff include the public information officer (PIO), the safety officer, and the liaison officer. The PIO provides the incident commander with advice on the media and dissemination of information and ensures that a clear and unified message is provided to the public. All public disclosures should be reviewed by the PIO. The safety officer provides the incident commander with advice on incident safety and ensures that operations conform to all applicable safety rules and regulations. The liaison officer serves as the contact point with all the agencies involved in supporting response operations. The five functional ICS areas (incident command, operations, planning, logistics, and finance) remain the same across organizations.

The ICS also applies to hospitals and other health care facilities. The Joint Commission requires all hospitals to use a command system that follows the principles and objectives of the ICS for dealing with both internal and external disasters. The hospital incident command system (HICS), which was created in the late 1980s by the California EMS Authority as an important foundation in preparing for emergencies, is used by many hospitals and health care agencies throughout the country.[20] As with incident command in the field, HICS provides common terminology to enhance communication and improve documentation. Duties are assigned by position and include a clear chain of authority and command. Health care workers must know their specific facility command structure and how they fit into its chain of command.

1.6.3.1   Emergency Operations Center

The emergency operations center (EOC) is the nerve center of disaster operations. The EOC is a central command and control location responsible for carrying out the principles of emergency management at a strategic level in an emergency. An EOC is the location for coordination of information and resources to support incident activities. It facilitates the safe, effective operation of the ICS at the scene (ie, coordinates information from the field-based incident command post) and ensures the continuity of operations for the affected region during and after the disaster. An EOC is the physical location where the leaders of a region or organization come together during an emergency or disaster to analyze response and recovery options, coordinate actions, and allocate resources. Generally, the EOC is not located within or adjacent to the disaster scene but rather at a safe distance to enable personnel to manage the challenges with minimal chaos and confusion. There may be levels of EOCs at the local, regional, or state levels, each with a coordinating function for ensuring the continuity of the chain of command. In a public health emergency, it is likely that a health EOC (HEOC) would be established to help coordinate medical and public health assets and maximize the health system response to the event.[21]

1.6.3.2   Disaster Communications

Getting accurate information to people quickly is a key component to saving lives during an emergency. A carefully prepared plan is needed to protect vital communication links among emergency responders and ensure that information interchange can continue. All agencies that may respond to a disaster in a community must cooperate in advance to identify those methods of communication that will persist under most conceivable conditions. In a disaster, the ability to establish and maintain open lines to communicate efficiently with health care facilities, public health agencies, emergency management agencies, public safety organizations, and citizens is crucial. All emergency responders must be able to communicate effectively with one another multidirectionally, in real time, using a common language, before, during, and after the event occurs. Information and communication networks should be secure and linked to the public health and health care systems for disease surveillance and timely information sharing. The redundant delivery of information via several sources can help fill communication gaps in the event of power outages or other interruptions in services.

NIMS prescribes interoperable communications systems for both incident and information management to standardize communications during a disaster. Disaster communication plans must be based on a clear understanding of the needs and perceptions of the target audience. This includes systems and protocols for communicating timely and accurate information to the public. Strategies need to consider how to reach persons of different cultures, races, and religions, as well as meet the needs of disabled (eg, blind, hearing-impaired) and disenfranchised (eg, homeless, impoverished) persons.

Crisis and emergency risk communication is a vital component of any disaster communication strategy.[22] Timely risk communication provides information for individuals and communities to support the best possible decisions to protect health, safety, and security. During emergencies, the public may receive information from a variety of sources. Effective communication of clear, concise, and credible information will help assure the public that the situation is being addressed competently. Public information must reach broad audiences to publicize both immediate and anticipated hazards, appropriate health and safety precautions, the need for evacuation or sheltering in place, and alternative travel routes. Under NIMS, state and local health authorities must have established procedures for providing the news media with timely and accurate public information. One way to ensure coordination and integration of public information across jurisdictions and agencies is through a centralized Joint Information Center. Risk communication is discussed further in Chapter 2, "Public Health Response to Disasters."

1.6.3.3 Logistical Support Services

By its very nature, a disaster or serious mass casualty incident requires the coordination of resources and assets from myriad public and private sector agencies and organizations. In a disaster, the response time, type, and amount of support can fluctuate significantly. The nature, size, and scope of a disaster, and the scene it creates, will dictate the prioritization of available resources and response assets to meet the needs of affected populations. Every disaster is unique in this regard. Effective disaster management hinges on the timely delivery of resources to where they are needed most. Support may not be given much thought until resources are depleted, by which time its arrival may be too late to help change the outcome.

Disaster support encompasses a spectrum of resources, from local volunteers to large federal programs. Some are available to assist in the early hours of disaster response. Others, such as the National Disaster Medical System (NDMS) teams, provide backup for depleted personnel and resources in the days after an event.[23] The Strategic National Stockpile (SNS) provides a national repository of emergency pharmaceuticals, medical supplies, and equipment that can be shipped anywhere in the United States in response to a national emergency.[24] The infrastructure for providing support under normal, day-to-day emergencies already exists in most communities through mutual aid agreements, in which resources in neighboring communities can be brought into the affected area to provide additional assistance. State-sponsored disaster teams can often respond faster than the federal system, but these assets vary widely from state to state.

Disaster response begins at the local government level. Once city and county government resources are depleted, local authorities request state assistance. When

---

Federal ESFs and the National Response Framework[25]

The National Response Framework (NRF) is the all-hazards response guide for the United States. It provides for coordination among federal, state, local, tribal, nongovernmental, and private-sector organizations. ESF Annexes delineated in the NRF group government and certain private-sector capabilities to provide support, resources, program implementation, and services.

➤ ESF 6, Mass Care, Emergency Assistance, Housing, and Human Services, provides for federal delivery of these services when local, tribal, and state response and recovery needs exceed their capabilities.

➤ ESF 8, Health and Medical Services, provides for coordinated federal assistance to supplement state and local resources in response to public health and medical care needs. This support function provides public health services, medical services, mental health services, and mass fatality management.

---

state resources are depleted, the governor asks for federal assistance. Part of the strategic capability of federal response planning involves a coordinating structure through the emergency support function (ESF) system.[26] The ESF system is designed to quickly mobilize needed resources to areas of need.

1.6.3.4 Disaster Forensics

When a disaster or mass casualty event is a result of criminal activity such as terrorism, part of the role of responders is to protect evidence. Clearly, the rescue and resuscitation of casualties is the first priority. However, one should be mindful of the need to protect possible sources of evidence and to not disrupt the crime scene by unnecessarily moving debris or leaving trash behind to contaminate the scene. First responders play a critical role in this process. Their initial responsibilities are to preserve the integrity of the scene and the evidence. Furthermore, they are responsible for the early documentation of the scene, its evidence, and all activities at the scene.

While there are general principles related to disaster scene investigations, local laws, rules, and regulations govern many activities of the investigation and forensic process. They relate to issues such as how to obtain authority to enter the scene, conduct the investigation, handle evidence (eg, the type of sealing procedure required), and submit physical evidence to the forensic laboratory. Failure to comply with existing laws, rules, and regulations can result in a situation in which the evidence cannot be used in court. It is therefore important for all personnel working at a disaster scene to be aware of, and ensure proper compliance with, these rules. If there is a conflict between preservation of evidence and the possibility of saving a human life, priority is always given to emergency medical care.

1.6.4 Health Care Facility Surge Management

Disasters can reduce the capabilities of local health care facilities by creating substantial additional demand for medical, surgical, and rehabilitation services. Nearly every disaster is accompanied by a surge of people with a variety of ailments. Many individuals require treatment for injuries that resulted directly from the disaster. Others seek medical attention for acute (eg, post-earthquake heart attacks and shelter-induced deep vein thromboses) and chronic conditions that can be exacerbated during stressful times. When a disaster forces a hospital to close and evacuate its patients, the influx of those patients will likely affect nearby facilities. Health officials need to plan for the provision of medical care in nonhospital environments if there is no capacity left in hospitals.

Disasters and mass casualty incidents can impact health care facilities in two ways: (1) health care facilities may become overwhelmed by the numbers of casualties encountered; or (2) these facilities may be the targets of acts of terrorism or impacted by natural disasters. An additional source of vulnerability for health care facilities reflects their dependence on outside resources. In a mass casualty event, the hospital closest to the disaster scene is most likely to be overwhelmed because of the "geographic effect," a well-observed phenomenon in which casualties go to the closest hospital, regardless of on-site direction.[27] Casualties do not distinguish the specialty characterization of hospitals (eg, adult vs pediatrics, cancer vs cardiac), so every health care facility should plan for reception of a demographic cross section of casualties.

It is paramount that hospitals be notified early to prepare for mass casualties. Many casualties will arrive at the hospital by private vehicle and thus without being decontaminated. In fact, the sarin incident in Tokyo demonstrated this reality when approximately four of five casualties presented directly to hospitals without the intervention of hazardous materials or other prehospital personnel. In most cases, individuals will not wait for emergency personnel to arrive on scene, as often their most realistic option is to self-evacuate from the scene. As a result, health care facilities will require decontamination facilities, personal protective equipment, antidotes, and disaster plans to respond to such incidents and must not rely on EMS for these actions. Early notification will allow the hospital to activate specific procedures and staff to prepare for the arrival of multiple casualties. In addition, this notification will allow various systems, such as surge capacity, to be in place.

The SNS provides many of the pharmaceutical agents and durable medical supplies that would likely be needed in a mass casualty situation. Additionally, the federal government and the military have the capability to mobilize and deliver medical teams and facilities that can care for and intern several thousands of patients. These supplies and facilities will take at least 24 hours, and in some cases up to 5 days, to be delivered and set up at the periphery of an incident. With the reality that supplies may not reach the scene for at least 24 hours, states should consider stockpiling of various pharmaceuticals and medical supplies that will be necessary in a large-scale disaster or public health emergency. This would include stockpiles of generic categories of routine medications used by patients on a daily basis, in addition to medications that would be specifically needed to treat victims of a biologic, chemical, or radiation emergency.

1.6.4.1 Space, Staff, and Supplies

Large-scale natural disasters and public health emergencies are often marked by a substantial increase in demand for health care services and a related decrease in the supply of resources available to provide such care. It is important to recognize this inequality in supply and demand as early as possible, and even more important to preemptively anticipate the likely areas in which shortages will be encountered. This requires that the health system has developed a meaningful surge capacity and capability strategy. In large-scale natural disasters, a framework for standards of care for health care facilities should be in place that includes consideration of crisis standards of care. Operational steps must be clearly identified and understood by all appropriate personnel.

Even though a health care facility may have escaped the worst of the disaster and may even have experienced no physical damage, it can still suffer reduced capabilities due to a surge in admissions. This surge (in both regular and emergency admissions) can result in serious shortages in personnel and supplies. Procedures to obtain additional capacity during a disaster must be both preestablished and flexible, with predetermined methods of activating these resources for different levels of response. Establishing surge capacity to meet increased health-related needs in a disaster consists of three primary medical support areas: human resources, facilities, and supplies. The availability of these resources is limited by the routine needs of a community and by the economics and logistics involved in creating and maintaining excess capacity from normal community requirements in a serious mass casualty event.

In a mass casualty situation, hospital staff will have to deal with an influx of people who need or think they need prompt attention. A challenge then becomes how to meet mass casualty demands while continuing to meet the needs of patients who were already receiving care in the facility before the event and the potential additional medical and trauma needs, unrelated to the event, that may present in the coming hours. Often, when health personnel must work through a disaster, they are very preoccupied with the safety of their homes, possessions, and loved ones. It is not unusual for nurses, physicians, health care administrators, and other health care providers to face a basic conflict between their professional and personal obligations during a disaster. Clearly, the personal stresses experienced by health personnel during times of crisis create an additional vulnerability for affected health care systems.

Although surge capacity is often touted as a solution, hard reality must intervene and point out that surge capacity beds must be staffed, provisioned, and supplied. Unless there is abundant staffing available, the local infrastructure may not be able to be expanded to treat more patients. Alternative health care facilities may have to be established within the affected area. Because of resource constraints, casualties will likely have to accept subtraditional levels of care. Local medical care surge capacity—including personnel, training, space, supplies, and equipment—must be strengthened.

Currently, US hospitals are simply unprepared to take on the tens to hundreds of thousands of mass casualties expected in the event of bioterrorism, a pandemic, or a nuclear event. Although surge expansion plans exist for use of Veterans Affairs, US Public Health Service, and even military medical assets, these plans often do not cover simultaneous multilocation outbreaks that may occur with pandemics. Appropriate management strategies also will have to be put into place to deal with the potentially large number of fatalities.

To adapt to changing resources (ie, space to deliver care, clinical staff availability, and the availability of key supplies), a surge capacity continuum has been proposed to

Surge Capacity Continuum for Health Care Facilities [8,9,28]

A surge capacity framework has been proposed to meet the challenges of dealing with a significant influx of casualties from a large-scale disaster. This framework can help health care institutions and communities plan for the spectrum of supply and demand challenges that may occur. The goal is always to maintain or return to conventional capacity.

➤ *Conventional capacity:* Traditional and normal patient care facilities and staff meet their normal goals in providing care.

➤ *Contingency capacity:* Minor adaptations are made that may have minor consequences for standards of care, but adaptations are not enough to result in significant changes to standards of care.

➤ *Crisis capacity:* A fundamental, systematic change takes place into a system in which standards of care are significantly altered.

help meet these challenges.[8,9,28] Surge capacity following a mass casualty event falls into three basic categories, depending on the magnitude of the event: conventional, contingency, and crisis surge capacity. As the imbalance increases between resource availability and demand, a health care facility will maximize conventional capacity, move into contingency, and, once that has been maximized, move finally into crisis capacity. The same event may result in conventional care at a major urban trauma center but require crisis care at a smaller, rural facility.

Concurrent with this transition along a surge capacity continuum is the realization that the accepted standard of care will shift in a disaster situation. This occurs primarily as a result of the growing scarcity of human and material resources needed to treat, transport, and provide patient care. The goal of the health care facility is to return as quickly as possible to conventional care by requesting resources or transferring patients out of the area and by drawing on the resources of partner or coalition hospitals and the greater health system. Every attempt must be made to maintain usual practices and the expected standard of care and patient safety.

1.6.4.2   Surge-Based Health Care Facilities

To supplement health system surge capacity, public health authorities may advise the public to seek care or reassurance in alternate settings so that hospitals and emergency care facilities can focus resources on those who need them most. The altered or alternative care environment (ACE) refers to the need to treat large numbers of casualties outside of a traditional setting because of limitations in existing traditional health care facility capacity. These may be established as mobile, temporary units to provide casualty care close to the disaster area. Often the mobile units are tent-like shelters or inflatable structures that can be easily transported and readily set up. An option in metropolitan areas is to use existing available buildings (eg, school gym or community center). Units are designed to admit, sort, and temporarily hospitalize casualties until they can be safely transported to more permanent health care facilities.

Federal, state, municipal, and academic authorities have grappled with developing consistent definitions for altered or alternative care for more than a decade. The essential issue is to provide lifesaving, stabilizing, and finally definitive care for more casualties than the traditional medical system can accommodate in any specific location near to the catastrophic incident. The problem posed by a serious pandemic or nuclear event is that local and regional health care capacity will immediately be overwhelmed by the large number of casualties. Additionally, the ability to move large numbers of people to distant locations for acute care is severely limited because of years of shrinkage of surplus EMS capacity.

A recent development has been the concept of providing a low to intermediate level of care for moderately injured or ill casualties in settings outside of a traditional care setting. The purpose of these facilities is to decompress traditional hospital settings by treating those individuals who are less than critically ill or injured. Additionally, the setting could provide support and stabilization of more seriously ill or injured people while awaiting transport to more advanced levels of care. In such a scenario, triage physicians at a central station would assess casualties and write standing treatment orders. Individuals would then be moved to community-based alternate care facilities (ACFs), staffed by a limited number of registered nurses and community volunteer support personnel. These facilities could be established in nursing homes, community health centers, schools, churches, malls, medical or dental professional offices, and other locations having adequate sanitary and support capabilities.

Surge-based health care facilities, such as ACFs, would be used during large-scale disasters or public health emergencies when the health system cannot rely solely on hospitals to care for the affected population. These sites can serve a variety of functions intended to relieve pressure on local health care systems. They may serve as triage stations or provide casualty care when local health care facility infrastructure is damaged. ACFs can be used to care for "overflow patients" transferred from hospitals and trauma centers to make room in these facilities for more acutely injured or ill people.

In addition to providing acute casualty care, an ACF can be staffed and equipped to provide long-term care services, distribute vaccines and other medical countermeasures, and provide for the quarantine, cohorting, or sequestration of potentially infected people in the context of an easily transmissible infectious disease. ACFs are most effective when they are identified and planned for in advance to ensure the capability and resources to provide adequate care. Trying to identify new space in the midst of the disaster is too late. ACFs also may have just-in-time applications. For example, a newly implemented large general-population shelter may benefit from on-site delivery of acute medical services, which can provide for more timely care, require less transportation resources, and prevent local emergency department surge for a community sheltering large numbers of displaced people affected by a disaster.

In the aftermath of Hurricane Katrina in September 2005, a large ACF was set up at the Pete Maravich Assembly Center in Baton Rouge, Louisiana, to provide medical care for New Orleans evacuees. Originally intended as a medical triage facility, it was transformed into a surge hospital and eventually served 6000 patients, thus becoming the largest acute care field hospital in US history.

1.7 RECOVERY AND BEYOND

Recovery begins from the moment a disaster occurs, as affected populations begin to restore their lives and the infrastructure that supports them. It is the final and usually longest phase of disaster management. There is no distinct point at which disaster relief changes into recovery and then into long-term sustainable development. The initial management of any disaster must address the long-term implications, costs, and impacts on all affected populations. Three to 7 days after the disaster, acute management of the injured and ill will be nearly completed, and reestablishment of local health care services becomes the primary focus. This includes ensuring services for people who may have postponed or avoided seeing their health care provider during the immediate response phase, patients who have lost their medications, those who have interrupted home health care service, oxygen-dependent patients who need supplies, diabetic patients who need their triglycerides brought under control, and a multitude of other patients with functional or access needs who will be seeking access to health care. This increased patient volume may be difficult for the local health care system to manage, especially if hospitals, clinics, and transportation options have been damaged or destroyed.

The reestablishment of local health and medical care infrastructure will be improved if the community preparedness planning includes the early recovery of local medical office-based practices. Preparedness elements that foster the early return of personnel, office-based facilities, supplies of medications and durable health care goods, as well as alternative facilities for displaced office-based practitioners and their staff are examples that support early recovery. By addressing and prioritizing short- and long-term recovery measures in advance, affected communities may avoid excess morbidity and mortality in a serious disaster or public health emergency. This includes a thorough evaluation of "what went right" and "what went wrong" in disaster response, which may reveal opportunities to mitigate or prevent health, environmental, economic, and societal effects of future disasters. Such evaluation also may highlight coping mechanisms that can be reinforced or encouraged for future events.

1.7.1 Continuity of Operations in Health Care Facilities

A fully functioning hospital consumes large amounts of energy; requires daily deliveries of food, medications, and other supplies; and depends on a highly skilled and specialized workforce. When the health care infrastructure is affected by an event, there must be a business continuity plan. Loss of electronic assets during a disaster complicates facility management, cuts off access to electronic medical records and diagnostics, and hinders communication among staff, all of which can compromise patient care. Having a continuity plan will both enable facilities to manage the patients currently being cared for and restore their vital operations as quickly as possible. When discussing the vulnerability of the health system, it is essential that facility disaster plans also consider the effects of a disaster on their most vital resource—their employees.

In addition to the immediate challenges of recovery, a disaster produces a variety of long-term challenges for affected health care facilities. Once a hospital has been evacuated and forced to close, for example, the process of reopening can be complex, time consuming, and resource intensive. This complexity extends to many of the external lifelines, such as water and sewerage access that may have been severed because of a disaster. When evacuated facilities are closed, other health care facilities in the region that remain open will be forced to accept the additional patient load. Even if the facility has been repaired and external services are available, personnel shortages can continue, especially if the disaster has destroyed a significant portion of the local infrastructure. Finally, emerging health threats can last for years and decades, a problem that emerges especially when the disaster results in large numbers of people being exposed to an environmental hazard created or exacerbated by the event.

Hospitals are important symbols of community health and well-being and have a critical role in providing psychosocial support for the community and hospital personnel. For a health care facility to recover and return to normal operations after a disaster, two important components must be taken into account and planned for adequately: first is the infrastructure, and second are the people. Facilities must reestablish their infrastructure, resume normal health care operations, and restore business continuity. Sustainment of community medical care may require assistance from outside the community, coordinated through public health authorities. Possibilities include state assets, such as the National Guard, and federal assistance through Disaster Medical Assistance Teams (DMATs) and the Medical Reserve Corps.

Continuity of operations refers to how quickly the health care facility can get back to business after a disaster.[29] Each health care facility must have a plan in place to allow it to resume normal functions as quickly as possible if it plans to remain a viable source of health care to the community it serves. To accomplish this, the facility's plan must address succession of management, payroll, accounting, contracts, vendor agreements, personnel issues, facility access issues, and patient discharge issues. This list is not exhaustive. Each health care facility must analyze its own operations and identify mission-critical functions that must be supported, enhanced, and returned to normal to ensure the continuity of operations and the success of the facility mission in delivering health care to its community. Recovery efforts will be affected if local and regional vendors are affected negatively by the event. Federal assets are best considered under recovery; the structure for federal engagement does not lead to federal deployment before 72 hours (and often longer). Recovery plans should provide mechanisms for procuring supplies from other outside vendors. Plans and resources should be in place to assist facility employees both physically and emotionally.

1.7.2   After-Action Review

A key element of disaster recovery is a critical analysis and review of the actual response. A structured method to accomplish this task is through an after-action review (AAR). This should be completed as soon as disaster response operations transition to recovery operations so as to not lose essential individuals and recollections of the event. The review should likely include all stakeholders involved in the response (health department, private-public hospitals, private-public EMS companies, emergency management, police, local government leadership) and should review the strengths and weaknesses of the response. Opportunities will likely be uncovered that need to be incorporated into future response planning and operations. This topic is covered in more detail in the ADLS® course (v3.0) and supporting course manual.

1.7.3   Preparation and Planning for Future Events

The AAR provides the basis for changing response plans and developing tabletop and full-field exercises to test the assumptions and recommendations made in the report. Communities and organizations will consider new or revised policies, plans, and procedures to enhance community and organizational preparedness for future events. State and local preparedness plans should contain clear guidelines on setting priorities for the use of scarce resources such as vaccines, health care providers, medications, ventilators, and hospital beds. To avoid overwhelming hospitals, community plans need to provide for the establishment of ACFs (such as schools and gymnasiums) to treat sick and exposed people. Community plans also should address the great need for local trained volunteers to work in these facilities because most health care personnel will remain in hospitals treating critically ill or injured patients. Plans need to be specific, practical, and practiced in tabletop and field exercises and reflect the unique characteristics and vulnerabilities of each community. State and local health authorities should review the plans continually, including capacities and capabilities for surveillance, laboratory testing, and communication.

The AAR also will likely identify gaps in knowledge, skills, and attitudes among response personnel and agency leadership. Disaster education and training programs are based on the experiences of others as detailed in AARs from past events and made applicable by evaluating the performance of those who participated in disaster relief operations. A continual process of revising education and training programs allows health professionals to prepare for and operate under the conditions most likely to be encountered in disaster management and assist them in accomplishing their mission, while at the same time helping them to protect personal health and safety and reduce the psychological stress associated with being away from their loved ones in a potentially fearful and chaotic environment. As appropriate, the BDLS® course and other NDLS™ courses will be revised to ensure that they comport with the best available scientific evidence and incorporate the experiences and best practices of health professionals and others who have worked on the front lines during major disasters and who have studied the impact and effectiveness of preparedness, response, and recovery operations.

Many resources, including this course, are now available to assist both military and civilian clinicians and public health professionals in planning for, and maintaining proficiency in, the management of real or threatened terror attacks. Moreover, electronic resources of a similar nature have been developed and multiple Web sites provide a wealth of training materials and information online. Numerous government, military, and civilian organizations have been organized, trained, and equipped to provide assistance and consultation to the clinician, first responder, and public health official faced with planning for and managing a mass casualty situation. It is assistance that should be incorporated into thorough planning efforts.

1.7.4 Building Community Readiness and Resilience for Future Events

Resilience is the sustained ability of communities to withstand and recover—in both the short and long terms—from adversity.[30-32] Communities build resilience by implementing policies and practices that ensure healthy conditions, gaining knowledge of and addressing the needs of at-risk individuals, and creating a culture of preparedness in which a "bystander response" is not the exception but the norm. Resilient communities are prepared to prevent, cope with, and mitigate the initial stress of an incident with limited expectation of external support, undertake recovery activities that restore the community to pre-incident levels of health and social functioning, and use knowledge gained from the incident to strengthen the ability of the community to withstand future events. Key components or "building blocks" of community resilience include the:

➤ Physical and psychological health of the population;

➤ Social well-being and connectedness of community members;

➤ Level of social integration of government and nongovernmental organizations in planning, response, and recovery;

➤ Individual attitudes of self-reliance and self-help;

➤ Effective risk communication; and

➤ Economic stability.

Services provided by public health, health care, and emergency response systems complement efforts to build community resilience. Strong public health, health care, and emergency response systems can help minimize and/or prevent some incidents from occurring; facilitate the rapid detection and characterization of a health incident; provide care to those affected, including behavioral health care; reduce the effects of the incident on the community; and help a community recover after an incident. Such systems must be resilient in that they should be durable, robust, responsive, adaptive to changing situations, efficient, and interoperable.

In the context of all-hazards disaster management, resilience has applicability to both deployed individuals and teams in improving their ability to complete the assigned mission and their readiness for redeployment. Through planning, training, and education, a team's function is enhanced, as are the expectations team members have of what to expect and what constitutes reasonable success. With such information, team members are better prepared intellectually, educationally, and operationally to face the challenges of a disaster or mass casualty environment. This will enhance their collective success and decrease the level of postevent stress they will encounter, thus enhancing their ability to redeploy.

1.8 SUMMARY

In light of recent global disasters, it is increasingly clear that all health professionals need to become more proficient in the recognition, diagnosis, and treatment of mass casualties under an all-hazards approach. They must be able to recognize the general features of disasters and public health emergencies, and be knowledgeable about how to report them and where to get more information should the need arise. Health professionals are on the front lines when dealing with injury and disease—whether caused by microbes, environmental hazards, natural disasters, highway collisions, terrorism, or other calamities. Early detection and reporting are critical to minimize morbidity and mortality through astute teamwork by public- and private-sector health and emergency response personnel.

Large-scale disasters and public health emergencies are marked by a sudden or gradual increase in demand for health care services and a related decrease in the supply of resources available to provide such care. Degradation of standards of care can occur as a result of widespread geographic destruction of health care systems and infrastructure. In such situations, health personnel may have to practice under less than desirable care conditions and service delivery methods. The standard of care owed to a patient by a health care professional depends on the circumstances. What is deemed to be "reasonable" care under normal circumstances may not be feasible during a serious disaster or public health emergency, in which large numbers of injured or ill persons overwhelm existing health system capacities and capabilities. Federal agencies and health organizations are developing guidance and policy related to adjusting the standard of care in a mass casualty event.

The best way to make communities safer is to be prepared before disaster strikes. Preparedness can be achieved through thoughtful planning and can ensure that if a disaster occurs, people are ready to respond safely and effectively. Preparedness reinforces the need for constant vigilance and planning to prepare for and respond to new and unexpected public health threats. To effectively prepare for and respond to an actual or threatened disaster, health officials and emergency management personnel must collaborate to:

➤ Identify the types of events that might occur in their communities;

➤ Plan emergency activities in advance to ensure a coordinated response to the consequences of credible threats;

➤ Build capabilities necessary to respond effectively to the consequence of those events;

➤ Rapidly assess the needs of affected populations;

➤ Implement the planned response quickly and efficiently; and

➤ Mobilize resources to recover from the incident.

The basic tenets of all-hazards disaster management are reinforced in the PRE-DISASTER Paradigm™ (*p*lanning and practice, *r*esilience, and *e*ducation and training) and the DISASTER Paradigm™ (*d*etection, *i*ncident management, *s*afety and security, *a*ssess hazards, *s*upport, *t*riage and treatment, *e*vacuation, and *r*ecovery).

1.9 DISCUSSION POINTS

All-Hazards Disaster Casualty Management: Putting the PRE-DISASTER Paradigm™ Into Practice

P	Planning and Practice	*Do your community and workplace have disaster plans? Do you have a personal and family plan? Are these plans practiced and evaluated regularly?* Various methods exist for planning and conducting useful disaster training exercises. To be useful, they don't have to be full-scale, field-based exercises. Useful exercises require that the "right" people are invited to participate, that clear objectives are established and tied to local threats and concerns, and that a practical approach is used to enable the group to learn and improve disaster plans and skills.
R	Resilience	*What measures are in place to help individuals and communities cope with physical and psychological trauma?* Resilience involves behaviors, thoughts, and actions that can be learned and developed in anyone. Resilience also refers to plans that return the infrastructure of a community back to normal as soon as possible after an event. Resilience can be enhanced through mitigation efforts to eliminate or reduce the probability of disaster occurrence or reduce the effects of unavoidable events.
E	Education and Training	*Are opportunities available for competency-based education and training in disaster medicine and public health preparedness to meet the needs of all health professionals?* Health professionals, regardless of specialty or area of expertise, should have a basic understanding of all-hazards disaster casualty management and how their various roles are integrated with other segments of the disaster response system. This includes the ability to recognize general features of disasters and public health emergencies; how to report a potential emergency; and where to get more information should the need arise. Health professionals also should know the ethical and legal structures that govern response to serious mass casualty incidents, while maintaining the highest possible standards of care under extreme conditions. This encompasses their rights and responsibilities to protect themselves and treat others.

All-Hazards Disaster Casualty Management: Putting the DISASTER Paradigm™ Into Practice

D	Detection	*Do needs exceed resources? Call 911.* Maintaining situation awareness via timely, credible, and reliable information is essential before, during, and after a disaster strikes. This includes up-to-date guidelines, recommendations, health alerts, and modern, standards-based information systems that monitor data on injuries and diseases and enable efficient communication among public and private health organizations, the media, and the public.

I	Incident Management	*What is your role? Who is the incident commander?* Incident management can be facilitated through the incorporation of standardized principles for managing time, personnel, and resources in any emergency or disaster. The importance of implementing a command structure from the very outset of an event cannot be overemphasized. Once an emergency situation has been detected, the safe and successful management of the event depends on the consistent application of core principles and proven response strategies. Disaster response includes basic elements that are similar in all events. The differences are the degree to which these elements are utilized in a specific incident and the degree to which outside assistance is needed.
S	Safety and Security	*Is the scene secure? Is it safe to enter?* Safety is always the top priority—personal safety followed by that of the response team. Report any recognized or suspected hazard to appropriate authorities. Do not enter any disaster scene or take any action until authorities determine it is safe. Protecting yourself from becoming a casualty is the number 1 priority.
A	Assess Hazards	*Fire? Hazardous materials? Radiation? Building collapse? Downed power lines? Secondary devices?* Actual and potential hazards related to a disaster must be assessed continually. Hazards will vary according to the situation encountered and the assignment given to the health responder. All disasters, regardless of the primary cause, create the possibility of secondary hazards capable of injuring anyone present at the scene, including responders.
S	Support	*What outside assistance is needed (eg, police, fire, emergency medical services, government, other)? Can adequate surge capability and capacity be established to meet local public safety and health needs and priorities?* Effective disaster management hinges on the timely delivery of resources to where they are needed most. Estimate when resources at hand will deplete and contact outside resources in advance giving them notice as to what your needs will be and when. Health responders should be knowledgeable about surge capacity assets in the public and private health response sectors and the extent of their potential assistance in an emergency.
T	Triage and Treatment	*Are protocols, procedures, and resources in place for the rapid triage and immediate treatment of casualties? What public health interventions are needed?* In a disaster, clinical responders should be prepared to apply and adapt their usual skill set and expertise to the triage and treatment of seriously injured or ill persons under crisis conditions, with limited situational awareness and resources. Triage systems will be used to guide casualty assessment and treatment at a disaster scene. Various public

		health actions and interventions also must be considered. The basics of risk communication and health messaging will be essential for communicating with affected individuals, their families, and the media regarding exposure risks and potential preventive measures, without contributing to public alarm, fear, and anxiety. Health responders should be familiar with clinical and mental health implications of natural and human-caused disasters and recognize that persons may have been exposed to nonconventional agents as the source of unusual presentations.
E	Evacuation	*Are enough transport units en route to the scene? Should affected persons evacuate or shelter in place?* Getting all potential survivors out of the scene as soon as possible during a disaster is usually the short-term goal. This may be challenging if the scene is deemed unsafe because of the presence of immediately life-threatening conditions.
R	Recovery	*What are the long-term mental and physical challenges facing the community? What are the financial and economic repercusions of the disaster?* Recovery is the longest phase of disasters. Recovery includes monitoring communities and first responder health weeks, months, and years after a disaster. Physical, psychological, social, and economic stress can prevent individuals and communities from recovering in a timely way. Effective preparation and planning can help build the resilience necessary for individuals and communities to withstand and recover from disasters and other tragic events.

REFERENCES

1. US Department of Health and Human Services (HHS). *National Health Security Strategy of the United States of America*. Washington, DC: HHS; 2009. http://www.phe.gov/Preparedness/planning/authority/nhss/Pages/default.aspx. Accessed March 25, 2011.

2. Burkle FM Jr, Greenough PG. Impact of public health emergencies on modern disaster taxonomy, planning, and response. *Disaster Med Public Health Prep*. 2008;2:192-199.

3. Burkle FM Jr. Public health emergencies, cancer, and the legacy of Katrina. *Prehosp Disaster Med*. 2007;22:291-292.

4. Sorensen BV. *Populations With Special Needs*. ORNL/TM-2006/559. Oak Ridge, TN: Oak Ridge National Laboratory; 2006. http://emc.ornl.gov/publications/PDF/Population_Special_Needs.pdf. Accessed March 25, 2011.

5. Phillips S, Knebel A, eds. *Mass Medical Care With Scarce Resources: A Community Planning Guide*. Publication 07-0001. Rockville, MD: Agency for Healthcare Research and Quality; 2007. http://archive.ahrq.gov/research/mce/. Accessed March 25, 2011.

6. Center for Health Policy, Columbia University School of Nursing. *Adapting Standards of Care Under Extreme Conditions: Guidance for Professionals During Disasters, Pandemics, and Other Extreme Emergencies*. Washington, DC: American Nurses Association; 2008.

7. Kanter RK, Andrake JS, Boeing NM, et al. Developing consensus on appropriate standards of disaster care for children. *Disaster Med Public Health Prep.* 2009;3:27-32.

8. Hick J, Barbera J, Kelen G. Refining surge capacity: conventional, contingency, and crisis capacity. *Disaster Med Pub Health Prep.* 2009;3(suppl 1):S59-S67.

9. Institute of Medicine. *Guidance for Establishing Crisis Standards of Care for Use in Disaster Situations*: A Letter Report. Washington, DC: National Academies Press; 2009.

10. Hun RC, Kapil V, Basavaraju SV, Sasser SM, McGuire LC, Sullivent EE. *Updated In a Moment's Notice: Surge Capacity for Terrorist Bombings.* Atlanta, GA: Centers for Disease Control and Prevention; 2010. http://www.bt.cdc.gov/masscasualties/pdf/CDC_Surge-508.pdf. Accessed March 25, 2011.

11. US Government Accountability Office (GAO). *Emergency Preparedness: States Are Planning for Medical Surge, but Could Benefit From Shared Guidance for Allocating Scarce Medical Resources.* GAO-08-668. Washington, DC: GAO; 2008. http://www.gao.gov/new.items/d08668.pdf. Accessed March 25, 2011.

12. Joint Commission on Accreditation of Healthcare Organizations (JCAHO). 2006 *Hospital Accreditation Standards.* Oakbrook Terrace, IL: JCAHO; 2006.

13. Comperatore C, Abernathy W. Situational awareness: what is it? *Crew Endurance Manage.* 2008;2:1-2. http://www.uscg.mil/hq/cg5/cg5211/docs/CEMSnlpubs/Vol_5_Issue2.pdf. Accessed March 25, 2011.

14. Nash D, Mostashari F, Fine A, et al, for the 1999 West Nile Outbreak Response Working Group. The outbreak of West Nile virus in the New York City area in 1999. *N Engl J Med.* 2001;344:1807-1814. http://www.nejm.org/doi/full/10.1056/NEJM200106143442401. Accessed March 25, 2011.

15. Semenza JC, Rubin CH, Falter KH, et al. Heat-related deaths during the July 1995 heat wave in Chicago. *N Engl J Med.* 1996;335:84-90. http://www.nejm.org/doi/pdf/10.1056/NEJM199607113350203. Accessed March 25, 2011.

16. Homeland Security Presidential Directive 5 (HSPD-5). *Management of Domestic Incidents.* Washington, DC: The White House; February 28, 2003. http://www.fas.org/irp/offdocs/nspd/hspd-5.html. Accessed March 25, 2011.

17. NIMS Resource Center, Federal Emergency Management Agency. http://www.fema.gov/emergency/nims/. Accessed March 25, 2011.

18. ICS Resource Center, Federal Emergency Management Agency. http://training.fema.gov/EMIWeb/IS/ICSResource/index.htm. Accessed March 25, 2011.

19. FIRESCOPE. http://firescope.org/. Accessed March 25, 2011.

20. California Emergency Medical Services Authority. *Disaster Medical Services Division—Hospital Incident Command System (HICS).* http://www.emsa.ca.gov/hics/. Accessed March 25, 2011.

21. Burkle FM Jr, Hsu EB, Loehr M, et al. Definitions and functions of health unified command and emergency operations centers for large-scale bioevent disasters within the existing ICS. *Disaster Med Public Health Prep.* 2007;1:135-141.

22. US Department of Health and Human Services (HHS). *Communicating in a Crisis: Risk Communication Guidelines for Public Officials.* Washington, DC: HHS; 2002. http://www.hhs.gov/od/documents/RiskCommunication.pdf. Accessed March 25, 2011.

23. *National Disaster Medical System.* Assistant Secretary for Preparedness and Response, US Department of Health and Human Services (HHS). http://www.phe.gov/preparedness/responders/ndms/Pages/default.aspx. Accessed March 25, 2011.

24. *Strategic National Stockpile.* Centers for Disease Control and Prevention (CDC). http://www.bt.cdc.gov/stockpile/. Accessed March 25, 2011.

25. *National Response Framework.* US Department of Homeland Security. http://www.fema.gov/pdf/emergency/nrf/nrf-core.pdf. Accessed March 25, 2011.

26. *Emergency Support Function Annexes: Introduction*; 2008. http://www.fema.gov/pdf/emergency/nrf/nrf-esf-intro.pdf. Accessed March 25, 2011.

27. Frykberg E. Principles of mass casualty management following terrorist disasters. *Ann Surg*. 2004;239(3):319-321.

28. Rubinson L, Hick JL, Hanfling D, et al. Definitive care for the critically ill during a disaster: a framework for optimizing critical care surge capacity: from a Task Force for Mass Critical Care summit meeting, January 26-27, 2007, Chicago, IL. *Chest*. 2008;133(5, suppl):18S-31S.

29. US Department of Homeland Security (DHS). *Ready Business: Continuity of Operations Planning*. http://www.ready.gov/business/plan/planning.html. Accessed March 25, 2011.

30. Norris FH, Stevens SP, Pfefferbaum B, Wyche KF, Pfefferbaum RL. Community resilience as a metaphor, theory, set of capacities, and strategy for disaster readiness. *Am J Community* Psych. 2007;41:127-150.

31. Gurwitch RH, Pfefferbaum B, Montgomery JM, Klomp RW, Reissman DB. *Building Community Resilience for Children and Families*. Oklahoma City: Terrorism and Disaster Center, University of Oklahoma Health Sciences Center; 2007. http://www.oumedicine.com/Workfiles/College%20of%20Medicine/AD-Psychiatry/CR_guidebook.pdf. Accessed March 25, 2011.

32. Blumenfeld M, Ursano RJ, eds. *Intervention and Resilience after Mass Trauma*. New York, NY: Cambridge University Press; 2008.

CHAPTER TWO

Public Health Response to Disasters

CHAPTER CHAIR

Frederick M. Burkle, Jr, MD, MPH, DTM

CONTRIBUTING AUTHORS

Jim Lyznicki, MS, MPH

Italo Subbarao, DO, MBA

2.1 PURPOSE

This chapter provides an overview of public health principles and practices for the management of communities and populations affected by time-limited disasters. The role of the public health system in the management of prolonged disasters and public health emergencies is discussed in the Advanced Disaster Life Support™ (ADLS®) course (v3.0) and supporting course manual.

2.2 LEARNING OBJECTIVES

After completing this chapter, readers should be able to:

➤ Explain the mission and core functions of the public health system.

➤ Discuss the roles and responsibilities of local, state, federal, and global health agencies and organizations in disaster management.

➤ Discuss emergency public health response actions that can be implemented in a disaster.

Learning Objectives for this chapter are competency-based, as delineated in Appendix B.

2.3   BACKGROUND

The immediate impact of large-scale disasters and public health emergencies on community and population health can be far reaching. Significant damage to public health infrastructure, widespread population displacement, and disruptions in health services can lead to secondary effects, which can contribute to excess and often preventable morbidity and mortality at rates exceeding those directly attributable to the event.

Preparedness and response plans need to be in place to monitor for additional increases in physical, mental, and behavioral problems resulting from disasters and other traumatic events. Integration of public health and the emergency care systems—first responders, emergency medical services (EMS), hospital emergency departments, trauma centers, and volunteers, among others—is critical to success.

In a major disaster, affected individuals and communities must have their basic physiologic and psychological needs met in a timely manner. Available resources will likely be challenged by a surge of people seeking medical and relief services. To meet this challenge, public health authorities must work with others to implement various measures to control the situation and help prevent further harm.[1-3] This includes establishing priorities, standards, and monitoring systems for water, food, sanitation, solid-waste removal, shelter, animal and vector control, and communicable disease control. Public health professionals will work with emergency response agencies to ensure that affected populations are aware of health and safety risks and how to either avoid them or prepare to deal with them. They will issue guidelines for the diagnosis, care, and reporting of injured and ill persons, as well as guidelines for the distribution of scarce medical resources to those who need them most. Throughout the event, public health personnel will focus on the bigger picture, that is, getting the community back to health.

2.4   THE PUBLIC HEALTH SYSTEM

The public health system protects the nation against injury, disease, and myriad environmental and occupational health hazards. The public health system focuses on populations—assessing and monitoring health problems, informing the public and professionals about health issues, developing and enforcing health-protecting laws and regulations, implementing and evaluating population-based strategies to promote health and prevent disease, and ensuring the provision of health care services. In 1988, the Institute of Medicine (IOM) defined the *public health system* as a complex network of individuals and organizations that, when working together, can represent what we as a society do collectively to ensure the conditions in which people can be healthy.[4] This system includes traditional partners, such as government public health agencies, the health care delivery system, and the public health and health sciences academia, as well as less-recognized partners such as community entities (eg, schools, religious groups, businesses) and the media.

The public health infrastructure is the underlying foundation that supports the planning, delivery, and evaluation of public health activities and practices. This infrastructure makes it possible to respond to disasters and public health emergencies, as well as to perform essential ongoing public health services.

The basic components of the public health infrastructure are maintained and protected by the public health workforce; surveillance, information and data systems; social protection agencies; and organizational capacities. These are the building blocks that support the work of the public health system to prevent epidemics and the spread of disease, protect against environmental and occupational hazards, prevent injuries, promote and encourage healthy behaviors and mental health, respond to disasters and assist communities in recovery, and ensure the quality

Public Health and Disasters

Mission

To promote physical and mental health and prevent disease, injury, and disability

Core Functions

➤ Prevent epidemics and the spread of disease

➤ Protect against environmental hazards

➤ Prevent injuries

➤ Promote and encourage healthy behaviors and mental health

➤ Respond to disasters and assist communities in recovery

➤ Ensure the quality and accessibility of health services

Essential Public Health Services

➤ Monitor health status to rapidly detect a public health emergency

➤ Identify and investigate health problems and health hazards in the community

➤ Inform, educate, and empower people about specific health issues

➤ Mobilize state and local partnerships to identify and solve health problems before, during, and after a disaster event or other public health emergency

Public Health and Disasters (continued)

➤ Develop policies and plans that support individual and community health efforts in preparing for and responding to emergencies

➤ Enforce laws and regulations to protect public health and safety

➤ Link people to needed personal health services in the course of a public health emergency

➤ Ensure a competent and trained public and personal health care workforce for rapid response to a disaster or other public health emergency

➤ Evaluate effectiveness, accessibility, and quality of personal and population-based health services available to respond to a public health threat or emergency event

➤ Participate in research for new insights and innovative solutions to health problems resulting from exposure to a disaster or other public health emergency

Source: Adapted from Essential Public Health Services Working Group of the Core Public Health Functions Steering Committee, US Public Health Service; 1994 (http://www.cdc.gov/nphpsp/essentialServices.html).

and accessibility of health services. The public health workforce is represented by a diversity of skill sets, educational backgrounds, and experience, including, redundant specialists in medicine, nursing, epidemiology, social work, health education, outreach, environmental health, laboratory science, and mental health and substance abuse counseling.

2.5   PUBLIC HEALTH AGENCIES AND ORGANIZATIONS

The capacity to respond effectively to a serious mass casualty situation depends on a well-prepared and flexible public health system at all government levels and on the vigilance of health care workers, who may be the first to observe and report unusual diagnoses. Public health agencies have a direct role in helping to ensure appropriate care for all populations through health monitoring, disease surveillance, and laboratory sciences. Additionally, they provide an expert system for tracking, predicting, and developing response tactics to curtail or mitigate disease outbreaks or other health threats.

2.5.1   Local Health Agencies

Local governments provide the bulk of public health services. In the United States, about 3000 local and state health agencies provide the programs and services that compose the "front line" of public health. Activities include conducting health education, providing environmental and personal health services, performing inspections, managing injury and disease control programs, and collecting health statistics. Local agencies may conduct these activities through school health centers, home health centers, nursing homes, mental health centers, and community clinics and health centers. Most public health agencies provide some personal health services to indigent, high-risk, or hard-to-reach populations. Such services may include home visits, primary care for underserved people, treatment for targeted conditions (eg, HIV/AIDS, alcohol and other drug abuse, mental illness), and clinical preventive services (eg, immunizations, family planning).

A complete directory of local public health agencies can be accessed at www.naccho.org/about/LHD/index.cfm.

2.5.2   State Health Agencies

States have the primary legal responsibility for protecting public health, which is carried out through state health agencies. In most states, public health agencies are freestanding entities; in others, public health functions are incorporated into superagencies, which may oversee a variety of health and social service activities. Responsibilities of state health agencies include the collection and analysis of health information; planning; setting health policies and standards; carrying out national and state mandates; managing and overseeing environmental, educational, and personal health services; and ensuring access to health care for underserved residents. Most states rely on local agencies for at least some aspects of public health service delivery. States rely on federal agencies for technical assistance, policy guidance, standard setting, and financial support.

A listing of state health departments can be accessed at www.cdc.gov/masstrauma/resources/state_departments.htm or www.statepublichealth.org.

2.5.3   Federal Health Agencies

Federal agencies establish and enforce laws and regulations that require a national scope. Most activities are conducted indirectly through funds distributed to states, localities, and private providers and organizations. Most federal public health activities, other than some aspects of environmental and occupational health, fall under the jurisdiction of the Department of Health and Human Services (HHS). Key federal health agencies are the following:

➤ Agency for Healthcare Research and Quality (http://www.ahrq.gov)

➤ Agency for Toxic Substances and Disease Registry (http://www.atsdr.cdc.gov)

➤ Centers for Disease Control and Prevention (CDC; http://www.cdc.gov)

➤ Food and Drug Administration (http://www.fda.gov)

➤ Heath Resources and Services Administration (http://www.hrsa.gov)

➤ Indian Health Service (http://www.ihs.gov)

➤ National Institutes of Health (http://www.nih.gov)

➤ Office of the Surgeon General (http://www.surgeongeneral.gov)

➤ Substance Abuse and Mental Health Services Administration (http://www
.samhsa.gov)

The HHS leads all federal public health and medical response to public health
emergencies and incidents covered by the National Response Framework (NRF;
http://www.fema.gov/emergency/nrf/). The Assistant Secretary for Preparedness and
Response (ASPR) serves as the principal advisor to the HHS Secretary on all matters
related to federal public health and medical preparedness and response to public
health emergencies. In particular, the ASPR coordinates with relevant federal officials to ensure integration of federal preparedness and response activities, as well as
coordinates with state, local, territorial, and tribal public health officials, health care
systems, and EMS systems.

2.5.4   Nongovernmental Organizations (NGOs) and Private Governmental Organizations (PGOs)

The American Red Cross serves governments as a PGO and supporting agency
for mass care functions. It also is sometimes listed along with the International
Committee of the Red Cross as a humanitarian NGO. The American Red Cross
(http://www.redcross.org) is a nonprofit humanitarian organization staffed mostly by
volunteers and has been providing disaster recovery assistance in the United States
since the 1880s. Although not a government organization, the American Red Cross
was given authority through a Congressional charter in 1905 to provide assistance
in disasters, both domestically and internationally. As a result, American Red Cross
chapters work closely with federal, tribal, state, and local governments to respond to
disasters. Some of the services offered by the American Red Cross in a disaster are
emergency first aid; health care for minor injuries and illnesses at mass care shelters
or other sites; supportive counseling for persons affected by a disaster; personnel to
assist at temporary infirmaries, immunization clinics, morgues, hospitals, and nursing homes; assistance with meeting basic needs (eg, food, shelter); and provision of
blood products.

In addition to the American Red Cross, it is likely that many other volunteer organizations will be involved in a response to a disaster or public health emergency.
The American Red Cross does not direct other NGOs but usually takes the lead in
the integration of efforts of the national NGOs and foreign NGOs that provide mass
care services during response operations. The National Voluntary Organizations
Active in Disaster (http://www.nvoad.org) is the forum in which organizations share
knowledge and resources throughout the disaster cycle (preparation, response,
and recovery) to help disaster survivors and their communities. This consortium of
approximately 50 national organizations and 55 state and territory equivalents sends
representatives to the Federal Emergency Management Agency (FEMA) national
response coordination center to represent the voluntary organizations and assist in
response coordination.

2.5.5   Global Health Agencies and Organizations

In most natural disasters, the majority of deaths occur in the first few hours or days, and likewise most of the lives that are saved are saved early on by local organized and volunteer efforts in disaster relief. A major disaster can overwhelm the resources of a poor country, destroy the emergency infrastructure itself, further compromise an already tenuous economic and social protective infrastructure of community-level resources, or overwhelm the system during a famine or outbreak of an infectious disease. Aid provided by global relief organizations immediately after the disaster can play a major role in averting health crises and reestablishing a functioning society.

Global health organizations are usually divided into three groups: multilateral organizations, bilateral organizations, and NGOs (also known as *private voluntary organizations*). The term *multilateral* means that funding comes from multiple governments (as well as from nongovernmental sources) and is distributed to many different countries. The major multilateral organizations are part of the United Nations (UN; http://www.un.org). Six UN organizations are involved directly in refugee and disaster relief:

➤ Food and Agriculture Organization (http://www.fao.org)

➤ Office of the UN High Commissioner for Refugees (http://www.unhcr.org)

➤ United Nations Children's Fund (http://www.unicef.org)

➤ United Nations Development Programme (http://www.undp.org)

➤ World Food Programme (http://www.wfp.org)

➤ World Health Organization (WHO; http://www.who.org)

The UN Office for the Coordination of Humanitarian Affairs ensures coordination among UN actors and key NGOs at the country level, serves as advocates for the victims of humanitarian crises, and mobilizes resources on behalf of the entire UN system through consolidated appeals and donor conferences. It has no postconflict or disaster recovery mandate, as this is the mandate of the UN Development Programme and the World Bank.

The WHO is likely the most recognized global health organization. The principal work of the WHO is directing and coordinating global health activities and supplying technical assistance to countries. It develops norms and standards, disseminates health information, promotes research, provides training in international health, collects and analyzes epidemiologic data, and develops systems for monitoring and evaluating health programs. The Pan American Health Organization (PAHO) serves as the regional field office for the WHO in the Americas and, because it predates WHO, carries on some additional autonomous activities.

Bilateral agencies are governmental agencies in a single country that provide aid to developing countries. The largest of these is the US Agency for International Development, under the US Department of State. Most industrialized nations have a similar governmental bilateral agency (eg, United Kingdom's Department for International Development and the Australian Government Overseas Aid Program).

While the UN agencies are probably the most recognized global relief organizations, there are many NGOs active in refugee and disaster relief. Outside the United States, the International Red Cross and Red Crescent Movement (http://www.icrc.org) and Medecins Sans Frontieres (http://www.msf.org) are examples of large humanitarian NGOs. Many are affiliated with faith-based organizations. In poor and underdeveloped countries, hospitals and clinics run by missionary societies provide essential care services in a disaster or other emergency. The global NGOs in the United States devoted to health are the International Medical Corps, International Rescue Committee, Mercy Corps, Save the Children, Samaritan's Purse, and Project Hope, among others.

2.6 PUBLIC HEALTH ROLE IN DISASTER RESPONSE

In a disaster, rapid and effective action is needed to save lives, protect health, and stabilize the situation to avoid making it worse. Critical public health actions include supplying basic life-sustaining commodities, such as food, water, and shelter; enhanced surveillance; distribution of vaccines and medications; implementation of environmental controls; legal interventions to restrict the movement of affected populations; emergency risk communication; and provision of essential treatment and preventive clinical services.[1,2,5-7] To respond rapidly, public health authorities must have the capacity to act on emerging information with the full range of necessary tools. These include the legal framework for action as well as adequate medical care facilities and treatment capabilities.

It is not possible to define a universally applicable order of priorities for emergency public health actions, as each situation demands a specific response. The large majority will fit within problems related to acute or chronic compromises in water, sanitation, access or availability of essential health services, adequate shelter, food, or energy to ensure heat during cold-related crises. The priorities following a population displacement in southern Africa, where a cholera epidemic may be imminent, are likely to be different from the priorities following a tornado in the United States. To make rational decisions about priorities, and to revise those priorities as the situation changes, means that an adequate assessment must be combined with basic public health and epidemiologic principles. In practice, several priorities usually need to be addressed simultaneously, as they are closely related, both epidemiologically and operationally. For instance, containing and disposing of human excreta is an important aspect of protecting water supplies from contamination; providing water collection and storage vessels and increasing water production are both needed to ensure the adequate collection and consumption of water for personal hygiene.

Overall public health priorities in the immediate response phase include ensuring access to food, shelter, health care, water supplies, and sanitation facilities; control of communicable diseases; public health surveillance; risk assessment and communication; containment or removal of chemical or radiologic contamination; and evacuation to ensure that people are no longer exposed to hazardous situations. Mass trauma experienced by disaster responders and affected populations can lead to widespread mental and physical health challenges. The public health system has a role in communicating coping strategies as well as information about self-care and evacuation or shelter-in-place strategies during a crisis. While immediate attention will be directed to the care of sick or injured casualties and the prevention of secondary mortality and morbidities, public health workers also coordinate with mortuary services to address the disposition of human remains and with animal care and control agencies for the care of live animals and the disposal of dead animals.

2.6.1 Emergency Public Health Powers

The power to implement measures necessary to protect the public's health is granted to each state under the US Constitution. These measures seek to balance individual rights and freedoms with the common welfare (eg, that of the general population). In a major disaster or public health emergency, states have authority to exert reasonable control over citizens to directly secure and promote the welfare of the state and its people. The power to act in the best interests of the people provides states and municipalities with broad discretion in how they respond to a disaster situation. This includes possible encroachment on civil rights of people in the affected area to promote the public welfare.

State statutes may provide for a declaration of a general emergency, disaster, or public health emergency, which is often broadly defined as an occurrence that immediately threatens public health and/or safety. Declaration of a state of emergency is a technical decision defined in most state laws and is carefully limited. Such declarations trigger emergency powers, the expenditure of emergency funds, the activation of emergency plans, and suspension of certain regulatory statutes. On the federal level, the HHS Secretary can declare a public health emergency under Section 319 of the Public Health Service Act. A declaration also may be made by the US President under the Stafford Act. Declarations under the Stafford Act can be either at the request of a state or unilateral (without the request of a state) if the United States has exclusive or preeminent authority (eg, federal facilities, tribal lands). A concomitant presidential declaration of emergency would enable the release and distribution of federal assets in support of the governor's declaration.

Emergency Public Health Powers

Once a disaster or an emergency situation has been declared, various orders may be issued on the basis of the police power available to the locality. These include: redundant

➤ Enforcing safety and sanitary codes

➤ Requiring health care professionals to report certain diseases to state authorities

➤ Establishing curfews

➤ Closing schools and businesses

➤ Ordering the evacuation of buildings, streets, neighborhoods, and cities

➤ Closing access to buildings, streets, or other public or private areas

Emergency Public Health Powers (continued)

➤ Imposing travel restrictions

➤ Suspending the sale or dispensing of alcoholic beverages

➤ Suspending or limiting the sale, dispensing, or transportation of firearms, explosives, or combustibles

➤ Authorizing the acquisition or destruction of property, supplies, and materials

➤ Issuing orders for the disposal of corpses

➤ Implementing medical protocols and procedures to limit the spread of a disease (eg, mandatory vaccinations)

➤ Issuing isolation and quarantine orders

➤ Issuing guidelines for access to and disclosure of protected health information

➤ Licensing of health care professionals

Section 361 of the Public Health Service Act authorizes the HHS to apprehend, detain, and examine persons to prevent the transmission of certain communicable diseases from individuals entering the United States from other countries or people moving across state lines. Containment of disease may also involve restricting the flow of animals, agricultural or food products, and other goods. Traditionally, courts have interpreted the authority of the states and the federal government broadly, giving great deference to public health officials. Still, even broad authority is not unfettered. Detained persons have a right to a court review of their detention's legality. Moreover, the US Constitution guarantees that protections and due process must be respected.

Special powers during a state of public health emergency also may be invoked to manage property. A disaster may create shortages in medical facilities and materials, impair access and control of health care facilities (eg, unruly mobs descending on emergency departments seeking medications), require overseeing safe disposal of infectious waste and human remains, require control of antibiotics and vaccines, necessitate just compensation for property seized for state purposes under emergency circumstances (eg, the government uses a private infirmary to treat or isolate patients), and require destruction of property eg, nuisance abatement. Similarly, the declaration of a public health emergency may require special powers to ensure the protection of persons. These include the power to examine, test, vaccinate, and treat patients; isolate and quarantine persons; access and disclose protected health information; and license and appoint health care providers. Not all states, however, have statutes that enumerate these public health powers over property and protection of persons in a consistent and uniform fashion.

Isolation and Quarantine

Isolation and quarantine are two of the oldest public health interventions, dating back centuries. The purpose of both interventions is to decrease the number of individuals exposed to a contagious disease.

➤ *Isolation* is the placement of persons known to have a communicable disease in a separate area where they will not expose others.

➤ *Quarantine* is the placement of persons exposed to a contagious disease, but currently asymptomatic, in a separate area where they will not expose others and can be monitored for the development of the disease. Quarantine is required for several infectious diseases, such as smallpox and severe acute respiratory syndrome (SARS), because individuals can be contagious before the development of the signs and symptoms of the disease. During this asymptomatic but contagious period, they can potentially infect a large number of people.

2.6.2   Epidemiologic Surveillance and Investigation

Epidemiology is the basic science fundamental to the practice of public health and preventive medicine. It is defined as the study of the distribution and determinants of health-related status and events in specified populations and the application of this study to the control of health problems. Epidemiologic studies are important for disease control, evaluation of program operation, and developing science-based policy. Public health surveillance and epidemiologic investigation are directed to the systematic, ongoing assessment of the health of a community. Epidemiologists at the local, state, and federal levels conduct investigations of suspected or confirmed patterns of disease, deaths, and injury in communities and populations. In some cases, an epidemiologist may suspect an outbreak by noticing unusual patterns or clusters of a disease in routine surveillance data. Well-developed epidemiologic expertise can improve community intervention strategies and lead to more effective prevention services; it is additionally essential to monitoring the effect of a disaster or public health emergency, managing public health concerns, and evaluating the impact of public health responses.

In a disaster or public health emergency, health assessment and monitoring programs increase dramatically. Public health readiness depends on timely and accurate situational awareness to inform mitigation and response strategies. In a disaster, situational awareness is the perception of environmental elements in a given time and space and the ability to comprehend their meaning and potential effects in the present and near-term future. Surveillance data and survey assessments of affected communities and health care systems may help to increase situational awareness by detecting the presence of new and expected risk factors and unexplained clusters of injury and disease.

Public health surveillance systems identify new health concerns, manage public information, and measure the effectiveness of ongoing interventions. They are generally established in sentinel sites, such as shelters, hospitals, or clinics, and collect data to:

➤ Reduce immediate injury, illness, and death associated with the event

➤ Track and document potential exposures

➤ Conduct long-term medical and mental health follow-up of affected individuals and populations

➤ Inform decisions regarding the safety and inhabitability of the affected area

Once a problem is identified, epidemiologists work with a multidisciplinary team to conduct a more comprehensive investigation; this team includes experts in clinical medicine, environmental health, microbiology, behavioral science, biostatistics, and health education. Part of their investigation involves interviewing affected individuals. These interviews provide epidemiologists with crucial data needed to map the spread of an outbreak (ie, source of the outbreak, mode of transmission). For example, by talking to affected individuals, epidemiologists may learn that all sick individuals attended the same event, which provides clues about how the outbreak started (eg, all ate the same food or drank from the same water source). Interviews also may allow epidemiologists to determine the "index case" (the first known case), which may be critical to determining the origin of the outbreak. Epidemiologists use focused interviews to identify the close contacts of each affected person (eg, family members, coworkers, close friends). In the case of a contagious disease, these people must be found and treated or isolated to prevent the spread of the illness. The "Achilles heel" of all infectious disease is that, by preventing its spread to other susceptible people, the outbreak will end.

Disease surveillance systems may be active or passive and are usually population-based rather than target specific. Passive systems do not rely on the initiative of public health surveillance personnel, but rather depend on other health care systems or providers to supply information without a specific request (eg, mailing reports of infectious diseases to the health department). Active systems require the initiative of public health surveillance personnel, for example by calling local hospitals to inquire about an uptick in case prevalence. In a disease outbreak, public health officials will use active surveillance to seek out infected and exposed persons. This includes making personal calls to health care professionals and interviewing infected people and their family members to identify contacts and other ill or exposed individuals.

Syndromic surveillance is a form of active surveillance that can give a more "real-time" report than traditional disease reporting by using indicators that are available before confirmed clinical or laboratory diagnoses. It relies on innovative approaches, perhaps by the monitoring and tracking of certain syndromic categories (eg, burns and trauma, respiratory failure, cardiovascular shock, neurologic toxicity), the sale of medications (both over-the-counter and prescription), or unexplained deaths (both human and animal). Within this system, public health agencies and first responders may be able to render more timely and clinically relevant treatment by detecting outbreaks and unusual clusters of disease before diagnoses are confirmed and reported. The outbreak of West Nile virus infection in the New York City area in 1999 is one example of successful syndromic surveillance, as monitoring of dead birds and horses detected an emergency situation that could potentially affect humans.

Two types of assessment are generally warranted: an initial rapid needs assessment (RNA) to establish the nature and scale of the emergency and the likely need for external assistance; and detailed sector assessments to plan, implement, and coordinate the response. Once information is gathered, it can be used to guide priority setting, decision making, and action planning aimed at reducing risk. Other types of assessment are required at various stages of the response, such as continual assessment (eg, monitoring or surveillance) and assessments for postdisaster rehabilitation and recovery (which actually is best assessed in the initial phase of the disaster).

Such assessments are important to establish objectives and indicators for immediate actions, as well as to ensure that any action undertaken is effective. Results of ongoing surveillance and assessment activities are used to modify relief efforts as appropriate. This will help to prevent a disproportionate response that leaves part or all of the affected population vulnerable for an extended period and to focus efforts where they will produce the greatest and most rapid health benefits.

Rapid Needs Assessment (RNA)

After a disaster, public health emergency response requires quick access to information about the magnitude of the event, the extent of the population's immediate needs, stability of the health care infrastructure, local health response capacity, and the impact on essential services (including potable water supply, sanitation services, food supply, sheltering facilities, and electricity). Performing an RNA can obtain objective and reliable information about population needs and capabilities, including the need for specialized emergency relief services.

RNA teams can assess availability of and access to essential services such as water, food, shelter, electric power, transportation, medications, and other supplies. They assess the local health care infrastructure, providing valuable information used for critical resource utilization decision making. Teams also may interview people in their homes or in shelters about their needs. Households to be interviewed are selected by means of statistical sampling to accurately assess community needs, and information is collected via a one-page standardized survey. Geographic information systems can assist with population-based sampling and are currently being used in large-scale natural disaster responses and complex humanitarian emergencies. They can additionally be used to monitor mortality rates, usually as crude rates, by querying local civic leaders or local health facilities. Collected data can be used to guide disaster response efforts to meet the identified needs of the community.

During the early aftermath of Hurricane Ike, RNA investigation teams queried multiple emergency departments in the Texas Medical Center and reported an immediate surge in patient encounters, namely a doubling of their usual daily census. These same facilities sustained an approximate 25% increase in patient surge for 2 weeks afterward. Combined with a reduced workforce attendance, this raised issues of worker safety, patient safety, and timely access to medical care. As a result of this RNA effort, decision making and resource allocation were improved significantly (R. Swienton, Texas Medical Assist Program Team Leader, personal communication, 2011).

An example of a field assessment form is available at http://www.who.int/hac/network/global_health_cluster/ira_form_v2_7_eng.pdf.

All public health surveillance systems must assure that individuals' privacy rights are not violated. A delicate balance exists between the "right to privacy" and the "need to know" regarding health-related data contained in individual medical records or maintained by the government. This balance must be addressed by health surveillance programs and is covered in state and federal legislation. The Health Insurance Portability and Accountability Act of 1996 (HIPAA), for example, provides for the disclosure of patient data to the appropriate authorities but requires confidentiality of communications and disclosure of only the minimum information necessary to achieve the intended purpose.

2.6.3   Enhanced Public Health Reporting

Every state has laws that require physicians to report certain diseases and injuries to a local or state health officer. Many extend this requirement to nurses, dentists, veterinarians, laboratories, school officials, institution administrators, and police officials. State laws require reporting of some or all communicable diseases, vital events such as births and deaths, cancer, and occupational and environmental conditions and injuries. Some state reporting systems are based on state laws and regulations adopted by the state board or department of health (which derives its authority from acts of the state legislature). Under certain emergency situations, surveillance activities may be initiated with additional reporting requirements that may be justified by the general charge to, and powers of, state and local public health agencies to protect public health. Many of these reporting programs form the basis of modern public health preparedness sentinel warning systems.

In a disaster, reporting to public health authorities is mandatory to provide information to best serve and protect community health. As such, reporting may include the number and types of casualties, suspected exposures and exposure routes, and therapeutic interventions such as the number of patients receiving mechanical ventilation. Such information will help guide public health authorities in issuing guidelines or directives to better serve the health care needs of affected individuals and populations.

States develop legal reporting requirements by using as a guide the list of communicable diseases recommended as part of the National Notifiable Disease Surveillance System (NNDSS), as well as state and local public health priorities. The NNDSS list is developed and revised periodically by the CDC and the Council of State and Territorial Epidemiologists (CSTE). Case definitions for each disease or condition are established and revised periodically by the CSTE and CDC. While most case definitions require laboratory test results to confirm a surveillance report, they have provisions to enable providers to report clinical cases without or in advance of laboratory confirmation. Case reports are usually considered confidential and are not available for public review.

➤ The current list of state reporting requirements is available from CSTE at http://www.cste.org.

➤ Current case definitions are available from the CDC Epidemiology Program Office at http://www.cdc.gov/osels/ph_surveillance/nndss/casedef/index.htm.

The list of notifiable diseases and conditions differs by state, which reflects the public health priorities and concerns of each state. In general, a disease is listed if it causes serious morbidity or death, has the potential to affect large numbers of people, and can be controlled or prevented with proper interventions. In addition to specific diseases or conditions that have been established as reportable within a given state, health department regulations commonly specify two additional circumstances that require reporting: (1) the occurrence of any outbreak or unusually high incidence of any disease; and (2) the occurrence of any unusual disease of public health importance.

Increasingly, basic surveillance efforts are being directed at collecting public health information in electronic formats such as from computerized clinical laboratory reports, medical record systems, and managed care databases. Despite these advances, the need for direct involvement of clinicians will continue for immediate reporting of clinical syndromes, unusual disease presentations, and disease clusters to trigger the necessary rapid public health response to prevent disease spread and to control diseases for which there are no confirmatory laboratory tests.

2.6.4   Incident Management

As discussed in Chapter 1, the National Incident Management System (NIMS) and its component incident command system (ICS) provide a standardized approach to command and control at an incident scene. Local officials use the ICS when responding to both natural and human-caused disasters. Depending on the incident management system that is in place for a particular situation and jurisdiction, state and local health departments, hospitals, and other health care entities can play leading, collaborative, or supportive roles. For instance, in a biologic event, such as an influenza outbreak or bioterrorism event, public- and private-sector health agencies will have a significant role in incident management.

2.6.4.1   Health System Integration

Local emergency management officials use the ICS when responding to both natural and human-caused disasters. Under the ICS, a designated official, typically the fire chief or the chief of police, serves as local incident commander. Incident command is most frequently employed on a daily basis to address fires, hazardous material spills, and other disasters with natural causes. The majority of these events are managed by non–health care/medical agencies. The integration of public health and clinical disciplines into the incident management framework presents several advantages:

➤ Timely input by public health and clinical authorities at decision-making levels regarding health and safety issues for non–health responders

➤ Ability to define public health and clinical response priorities across all aspects of an incident and incorporate them into a single cohesive strategy

➤ Promotion of a proactive rather than a reactive response by public health agencies and health care organizations, which can help ensure the continuity of health-related operations during an incident

➤ Hands-on instruction for public health and clinical authorities by jurisdictional emergency managers who have extensive incident management experience.

In a biologic disaster, public health and clinical disciplines must assume a leadership role in incident management. If an outbreak proves to be the result of terrorism, or if the scope of the outbreak overwhelms local resources, a regional or national response becomes imperative. Public safety agencies, which traditionally are the lead agencies in community response, would provide support. This represents a significant adaptation for medical and public safety groups from their traditional roles in large-scale incident management. An effective unified command team, with a medical or health incident commander as the lead, may be the most effective way to accomplish this important task.

In a biologic disaster, public health officials will focus on identifying and treating exposed persons (ie, persons who may have had contact with the pathogen but who do not yet have signs or symptoms of disease) and preventing the spread of disease. Public health officials usually have the role of notifying law enforcement officials once a suspicion has arisen regarding a crime involving the deliberate use of biologic agents. In any infectious disease outbreak, public health authorities are responsible for developing community strategies to prevent or limit the spread of the disease. These include the following:

➤ Issuing guidance for the distribution of scarce medical resources and for the management of all exposed and infected people. This includes guidance on isolation and quarantine measures.

➤ Establishing sites for the mass distribution of medications and vaccines in various community settings.

➤ Coordinating efforts for the management of mass fatalities.

➤ Implementing surveillance and monitoring systems to protect human and environmental health and safety.

2.6.4.2   Multiagency Coordination

Large-scale disasters require integration of the capabilities and resources of various governmental jurisdictions, NGOs, and the private sector into a cohesive, coordinated, and seamless response system. Evidence supports that the health of both nations and communities during health-related crises is dependent on their capacity and capability to work in a multidisciplinary and multiagency environment. Multiagency coordination is a process that allows all levels of government and all professions to work together more efficiently and effectively. Multiagency coordination occurs across the different disciplines involved in incident management, across jurisdictional lines, and across levels of government.

In a disaster, all response personnel must be able to work together in their appropriate function and avoid duplication of effort. Interoperability of the diverse professions and disciplines involved in disaster response must be ensured to increase efficiency, as well as to protect the safety of the affected community and response workforce. All potential responders and response agencies must be aware of their roles before an event and understand how they fit into the disaster management system. For example, a local emergency operations center established in response to a bioterrorism incident would likely include a mix of law enforcement, emergency management, public health, and clinical personnel (eg, local, state, or federal public health officials; representatives of health care facilities and EMS agencies).

To enhance community preparedness for disasters and public health emergencies, the HHS supports the creation of health care coalitions and geographically regionalized health care systems.[8,9] This may include plans for the establishment of regional Health Emergency Operations Centers (HEOCs), which can be activated to coordinate local health care assets in the private and public sectors and provide additional regional support for the response.[10] The composition and function of HEOCs is discussed in greater detail in the ADLS® course (v 3.0) and supporting course manual.

2.6.5 Crisis and Emergency Risk Communication

An essential component of any public health system is a robust information and communication system able to disseminate timely, credible, and reliable information before, during, and after a disaster. It is imperative to share up-to-date guidelines, recommendations, surveillance data, and health alerts with public and private health organizations, the media, and the population at-large. Because disasters can cause great fear and uncertainty in the population, public health officials need to provide appropriate and complete information as quickly as possible and involve the public in any decision making that will affect their health, safety, and well-being.

Sound and thoughtful risk communication can allay fears and help public health officials mitigate the effects of fear-driven and potentially damaging public responses to events such as infectious disease outbreaks and acts of terrorism. When delivered appropriately, public health risk communication can foster public trust and confidence and subsequently improve health outcomes related to the disaster. In a disaster, the HHS and CDC will issue guidance and announcements to advise health professionals and the public on the best course of action by using television, radio, print, and the Internet. During a pandemic, the HHS serves as the focal contact point for the states to send outbreak data required by the International Health Regulations (http://www.who.int/ihr/en/). The HHS also serves as the contact point with the WHO and works closely with the CDC in decision-making responsibilities.

The CDC has developed several national networks to encourage and facilitate the sharing of information within the health community. One of these networks, the Health Alert Network (HAN; http://www2a.cdc.gov/han/index.asp), is a nationwide, integrated electronic information and communications system for the distribution of health alerts, prevention guidelines, national disease surveillance, and laboratory reporting. The HAN represents a collaboration between the CDC, local and state health agencies, and national public health organizations. It allows for the sharing of information among state, local, tribal, and federal health agencies as well as hospitals, laboratories, and community health providers. The HAN is designed to assist public health and emergency response during a disaster or other public health emergency. It provides early warnings by broadcast fax and e-mail to alert officials at all levels about urgent health threats and appropriate actions. Many states have developed their own HANs.

Because of the varied psychological, psychosocial, and behavioral effects of traumatic events, it is not sufficient to give facts about a situation and tell the public what to

Seven Cardinal Rules for the Practice of Risk Communication[12]

Crisis and emergency risk communication can empower individuals, stakeholders, or communities to make good decisions to protect health and safety. Effective communication of clear, concise, and credible information is essential to reassure the public that the situation is being addressed competently. Effective public information must reach broad audiences to publicize both immediate and anticipated health hazards, appropriate health and safety precautions, the need for evacuation or sheltering in place, and alternative travel routes. Effective risk communication efforts should:

➤ Accept and involve the public as a legitimate partner.

➤ Be planned carefully and evaluated systematically.

➤ Be responsive to the specific concerns of the public and correct misinformation.

➤ Be honest, frank, and open.

➤ Coordinate and collaborate with other credible sources.

➤ Meet the needs of the media.

➤ Involve clear and compassionate messaging.

do, and expect that they will actually process the information and take recommended protective actions. High distress levels can keep people from engaging in protective behaviors. Effective crisis and emergency risk communication aims to help people channel distress into productive and protective behaviors rather that destructive ones. People will be more able to make appropriate decisions about safeguarding their health and safety when their concerns and fears are acknowledged than when they are told not to be fearful.[11] Some things that people need to know are not easy for them to hear: that people are dying, that the risks and severity are not really understood, that it is not known when the emergency will be over, and that decisions may have to be made with imperfect information.

2.6.6 Community Evacuation Considerations

Evacuation involves the temporary transfer of a population (and, to a limited extent, property) from areas at risk of disaster to a safer location. Effective public health emergency management requires planning for individual and community evacuation needs, understanding the target population, their concerns and nuances, and where they can be safely relocated to during a disaster. The number of people to be evacuated, the available modes of transportation, and the rapidity with which the evacuation occurs vary with each disaster situation. Evacuation plans must account for complex scenarios, such as the evacuation of schools, high-rises, hospitals, critical-care ventilator–dependent patients, and long-term care facilities (eg, nursing homes, rehabilitation facilities). Mechanisms must be in place to help relatives, neighbors, and emergency management personnel identify persons who may still be in danger and require assistance. This includes mechanisms to help reunite families and loved ones after an event, as well as assist efforts to identify missing persons.

If a disaster can be monitored or predicted, local authorities can order and execute an evacuation before the event occurs, usually on the advice of emergency managers. This will allow individuals to escape unharmed in a timely fashion and allow a more orderly evacuation as routes and resources may not yet be limited by the event. Examples include a forest fire encroaching on a neighborhood several miles away or a distant hurricane. For many other disaster situations, such as earthquakes, chemical releases, bombings, and nuclear explosions, there is no advance warning, and the disaster may be completely unexpected. If potentially hazardous exposures are immediately present (eg, exposure to chemical or radiologic materials), local authorities may provide instructions for people to shelter in place (at home, work, school) for a specified period of time.

Government agencies, the American Red Cross, the Salvation Army, and other disaster relief organizations will assist by providing temporary shelter and emergency supplies.

Determinations need to be made about the safety of evacuation routes to facilitate the movements desired. Questions that need to be addressed include the following:

➤ Is evacuation the best course, or should shelter in place be considered?

➤ Where will populations be evacuated to?

➤ How will they get there?

➤ Who will manage and communicate updates to them while they are temporarily housed?

➤ What about companion animals? (Many people simply will not leave without the family pet.)

Special provisions need to be made to move disabled, elderly, and dispossessed (eg, homeless) persons, children, and institutional populations such as those in schools, hospitals, and prisons. Hospital evacuations are often facilitated by predetermined mutual aid agreements with other community medical facilities. These agreements may increase capacity for personnel, equipment, or space for evacuated patients. Hospital evacuation challenges are compounded when the structure is a high-rise. The evacuation of a "stable" ventilator-dependent patient from an intensive care unit, down several flights of stairs, using manual or portable means to provide respiratory support, while continuing critical intravenous medications is extremely challenging. The potential for increased morbidity, mortality, and liability in these situations is significant.

2.6.7 Population-Based Surge Management

Large-scale disasters and public health emergencies inherently cause a scarcity of available resources and disproportionately affect populations with functional and access needs (eg, pregnant women, children, those with chronic disease, the elderly, the disabled, and the dispossessed). Facility-based or "surge-in-place" solutions maximize health care facility capacity for patients during a disaster. When these resources are exceeded, community-based solutions, including the establishment of off-site hospital facilities, may be implemented. The only method to mitigate such an impact is to have plans in place that effectively allocate scarce resources among casualties, based on need, availability of resources, and anticipated outcomes.[8,9,13] Many states and communities now recognize and plan to access satellite health care facilities such as dental, podiatric, and veterinary surgery centers, which normally have surgical supplies and equipment. These satellite offices can serve as critical force multipliers when primary and regional hospital infrastructures are overwhelmed. Population-based surge strategies are discussed further in the ADLS® course (v 3.0) and supporting course manual.

It is imperative that communities prepare for cooperation and joint response to a large incident. The first response to any disaster is always the local response. Local fire, police, and EMS personnel are usually the first to respond to disasters with immediate impact (eg, explosions, large fires, earthquakes). Similarly, local public health agencies are typically the first to be involved in disease outbreaks, including possible acts of bioterrorism. However, many incidents may be beyond the scope of the local community's capacity to respond alone, and local resources may be rapidly depleted. For disasters that exceed regional capacity, state and federal assistance may be obtained through the Emergency Management Assistance Compact (http://www.emacweb.org). Interstate compacts involve prearranged agreements to offer assistance to other states, including fire, police, and health care assets. It is essential that these compacts, and the personnel who will implement them, be in place and well drilled before a disaster strikes.

Federal response consists of 15 emergency support functions (ESFs), which are delineated in the NRF (http://www.fema.gov/pdf/emergency/nrf/nrf-esf-all.pdf). The ESF structure includes mechanisms used to provide federal support to states and federal-to-federal support, both for declared disasters and emergencies under the Stafford Act and for non–Stafford Act incidents as defined in Homeland Security Presidential Directive 5. The ESF structure provides mechanisms for interagency coordination during all phases of incident management. Some departments and agencies provide resources for response, support, and program implementation during the early stages of an event, while others are more prominent in the recovery phase. The purpose of ESF 8, Public Health and Medical Services, is to provide US government assistance to supplement state and local responses in responding to public health and medical care needs after a disaster or a public health emergency, such as a pandemic. These resources are provided when state and local assets are overwhelmed and federal assistance has been requested. ESF 8 is coordinated by HHS, principally through the Assistant Secretary for Preparedness and Response. ESF 8 resources can be activated through the Stafford Act or the Public Health Service Act (pending the availability of funds).

Federal assets include the National Disaster Medical System (NDMS), the US Public Health Service (USPHS) Commissioned Corps, and the Medical Reserve Corps (MRC). In addition, HHS may reach out to the Department of Veterans Affairs and the Department of Defense if more medical personnel are needed.

➤ The NDMS (http://ndms.dhhs.gov) is a federally coordinated system that provides medical services to help local and state agencies respond to major disasters and public health emergencies. The NDMS is composed of community-based health professionals who are specially trained and volunteer their services in case of an emergency as a supplement to local hospital systems.

➤ The USPHS Commissioned Corps (http://www.usphs.gov), led by the Surgeon General, is one of the seven uniformed US services. It is composed of 6000 public health professionals (ordinarily working in a range of agencies) who are available to respond rapidly to urgent public health challenges and health care emergencies.

➤ The MRC (http://www.medicalreservecorps.gov) consists of groups of specially trained volunteers whose goal is to improve the health and safety of communities across the country by organizing and utilizing public health, medical, and other volunteers. MRC units are community based and function as a means to locally organize and utilize volunteers who want to donate their time and expertise to prepare for and respond to emergencies and promote healthy living throughout the year. MRC volunteers supplement existing emergency and public health resources. The MRC program is administered by the Office of the US Surgeon General.

In response to a public health emergency, the federal government also may dispatch personnel from the Epidemic Intelligence Service (EIS). The EIS (http://www.cdc.gov/eis) is a 2-year postgraduate program of service and on-the-job training for health professionals interested in epidemiology. Managed by the CDC, the EIS was

Disaster Medical Assistance Teams

Disaster Medical Assistance Teams (DMATs) are groups of professional and paraprofessional medical personnel (supported by a cadre of logistical and administrative staff) designed to provide medical care during a disaster or other event. The NDMS recruits personnel for specific vacancies, plans for training opportunities, and coordinates the deployment of the team. To supplement the standard DMATs, there are highly specialized DMATs that deal with specific medical conditions such as crush injury, burns, pediatric emergencies, and mental health emergencies. DMATs are designed to be a rapid-response element to supplement local medical care until other federal or contract resources can be mobilized, or the situation is resolved.

DMATs deploy to disaster sites with sufficient supplies and equipment to sustain themselves for a period of 72 hours while providing medical care at a fixed or temporary medical care site. Generally, the personnel are activated for a period of 2 weeks. In mass casualty incidents, their responsibilities may include triaging patients, providing high-quality medical care despite the adverse and austere environment often found at a disaster site, patient reception at staging facilities, and preparing patients for evacuation. DMATs are principally a community resource available to support local, regional, and state requirements. However, as a national resource they can be federalized.

For more information, see http://www.dmat.org.

Strategic National Stockpile

The Strategic National Stockpile (SNS; http://www.bt.cdc.gov/stockpile) is a national repository of critical medical supplies and equipment designed to supplement and resupply state and local inventories in the event of a national emergency anywhere and at any time within the United States or its territories. It is managed by the CDC working with states and communities, which have responsibility for developing plans for the receipt and distribution of SNS supplies and equipment. The SNS contains multiple caches of medical supplies and equipment stored in warehouses across the country. These include antibiotics, chemical antidotes, antitoxins, life support medications, intravenous administration supplies, ventilators, airway maintenance supplies, and various medical and surgical items. Items included in the SNS are based on threat assessments and availability and ease of distribution of supplies.

SNS supplies may be sent in a "12-hour push package," which contains a broad range of products potentially needed in the early hours of an emergency to support mass treatment or prophylaxis. Push packages are maintained in a ready state for loading on trucks or aircraft. Supplies would be distributed to predesignated receiving, staging, and storage sites, depending on the situation and plans already made by the affected community.

developed more than 50 years ago to defend the nation against biologic warfare. EIS staff provide surveillance and response units for all types of outbreaks. They include physicians, researchers, and scientists who study infectious diseases and outbreaks, under the supervision of experienced epidemiologists at the CDC and at local and state health departments.

2.6.8   Communicable Disease Prevention and Control

The potential impact of communicable diseases is often presumed to be high following a disaster. Increases in endemic diseases and the risk of outbreaks depend on many factors that must be evaluated systematically. This allows the prioritization of interventions to reduce the post-disaster impact of communicable diseases:

➤ Diarrheal disease outbreaks can occur following contamination of drinking water and have been reported following flooding and disaster-related population displacement.

➤ Natural disasters, particularly weather-related events (eg, cyclones, hurricanes, flooding) can affect vector breeding sites and vector-borne disease transmission. The risk of vector-borne disease outbreaks (eg, malaria, dengue) can be influenced by other complicating factors, such as changes in human behavior (increased exposure to mosquitoes while sleeping outside, movement from non-endemic to endemic areas, a lapse in disease control activities, overcrowding), or changes in habitats that promote insect breeding (landslide deforestation, river damming and re-routing).

➤ Crowded living conditions, as is common among people displaced by natural disasters, facilitate disease transmission and necessitate attention to immunization coverage levels (eg, measles, hepatitis) to prevent outbreaks.

➤ Tetanus is not transmitted from person to person but is caused by a toxin released by the bacterium *Clostridium tetani*. Contaminated wounds, particularly in populations in which routine vaccination coverage levels are low, are associated with morbidity and mortality from this disease.

➤ Power outages related to disasters may disrupt water treatment and supply plants, thereby increasing the risk of water-borne diseases. Lack of electric power also may affect proper functioning of food storage facilities, increasing the likelihood for spoilage and microbial contamination.

Ensuring uninterrupted provision of safe drinking water is the most important preventive measure to be implemented following a disaster. Chlorine is widely available, inexpensive, easily used, and effective against most waterborne pathogens. Shelter and settlement planning must provide for adequate access for water and sanitation needs and meet minimum "per person" space requirements, in accordance with international guidelines.[7] The risk of transmission of endemic communicable diseases, such as acute respiratory and diarrheal diseases, is increased in displaced populations due to associated crowding, inadequate water and sanitation, and poor access to health care. Access to primary care is critical to prevention, early diagnosis, and treatment of a wide range of diseases, as well as providing an entry point for secondary and tertiary care.

Rapid detection of potential epidemic diseases is essential to ensure rapid control. Improved detection and response to communicable diseases is important to monitor the incidence of diseases, to document their impact, and to help quantify the risk of outbreaks following disasters. The detection of a biologic or other potentially hazardous agent begins with a high index of suspicion, which then needs to be confirmed through epidemiologic and clinical investigation. Public health surveillance and early warning systems should be established quickly to detect outbreaks and monitor priority endemic diseases.

Guided by epidemiologic data, state and local public health authorities will implement the most appropriate measures to minimize disease transmission. This includes the Internet, television and radio station news broadcasts, and public service announcements to transmit health-related information, stressing the importance of personal prevention and protective measures. Local health authorities will work closely with clinicians and community leaders to develop dedicated community hotlines and communication systems to advise local residents about the situation as it evolves. If agents of transmissible (contagious) diseases are involved, basic hygiene and infection control measures (eg, washing hands after contact, avoiding direct contact with secretions from infected individuals, keeping exposed persons away from public places, and isolating suspected or symptomatic cases) may be essential in limiting secondary spread. The communication of even this basic information on infection control precautions to health care providers and the public will be an important public health control strategy.

2.6.9 Laboratory Services

State and local health authorities have a responsibility to ensure access to laboratory services for diagnostic testing required to support emergency health and medical services in a time-sensitive manner. In most cases, local and state laboratories can manage testing for localized outbreaks or other local public health emergencies. This includes various hospital, commercial, and public health laboratories, which support public health surveillance activities. Many local agencies and medical facilities, however, lack the resources and expertise to isolate or confirm suspicious disease agents. To facilitate sample collection, transport, and testing and training for laboratory readiness, the CDC, the Association of Public Health Laboratories (http://www.aphl .org), and the Federal Bureau of Investigation (FBI; http://www.fbi.gov) established the Laboratory Response Network (LRN), composed of local, state, and federal laboratories (http://www.bt.cdc.gov/lrn).

Most US laboratories have only the minimum-defined LRN capabilities, which can limit their ability to identify chemical and biologic terrorism agents. The state public health laboratory is typically the most appropriate laboratory to which to submit specimens for higher-level testing. The LRN has two major components: a network of epidemiologists and public health laboratories dealing with biologic agents and a network of public health laboratories dealing with chemical agents.

2.6.10   Mass Care Services

After a disaster, mass care involves the coordination of non-medical services including sheltering of displaced persons, food and water distribution, provision of emergency first aid, communication regarding casualties and the missing, and bulk distribution of emergency relief items. It also includes human services such as mental health counseling, identification and provision of services for people with access and functional needs, the processing of claims, and expediting of mail services in affected areas.

Sheltering, food, and water are often the most immediate and essential needs of populations affected by a disaster. Adequate housing involves the provision of short- and long-term housing options for displaced persons. As designated in the National Response Framework (NRF), FEMA (under ESF-6, Mass Care, Emergency Assistance, Housing, and Human Services) is the primary federal agency responsible for leading the federal response for mass care and related human services, in close coordination with other federal agencies, states, localities, and volunteer organizations.

The American Red Cross is the primary agency charged to assist FEMA with mass care efforts. During the outbreak of severe acute respiratory syndrome (SARS), the Canadian Red Cross was instrumental in moving its in-shelter expertise to serving more than 20,000 people in the most vulnerable populations within their homes with health packets that contained critical information, protective masks, thermometers, medications, and other essentials to keep them safe and isolated from the infectious agent. In a pandemic, placing large numbers of people in shelters is generally contraindicated because the close proximity of individuals may increase transmission of the infectious agent.

2.6.11   Environmental Health Services

Nearly every disaster requires some level of environmental health assessment and response. Public health authorities provide needed services for the monitoring and evaluation of human and environmental health hazards and for ensuring that appropriate actions are taken to protect the health and safety of responders and affected populations. These include the provision of shelter, water supplies, sanitation, vector control (control of insects and rodents), and the burial of the dead, as well as measures to protect food, control epidemics and communicable disease, limit exposure to chemical and radiation hazards, and remediate contaminated environments. When critical infrastructure such as water and waste systems are affected, public health workers ensure that temporary or alternative systems are in place and operational to prevent disease outbreaks.

Proper management of human waste is a public health priority for affected individuals and emergency response personnel. Sanitation efforts are focused on reducing fecal contamination of food and water supplies to control disease spread. Disease outbreaks can result from breakdowns in environmental safeguards, crowding in temporary shelters or camps, malnutrition, inadequate surveillance, and limited availability of medical treatment services. Communicable diseases can be transmitted directly from person to person or indirectly through contaminated food and water or disease vectors. Children are particularly vulnerable to dehydration from diarrheal illness characteristic of postdisaster gastroenteritides. Public health authorities will take necessary action to prevent or control disease vectors such as flies, mosquitoes, and rodents and to inspect indoor and outdoor environments for health hazards.

Although the most effective environmental health measure in most disasters, in terms of public health impact, is ensuring safe water and sanitation for the affected population as a whole, serving hospitals and feeding centers may be more urgent when a large number of people are injured or ill or when a significant portion of the population depends on mass feeding centers. Refuse collection and disposal, drainage, and vector control are usually lower priorities than water supply and waste disposal. Infectious diseases, such as malaria and cholera, may rapidly become the most important health risks after a disaster, and environmental and human health surveillance systems should be established to enable a rapid response to disease outbreaks.

Community emergency plans must address the delivery of food and water to support clinical facilities, feeding centers, and other public health activities. Priorities will differ from situation to situation and will change for each disaster as it evolves. This underscores the need to adhere to sound public health epidemiologic and surveillance principles and practices.

2.7   RECOVERY AND BEYOND

After a disaster, the affected community needs to be brought back—hopefully, by applying lessons learned, to a better state preparedness. There will be many opportunities during the recovery period to enhance prevention and increase preparedness, thus reducing vulnerability to future events. Recovery measures, both short and long term, include returning vital life-support systems to minimal operating standards; sheltering and housing; public information; health and safety education; reconstruction; counseling programs; and impact studies. The reconstruction of housing, water supply, sanitation, and other environmental systems (eg, heating, ventilation) are priorities. Once damaged systems have been repaired and services to the disaster-affected population are adequate for protecting safety and health, longer-term reconstruction should be planned. A critical element in community recovery is reestablishing public health and health care infrastructures and ensuring access to preventive, treatment, and rehabilitative programs and services.

Increasing the capacity of people to offset risk, absorb tragedy, and meet contingencies is central to the goal of sustainable recovery. Reconstruction of a damaged area is not limited to the construction of new buildings. An integrated development process is required that should embrace the full redevelopment of the affected area according to the needs of the affected population. Long-term recovery from a major disaster is inevitably a slow and difficult process. No society is ever the same after a disaster, nor should it be. Disasters reveal weaknesses and deficiencies in a community's ability to protect itself, especially its more vulnerable members.

Public health personnel will participate in after-action reviews to evaluate overall response operations and identify strategies to enhance the resilience and responsiveness of community health systems and infrastructures. This includes drawing out the more general lessons that will result in prevention and mitigation to enhance preparedness for future events. Disasters and public health emergencies often provide an opportunity for new voices to be heard (eg, emergent community-based organizations expressing the needs of disaster-affected people) and can become a force for societal change, catalyzing a more rapid and effective transition from the emergency phase to sustainable development once the event subsides.

After major disasters, government officials often introduce new legislation and establish new institutions and programs. These may include adoption of new or revised building codes; regulations for land use; controls on dangerous industrial processes and the transportation of toxic chemicals; insurance provisions to reduce vulnerability; improved early-warning systems; increased preparedness efforts; and improved coordination of emergency response functions. All these initiatives and changes offer public health planners and administrators opportunities to promote community health and safety, and all are part of the overall recovery process.

2.8 SUMMARY

Early detection and control of a disaster depends on strong and flexible public health systems at the local, state, and federal levels and on the vigilance of health professionals, who may be the first to observe and report unusual illnesses or injuries. Local health officials perform routine epidemiologic surveillance to develop a community health profile with baseline health statistics. Hazard and vulnerability assessments are used to determine which hazards merit special attention, specific populations that may be at increased risk, what actions must be planned for, what resources are likely to be needed, and the probable effects. This includes contingency planning for populations with functional and access needs such as children, the elderly, pregnant women, and individuals with chronic health conditions who may be more vulnerable to the adverse health effects of disasters.

Health professionals should be knowledgeable about when and where to report suspicious cases of disease and be aware of the need to collect and send specimens for laboratory analysis, as well as the criteria used to launch a public health investigation. To respond effectively, health professionals should ensure that they understand their particular roles, responsibilities, and contributions to the public health system.

In a major disaster or public health emergency, affected individuals and communities must have their basic physiologic and psychological needs met in a timely manner. Available resources will likely be challenged by a surge of people seeking medical and relief services. To meet this challenge, public health authorities work with others to implement various measures to control the situation and help prevent further harm. This includes establishing priorities, standards, and monitoring systems for water, food, sanitation, solid-waste removal, shelter, redundant and potentially confusing vector control, and communicable disease control. Guidelines will be issued for the diagnosis, care, and reporting of injured and ill persons, as well as for the distribution of scarce medical resources to those who need them most. Throughout the event, public health personnel will focus on the bigger picture, that is, getting the community back to health.

2.9 DISCUSSION POINTS

Public Health Response to Disasters: Putting the PRE-DISASTER Paradigm™ into Practice		
P	Planning and Practice	Ongoing testing of public health emergency response plans, policies, and procedures during exercises and drills is an important part of disaster preparedness. This allows participants to apply knowledge and skills and, at the same time, allows them to identify opportunities for improvement and develop action plans to fix identified gaps. All exercises should be followed by a detailed evaluation and the development of an action plan for improvement.
R	Resilience	Depending on the type of event that occurred, there may be long-term health effects, economic problems, and infrastructure issues for the community as a whole. Specific individuals and populations may be disproportionately affected. Public health officials will take steps to promote postcrisis resilience and recovery for all affected persons.
E	Education and Training	Federal, state, and local public health personnel have an obligation to maintain proficiency in the management of disasters and public health emergencies. Health professionals must know when and where to report suspicious cases of disease and be aware of the need to collect and forward specimens for laboratory analysis and the criteria used to launch a public health investigation. Education should ensure that they understand their particular roles and responsibilities in the health response system and are aware of available resources and support services.

Public Health Response to Disasters: Putting the DISASTER Paradigm™ into Practice

D	Detection	Effective information and communications systems are vital for disease surveillance. These link initially rare events to a common source and then communicate this information quickly to frontline workers. Detecting an outbreak early allows preventive measures to be initiated earlier, mitigating the effect of the disaster. Well-designed public health surveillance systems provide essential data to support epidemiologic investigation and inform public health decision making. Public health surveillance provides information necessary to ensure accurate diagnosis and appropriate treatment of an individual with a disease, injury, or condition of public health importance; identify and address the cause of the problem; monitor the health status and trends in the community; and determine the need for and effectiveness of public health programs at the community level.
I	Incident Management	Depending on the incident management system that is in place for a particular situation and jurisdiction, the local public health agency can play a leading, collaborative, or supportive role. In a biologic event, to include influenza outbreaks or bioterrorism events, public- and private-sector health agencies will have a significant role in incident management. Multiagency coordination occurs across the different disciplines involved in incident management, across jurisdictional lines, and across levels of government.
S	Safety and Security	Guided by epidemiologic data, state and local public health authorities will implement the most appropriate measures to maximize protection of public health and safety and minimize effects on individual freedom of movement. Federal health officials will provide assistance as requested.
A	Assess Hazards	During a disaster, public health assessment activities increase dramatically and are targeted at reducing immediate injury, illness, and death associated with the event; documenting exposures; working with physicians and other health professionals to identify people with exposure-related illnesses and injuries; conducting long-term medical and mental health follow-up of affected individuals and populations; and determining when it is safe to return to the affected area.
S	Support	Local public health agencies are typically the first to be involved in disease outbreaks, including possible acts of bioterrorism. However, many incidents may be beyond the scope of the local community's capacity to respond alone, and local resources may be rapidly depleted. It is imperative that local municipalities and states prepare for cooperation and joint response to a large incident.

T	Triage and Treatment	Population-based surge strategies recognize that overall mortality and morbidity are dependent on the accuracy and interoperability of four distinct stages of casualty population contact: at the community level through risk communication; at the pre-hospital level; at the hospital level; and at the regional or state level. The process is inherently dynamic, with casualty prioritization based on the accuracy and timeliness of situational awareness, the availability of resources, and the efficacy of risk communication. Through the use of valid and reliable clinical assessment methods, health responders will assess survivors; identify vulnerable, at-risk individuals and groups; and provide referral or emergency hospitalizations when indicated. In a disaster, critical public health actions include supplying basic life-sustaining commodities, such as food, water, and shelter; enhanced surveillance; distribution of vaccines and medications; implementation of environmental controls; legal interventions to restrict the movement of affected populations; emergency risk communication; and provision of essential treatment and preventive clinical services.
E	Evacuation	Effective public health emergency preparedness requires planning for individual and community evacuation needs, understanding the target population and its concerns and nuances, and determining where affected individuals can be safely relocated during a disaster. Special provisions need to be made for individuals with access and functional needs, dispossessed (eg, homeless) persons, children, and institutional populations such as those in schools, hospitals, and prisons.
R	Recovery	After a disaster, the provision of housing and of water-supply and sanitation systems is a public health priority. Once damaged systems have been repaired and services to the disaster-affected population are adequate for protecting safety and health, longer-term reconstruction should begin. A critical element in community recovery is reestablishing public health and health care infrastructures and ensuring access to preventive, treatment, and rehabilitative programs and services. During the recovery process, the affected community can apply lessons learned to reduce vulnerability to future events.

REFERENCES

1. *The Johns Hopkins and Red Cross Red Crescent Public Health Guide in Emergencies.* 2nd ed. Geneva, Switzerland: International Federation of Red Cross and Red Crescent Societies; 2008. http://www.jhsph.edu/bin/s/c/Forward.pdf. Accessed April 11, 2011.

2. Landesman LY. *Public Health Management of Disasters: The Practice Guide.* 3rd ed. Washington, DC: American Public Health Association; 2011.

3. Burkle FM Jr, Greenough PG. Impact of public health emergencies on modern disaster taxonomy, planning, and response. *Disaster Med Public Health Prep.* 2008;2:192-199.

4. Institute of Medicine. *The Future of Public Health*. Washington, DC: National Academy Press; 1988.

5. Centers for Disease Control and Prevention (CDC). *Public Health Emergency Response Guide for State, Local and Tribal Public Health Directors*. Version 2.0. Washington, DC: US Department of Health and Human Services. http://www.emergency.cdc.gov/planning/pdf/cdcresponseguide.pdf. Accessed April 11, 2010.

6. Carmona RH, Darling RG, Knoben JE, Michael JM. *Public Health Emergency Preparedness and Response: Principles and Practice*. Washington, DC: Public Health Service Commissioned Officers Foundation for the Advancement of Public Health; 2010.

7. The Sphere Project. *The Sphere Project: Humanitarian Charter and Minimum Standards for Disaster Response*. Geneva, Switzerland: The Sphere Project, 2011. http://www.sphereproject.org. Accessed April 11, 2011.

8. Barbera J, Macintyre A. *Medical Surge Capacity and Capability: A Management System for Integrating Medical and Health Resources During Large Scale Emergencies*. 2nd ed. Washington, DC: US Department of Health and Human Services; 2007. http://www.phe.gov/Preparedness/planning/mscc/handbook/Documents/mscc080626.pdf. Accessed April 11, 2011.

9. Barbera J, Macintyre A. *Medical Surge Capacity and Capability: The Healthcare Coalition in Emergency Response and Recovery*. Washington, DC: US Department of Health and Human Services; 2009. http://www.phe.gov/Preparedness/planning/mscc/Documents/mscctier2jan2010.pdf. Accessed April 11, 2011.

10. Burkle FM, Hsu EB, Loehr M, et al. Definitions and functions of health unified command and emergency operations centers for large-scale bioevent disasters within the existing ICS. *Disaster Med Public Health Prep*. 2007;1:135–141.

11. US Department of Health and Human Services (HHS). *Communicating in a Crisis: Risk Communication Guidelines for Public Officials*. Washington, DC: HHS; 2002. http://www.hhs.gov/od/documents/RiskCommunication.pdf. Accessed April 11, 2011.

12. Covello VT, Allen FH. *Seven Cardinal Rules of Risk Communication*. OPA-87-020. Washington, DC: US Environmental Protection Agency;1988.

13. Burkle FM. Population-based triage management in response to surge-capacity requirements during a large-scale bioevent disaster. *Acad Emerg Med*. 2006;13:1118-1129.

CHAPTER | THREE

Population Health and Mental Health in Disasters

CHAPTER CHAIR

Frederick M. Burkle, Jr, MD, MPH, DTM

CONTRIBUTING AUTHORS

Jim Lyznicki, MS, MPH

Arthur Cooper, MD, MS

Lauren Walsh, MPH

Italo Subbarao, DO, MBA

3.1 PURPOSE

This chapter discusses disaster-related health issues and challenges faced by children, women, individuals with chronic illness, and people with access and functional needs. It also discusses mental and behavioral health consequences of disasters on all affected ages and populations.

3.2 LEARNING OBJECTIVES

After completing this chapter, readers should be able to:

➤ Describe pediatric vulnerabilities and challenges that need to be addressed in all-hazards disaster preparedness and response planning.

➤ Discuss women's health issues that need to be addressed in all-hazards disaster preparedness and response planning.

➤ Discuss the potential effects of disasters on individuals with chronic illnesses.

➤ Explain the rationale for a function- and access-based definition to address all individuals who may be more vulnerable to adverse health effects in a disaster or public health emergency.

➤ Discuss mental and behavioral health consequences for children and adults affected by a disaster or public health emergency.

➤ Discuss clinical interventions that can help individuals cope with the psychological impact of disasters and public health emergencies.

Learning Objectives for this chapter are competency-based, as delineated in Appendix B.

3.3 BACKGROUND

Large-scale disasters and public health emergencies disproportionately affect at-risk populations such as infants and children, women, populations with functional and access needs, and those with chronic disease. The medical care, support services, and sheltering needs of these populations require considerable resource utilization readiness. Issues regarding the triage and treatment of vulnerable populations such as children, pregnant women, the frail elderly, and individuals with functional and access needs should be addressed well in advance of a disaster. Strategic and operational planning for meeting the needs of these vulnerable populations is crucial. General population sheltering, for example, must provide reasonable accommodations to meet the needs and fulfill the activities of daily life requirements of these groups. Disaster plans can help forecast the health-related needs of all ages and populations in the community, anticipate and assign resources, and develop strategies to deliver resources to those groups for different disaster scenarios.

3.4 CHILDREN AND DISASTERS

Children are uniquely vulnerable to disasters and traumatic events because of anatomic, physiologic, developmental, and psychiatric factors. Pound for pound, because of their higher metabolic rates compared with adults (ie, 6 to 8 mL O_2/kg/min vs 3 to 4 mL O_2/kg/min), they breathe, drink, and eat more than adults. Thus, they are more vulnerable both to ambient weather conditions and to toxic exposures and doses, both directly via inhalation or ingestion (their shorter stature keeps children living "closer to the ground" where potentially toxic, heavier-than-air gases and other such substances tend to accumulate) and indirectly via ingestion (through consumption of foodstuffs or breast milk containing toxic agents). In addition, they may lack the motor skills to escape from a disaster scene as well as the cognitive ability to comprehend risk or seek a viable escape route. Even worse, they may actually migrate toward the event out of curiosity to see the gas, colored agent, or other effects. Young children also will be unable to self-identify and may not be able to provide reliable exposure histories, effectively communicate their symptoms, or even localize pain. They are likely to be afraid of health care providers wearing personal protective equipment (PPE), especially masks and goggles, and will therefore need constant reassurance that such providers are there to help. They may be unable to walk through decontamination lines or pass through decontamination corridors on their own. They typically need constant adult supervision to avoid harming themselves, and, of course, they are unable to legally consent to their own medical care.

It is beyond the scope of the BDLS® course to provide detailed instructions to health care providers in the fundamentals of pediatric resuscitation and care. However, public health and health care professionals who care for children in disasters must be well schooled in such principles before accepting assignment to a disaster zone. Medical and surgical pediatricians and pediatric nurses knowledgeable in disaster health care are clearly best suited to provide such care and may need to be deployed to coach or supervise adult-oriented providers. Because pediatric health professionals will likely be in short supply, adult-oriented health care providers must be able to provide such care in their stead. Numerous courses are available to prepare them to provide initial or ongoing care to infants, children, and adolescents after a mass casualty event.[1-9] Numerous resources have been developed to assist health care providers in meeting the needs of pediatric casualties; all of these resources are available on the Internet.[10-14] It should be noted that, for the first time, the *SPHERE Handbook* (2011 edition), which provides minimum standards in disasters and humanitarian assistance, now includes a chapter for the assessment, response, targeting, monitoring, evaluation, staff competency, and management of children.[15]

3.4.1 Pediatric Vulnerabilities in Disasters

It is axiomatic that children are not small adults. Their immature anatomy, developing physiology, the different mechanisms of illness and injury to which they are subject, and the distinct patterns of illness and injury all require a working knowledge of emergency pediatrics to facilitate optimal outcomes in disasters, no less than during routine emergency medical care. Yet, despite these facts, few jurisdictions at this time have made special provisions for the care of infants, children, and adolescents in disasters. Most terrorist events are planned to occur in public spaces, where children tend to be of school age or above. Disasters and public health emergencies do not discriminate by age. It is therefore imperative that public health and health care professionals be familiar with the special needs of children, who may account for as many as 40% of the casualties in natural disasters; this was vividly illustrated in the aftermath of the 2010 earthquake near Port-au-Prince, Haiti, which continues to devastate that nation.[16]

3.4.1.1 Anatomic Considerations

Children are smaller than adults and vary in size depending on stage of growth and development. This makes them more vulnerable to exposure and toxicity from agents that are heavier than air, such as sarin gas and chlorine. These agents accumulate close to the ground in the breathing zone of infants, toddlers, and children. Children's smaller mass also means that they are more susceptible to blunt trauma, because greater force is applied per unit of body area. The energy imparted from flying objects, falls, or similar injury mechanisms is transmitted to a small body with less fat, less elastic connective tissue, and closer proximity of chest and abdominal organs. The result is a higher frequency of multiorgan injuries. Additional anatomic considerations for children include:[10]

Body surface area (BSA): Children have a higher percentage of BSA devoted to the head relative to the lower extremities. The ratio of BSA to mass is highest at birth and gradually diminishes as the child matures. The large percentage of BSA devoted to a child's head accounts for significant heat loss. This should be considered when determining the percentage of BSA involved in burn injuries and in treating or preventing hypothermia. The higher BSA-to-mass ratio also leads to more rapid absorption and systemic effects from toxins that are absorbed through thinner, less keratinized, highly permeable skin.

Central nervous system: The brain doubles in size in the first 6 months of life and achieves 80% of its adult size by age 2 years. During childhood, there is ongoing brain development (eg, hyalinization, synapse formation) and biochemical changes. Injury to the developing brain can affect or arrest these processes, resulting in permanent changes.

Circulatory system: Children have a smaller circulating blood volume (on average 80 mL/kg) and less fluid reserve than adults. Blood loss that would be easily handled by an adult can result in hemorrhagic shock in a child. Because children become dehydrated easily and possess minimal reserve capacity, they are at greater risk than adults when exposed to agents that may cause diarrhea or vomiting. Infectious agents that cause mild symptoms in adults (ie, vomiting and diarrhea) could lead to hypovolemic dehydration and shock in infants, small children, and children with special health care needs. Also, the mediastinum is very mobile in children. Consequently, a tension pneumothorax can quickly become life threatening when the mediastinum is forced to the opposite side, compromising venous return and cardiac function.

Respiratory system: Children's lungs are smaller and more delicate and therefore subject to barotrauma, resulting in pneumothorax with inappropriate ventilation. The airway also differs between children and adults. The tongue is relatively large compared with the oropharynx, which creates the potential for obstruction of a poorly controlled airway. The larynx is higher and more anterior in the neck; the vocal cords are at a more anterocaudal angle. The epiglottis is omega (Ω)-shaped and soft. Unlike adults, the narrowest portion of the airway is the cricoid ring, not the vocal cords.

Skeletal system: A child's skeleton is incompletely calcified with active growth centers that are more susceptible to fracture. Serious internal organ damage (eg, lung, cardiac) can occur without a skeletal fracture. Head injury is common in children. A child's head is supported by a short neck that lacks well-developed musculature. The skull cap (calvarium) in children is thin and vulnerable to injury, thus allowing greater transmission of force to the growing brain of a child. The thoracic cage of a child does not provide as much protection of upper abdominal organs as that of an adult. Hepatic or splenic injuries from blunt trauma can go unrecognized and result in significant blood loss leading to hypovolemic shock.

3.4.1.2 Physiologic Considerations

Children also differ from adults physiologically in many ways.[10] They can compensate and maintain heart rate during the early phases of hypovolemic shock; this false impression of normalcy can lead to administration of too little fluid during resuscitation. This can be followed by a precipitous deterioration with little warning. Vital signs, including heart rate, respiratory rate, and blood pressure, vary with age. Caregivers should be able to quickly interpret whether a child's vital signs are normal or abnormal for age. Temperature is an often forgotten but important vital sign in injured children. The child's ability to control body temperature is affected not only by the BSA-to-mass ratio but also by thin skin and lack of substantial subcutaneous tissue. These factors increase evaporative heat loss and caloric expenditure. In fact, hypothermia is a significant risk factor for poor outcomes in many illnesses and injuries. Considerations of methods to maintain and restore normal body temperature are critical to the resuscitation of children. These can include thermal blankets, warmed resuscitation rooms, warmed intravenous fluids, and warmed inhaled gases.

Children have a unique respiratory physiology in that they have a higher minute ventilation per kilogram of body weight than adults. Many of the agents used for chemical and biologic attacks are aerosolized (eg, sarin, chlorine, or *Bacillus anthracis* spores). Because children have higher respiratory rates than adults, they are exposed to relatively greater dosages and will suffer the effects of these agents much more rapidly than adults. Children also will potentially absorb more of the substance before it is cleared or diffuses from the respiratory tissues. Many chemical agents have a high vapor density and are heavier than air, which means that they "settle" close to the ground, in the air space used by children for breathing. In a nuclear detonation, fallout also will settle to the ground, resulting in a higher concentration of radioactive material in the space in which children live and breathe.

Some biologic and chemical agents are absorbed through the skin. Recognizing that children have more surface area relative to body mass than adults, and because young children (especially those younger than 6 months) have more permeable skin, they receive proportionally higher doses of agents that either affect the skin or are absorbed through the skin. In addition, because the skin of children is poorly keratinized, vesicant and corrosive chemicals can result in greater injury to children than adults.

3.4.1.3 Immunologic Considerations

Children have an immature immunologic system, which places them at higher risk of infection. Infants rely on placentally transmitted antibodies (immunoglobulins) during the first 6 months of life. Afterward, children must rely on their own developing immune systems. Because infants and young children are relatively immunologically naïve, not having been exposed to the wide range of pathogens to which older children and adults have been subject, they lack the faster, secondary "amnestic" response found in the latter. Therefore, their immunologic responses will be slower. As a result, infants and children are more susceptible to novel biologic agents (eg, "emerging" infectious diseases), including shifting strains of pandemic influenza and unusual biologic agents used to terrorize a population.

3.4.1.4   Developmental Considerations

Neonates and infants (birth to 12 months), toddlers and preschoolers (1 to 5 years), school-agers (6 to 12 years), and teenagers (13 years and older) all have developmental tasks to accomplish before they can progress to the next stage of life. Neonates and infants eat, sleep, and grow; toddlers and preschoolers watch, explore, and play; school-agers learn, compete, and socialize; teenagers think, test, and mature. While a specific iteration of developmental milestones is beyond the scope of the BDLS® course, it is important to recognize that communicating with ill and injured children in a disaster, as in routine emergent and acute health care, is rooted in a working knowledge of normal growth and development. General strategies include allowing parents to remain with children; approaching ill, injured, or frightened children calmly and slowly; using a quiet, soothing voice; positioning oneself at the child's eye level; using words the child can understand; being honest; and explaining any procedures.

> **Communicating with Children in Disasters**
>
> While it is useful to know the chronological age of the child being treated, it is far more important to recognize his or her approximate developmental age; in other words, if a child "looks like" an infant or toddler, he or she should be approached as if an infant or toddler. The best advice is to go with the age that their actions portray, not their stated age.

Note that if children are ill, injured, or frightened, they may developmentally regress, acting younger than their developmental ages or stages. A very sick toddler with excellent walking skills may sit on the ground and refuse to move unless carried; an outgoing, friendly preschooler with pain and fever may act fearful and anxious, clinging to the parent; a talkative school-ager who has had a major injury resulting in a fracture may revert to baby talk or silence; an overconfident teenager who has been involved in a blast disaster may sob uncontrollably and resist all help.

3.4.1.5   Mental and Behavioral Health Considerations

Children are particularly vulnerable to the impact of disasters and lack the experience, skills, and resources to independently meet their mental and behavioral health needs. Unlike adults, children have little experience to help them place tragic events into perspective. As discussed in Section 3.8.5 of this manual, each child responds differently to tragedy, depending on his or her understanding and maturity.

3.4.2   Pediatric Casualty Care

The role of the health care provider or responder is to assess the child and family, and to provide clinical and emotional support and reassurance to them. Emotional considerations begin with the recognition that pediatric disaster victims are usually normal children who have experienced stress from trauma and loss. Stress can produce a variety of symptoms in children including headaches, abdominal pain, chest pain, vomiting, diarrhea, constipation, changes in sleep, and changes in appetite. Even so, parents may be so upset that they are unaware of the effect of the event on their children. The main goals are to keep the family together, to provide support, and to encourage communication.

Children are generally resilient; nevertheless, they need the reestablishment of order when their routines have been disrupted. Health care providers should emphasize the importance of establishing a routine and getting back to normal as much as possible.

The most important point to keep in mind for any child in a disaster is that the child and the family can be helped to recover through working together, with the assistance of the health care provider, as they deal with a traumatic situation.

3.4.2.1 Communicating with Children

Children come as part of a family unit. Treating the child means treating the family as well. General treatment strategies are based on developmental assessment. The child should be treated as a person. Health care providers should introduce themselves, talking to the child as they would their own. Parents should be allowed to remain with their children as appropriate. Providers should project authority, but respect the parents' knowledge of and experience with their own child. A child should be separated from parents during resuscitation, but otherwise the provider should interview and examine the child and parents together. For newborns and infants, parents should be questioned while the baby is being examined; for toddlers and preschoolers, most questions should be directed to the parent and a few to the child; for school-agers, providers should direct about half of their questions to the parent and half to the child; and for teenagers, most questions should be directed to the child and a few to the parents, although the parent should still be addressed first.

It is important that the health care provider talk to the verbal child. The child's view of what happened may be very different from a parent's, guardian's, or other adults' perceptions. The provider should listen carefully to the child, thus legitimizing and validating his or her fears and grief. This also helps parents realize that what they and their child are experiencing is not abnormal. Key age-specific strategies in communicating with children are listed in Table 3-1.

TABLE 3-1 Communicating with Children

Infants/Toddlers (Birth to 12 months)	Toddlers/ Preschoolers (1 to 5 years)	School-Agers (6 to 12 years)	Teenagers (13 years and older)
Smile and be caring	Keep child in contact with parent	Smile and be friendly	Treat teenagers as adults
Speak softly and quietly	Speak to child, parent before contact	Start by introducing yourself	Start by introducing yourself
Use the child's name	Use the child's name	Speak directly to child	Speak directly and respectfully
Warm your hands first	Let child hide face	Use child's name	Explain your actions in adult terms
Use a gentle touch; tender caresses may help	Give praise and rewards	Always tell the truth	Maintain appropriate parental involvement
	Offer choices if possible	Respect the child's modesty	Let friends comfort patient if possible

3.4.2.2   Communicating with Parents

Communicating with aggrieved parents can be challenging. It is wise to remember, especially in a disaster, that parents are afraid and feel guilty, rightly or wrongly, about their child's illnesses or injuries ("If only I had not taken my child to the day care center"; "If only I had not let my child go to the store with friends"; "If only I had kept my child home from school today"; and myriad other "what if"s.). In addition, they may feel both helpless and powerless to protect their children or to provide appropriate emergency health care. As such, some will resort to primitive defenses. Denial and anger always come first, so health care providers should be prepared for displaced rage. Bargaining, depression, and acceptance will come much later, after the providers are gone.

General strategies for dealing with aggrieved parents include acknowledging their fears. Parents should be told that the situation was not their fault. They should be allowed to assist in the treatment. Most important, health care providers must not respond to angry behavior, but should maintain a professional demeanor. Parents should be reminded that health care providers are trained to help, which includes explaining what is happening and why. It is important to remember that parents may regress, too. Speaking in clear, simple, unambiguous phrases will help. Defusing angry parents can be especially challenging. Health care providers should stay calm and project authority. If possible, an angry parent should be drawn away from the child, letting the other parent stay with the child. Health care providers should speak to the parent first, then the child. Parents should be addressed formally, using their titles and last names. Parents should be allowed to show their emotions. Appropriate adult behaviors should be praised. If all else fails, immediate police assistance should be requested, if available.

3.4.2.3   Decontamination

As discussed in Chapter 4, the best general advice regarding pediatric decontamination is to keep parents with their children whenever possible. This will decrease anxiety, improve supervision, and reduce staffing needs. To the extent feasible, the need for decontamination should be determined as soon as possible. If the contamination threat is nonexistent or minimal, infants and children will be better served by avoiding decontamination entirely, thereby minimizing the attendant risks of worsening respiratory distress and hypothermia. Ideally, hazardous materials teams at the scene will establish a pediatric decontamination corridor through which parent-child teams will be funneled, allowing parents to carry infants and children through the decontamination line. Special attention must be directed toward airway protection, while all pediatric casualties should be dried and warmed immediately to avoid the subsequent development of hypothermia.

Another concern in children, because of their relatively large surface area in relation to body mass, is that they lose heat quickly when showered. Consequently, skin decontamination with water may result in hypothermia unless heating lamps and other warming equipment are used. Another decontamination challenge is the handling of infants by workers in PPE. Protective gear limits vision, mobility, and dexterity, making it difficult to handle small children and infants.

3.4.2.4 Pediatric Medications, Equipment, and Supplies

Fluid resuscitation, drug dosages, and equipment sizes are based on the child's weight. Estimating the weight of a child can be difficult, particularly for health care providers with limited pediatric experience. Basic pediatric drug doses and fluid resuscitation volumes can be found in all pediatric resuscitation courses cited in this chapter, as well as on commercially available length-based pediatric resuscitation tapes, such as the Broselow Pediatric Emergency Tape (http://www.armstrongmedical.com/index. cfm/go/product.detail/sec/3/ssec/14/fam/2371).[1-9,17] Basic pediatric disaster drugs and dosing for chemical, biological, radiologic, and nuclear agents can be found in several pediatric disaster resources.[12,18] Information regarding specific drugs and dosages, including their indications, also can be found in Chapters 7 through 9 of this manual.

In addition to chemical, biologic, and radiologic antidotes and medications, ambulances and emergency departments should carry all equipment listed in the standard guidance documents.[19,20] Both documents describe the minimum equipment necessary for resuscitation of infants and children, listing all supplies needed for respiratory and circulatory support. Ambulances, clinics, and hospital emergency departments typically carry only limited quantities of pediatric equipment. Sufficient supplies and equipment should be readily available to treat large numbers of pediatric casualties. Because equipment choices and drug dosages, including intravenous rates, depend on the child's size, a quick, convenient system to guide appropriate choices should be in place. From experience in the developing world where laboratory assessment of electrolyte status and other parameters are unavailable, in general, practitioners will assume that the child is isotonic in fluid and electrolyte balance and treat accordingly while keeping an eye on other physical, electrocardiographic, and behavioral changes that may alert them to suspect an electrolyte imbalance. Whatever system is used should be comprehensive enough to include dosages for antidotes and other medications that may be relevant during a mass casualty event.

A surge in pediatric casualties can quickly overwhelm hospital, regional, and even state pediatric capacity, so strategies should include solutions that involve hospital, regional, state, and federal planning to manage such surges. Plans should consider that pediatric casualties will present as families when injured adults refuse to be separated from their children. As part of a community population vulnerability assessment, emergency planners should address the need for medical supplies and resources to support pediatric care. State, territorial, tribal, and local governments should develop preagreements for pharmaceuticals and durable medical equipment, keeping in mind that they might need supplies not typically found in emergency facilities or on ambulances.

3.4.3 Family Identification and Reunification

In most disasters involving large segments of a population, but especially natural disasters, large numbers of children may be separated from their families and caregivers, who in some cases may be deceased. Many of these children will present for treatment at emergency departments or be evacuated to relocation sites. Depending on their age, some children may not be able to give their names or may be too frightened to give any information, making identification difficult. At the same time, parents will instinctively rush to hospitals to find their children. In the process, parents may unintentionally obstruct medical care, overwhelm an already stressed staff, and violate patient privacy as they frantically search for their children. As such, a critical aspect of pediatric disaster response is to effectively address the needs of children who have been displaced from their parents or guardians.

An inherent goal and imperative is to rapidly identify and protect displaced children to reduce the potential for maltreatment, neglect, exploitation, and emotional injury. Aligning pediatric casualties with family members is ideal. However, absent family involvement, efforts should be taken to create a system whereby children are matched to other volunteers or care providers. Where infant feeding is necessary, a 1:1 or 1:2 infant-to-provider ratio is desirable and, where wet nurses are not available, appropriate and safe breast milk substitutes are needed. Without a history of allergies, potential for allergic reactions must be monitored. Consideration must be given to environmental safety and security, as children can wander off or be harmed by hazards created in a disaster. Shelter facility planners should implement necessary safeguards and arrangements to secure children in appropriately designated areas, as intentional or unintentional injury could occur. Effective systems are needed in the United States that expedite the reunification of children with their families when children cannot be identified by health care or public health personnel.

The key element in such systems is tracking. Unaccompanied children and adolescents must be photographed and assigned unique identifiers that will follow them as they are transported to distant sites for ongoing health care. A central registry of tracking information must be established to which aggrieved parents can turn for information about their missing children. If parents cannot ultimately be located, relief agencies will need to provide for the needs of unaccompanied children and adolescents until such time as local social services agencies can institute placement.

3.4.4   Pediatric Health Challenges

In disasters, children are predisposed to multiple risk factors. At the same time, children must rely on parents or other caregivers for food, clothing, and shelter. Children of different ages or stages of development also interpret the world differently and at their own pace. This influences their responses to disasters or catastrophic events. In a disaster, adult caretaker supervision may be lacking, and the usual resources of school or child care may be unavailable. Caregivers may even be injured, killed, or simply not present. Infants especially are vulnerable when their food sources are eliminated or contaminated. Younger children are unable to take care of their needs for activities of daily living, so an adult caregiver must oversee them.

The unique health needs of children have only recently begun to be considered and understood in disaster planning. This includes consideration of children who are at home, in school, in child care, or in transit; children who cannot be reunited with their families; and children with special health care needs who cannot perform activities of daily living or provide necessary medical interventions by themselves. It should also include recognition of the toll that care for pediatric casualties of major disasters may take on first responders and first receivers themselves.

3.4.4.1 Lodging and Shelter

Families and communities affected by disasters prefer to stay together. In cases where this is impossible, children and families should be hosted by other family members, or people who share historical, religious, or similar cultural ties. Children typically form the largest part of populations housed in disaster shelters. In addition to malnutrition and infection, they are more vulnerable to exploitation, such as abduction and all forms of sexual violence, as well as exclusion from provision of essential humanitarian services. Safe play areas should be made available for children. Although school buildings are often used as temporary shelters, alternative structures should be sought wherever possible to enable schooling to continue.

The unique needs of children in shelter situations include the need for special supplies and services, such as foods (eg, formula), clothing and sanitation (eg, diapers), and sleeping accommodations (eg, cribs), as well as games and other distractions for children. Staffing is an issue with regard to supervision. Shelters should be child-proofed to promote safety for children as well as the elderly. Sick children should be isolated. Children should be protected from environmental hazards such as weapons, alcohol, and cigarette smoke. Children with special health care needs, especially those who depend on technology for survival, are particularly vulnerable and should be considered in shelter planning. Also, parents with sick children cannot be caregivers simultaneously for both a hospitalized child and nonhospitalized, sheltered children.

Efforts to distract, entertain, comfort, and even separate families with crying newborns and toddlers will help calm other evacuees in the shelter who find these sounds discomforting. Planning for special medical needs and for mental health care that focuses on children's unique developmental stages also is critical. Detailed guidelines are available for disaster shelters to ensure that the needs of children and families are addressed and accomodated.[15,21,22]

3.4.4.2 Environmental Health, Nutrition, and Communicable Disease Control

Environmental hazards can be increased from collapsed buildings, downed power lines, and hazardous debris. Increased stress on adults might lead to a higher risk of domestic violence or child abuse. Infectious agents present in the community, especially respiratory and gastrointestinal tract infections, may spread rapidly in group shelters. Contaminated food or water can lead to epidemic outbreaks of infectious diseases, resulting in vomiting, diarrheal illness, and dehydration. Changes in the environment can lead to heat-related illness or hypothermia. The use of generators or alternative sources for heating can lead to carbon monoxide exposure.

Children are at high risk for communicable and vaccine-preventable diseases, especially measles, diarrhea, acute respiratory infections, and malaria. Acute malnutrition worsens survival in children with these and other common diseases, such as meningococcal meningitis, yellow fever, viral hepatitis, and typhoid. Measles vaccination is a critical element in communicable disease control in disasters, in addition to routine supplementation with vitamin A, especially for young children. Attention to standard sanitation and hygiene practices is critical to ensure that children's feces are disposed of safely to avoid cross-infection of other children and other families.

Breastfeeding is the ideal method for feeding infants in disasters, even for infants of HIV-infected mothers, unless the safety and sustainability of bottle feeding can be ensured. Breastfeeding should continue for at least the first 2 years of life in prolonged disasters, although supplementation with energy-dense foods should begin at 6 months of age. Vitamin A supplementation should be provided to all children aged 6 months to 6 years. Powdered milk, or liquid milk distributed as a single commodity, should not be included as part of a general food distribution, because of improper dilution and microbial contamination.

3.4.4.3   Children with Chronic Illness and Injury

Chronically ill pediatric patients (referred to as *children with special health care needs*) are particularly vulnerable in major disasters, especially if their survival depends on mechanical devices (*technology-assisted children*). Children with asthma, for example, may have acute exacerbations due to stress or exposure to environmental contaminants. Upon evacuation, children may not have access to their prescription medications, or the supply may be exhausted, resulting in exacerbations of chronic illnesses. Their parents are often their primary caregivers and will not, nor should they, evacuate without them. In addition, many of these children are cared for at home rather than in an institutional setting. Evacuation efforts will be challenged if response agencies are not aware of the location of these children. It is incumbent on emergency managers and health planners to identify these children in advance by partnering with local pediatricians, pediatric-capable hospitals, and transport services to ensure that workable plans are in place to evacuate children with special health care needs on a priority basis.

3.4.4.4   Pediatric Health Care Access in Disasters

Women and children are primary users of health services in disasters. In addition, women are the primary caregivers to children. As such, health services for both population groups should be widely available. In the developed world, comprehensive pediatric specialty care is available at most large general and university hospitals. Free-standing children's hospitals are ideal for providing for the special needs of children but may not be readily available outside large metropolitan areas. It is incumbent on emergency managers and health planners in every region to partner with existing pediatric health resources in developing a plan that facilitates primary transport of critically ill or injured children to health care facilities able to care for them, yet provides for secondary transport of ill and injured children to pediatric-capable health care facilities in the event they are initially transported elsewhere. Even so, every health care facility should be able to resuscitate and stabilize a critically ill or injured child, in preparation for subsequent transfer to a pediatric-capable health care facility.

The *Pediatric Hospital Disaster Toolkit* of the New York City Department of Health and Mental Hygiene, currently in its third edition (http://www.nyc.gov/html/doh/html/ bhpp/bhpp-focus-ped-toolkit.shtml), is available to provide nonpediatric hospitals with detailed instructions on a variety of issues relevant to pediatric disaster care, including security, dietary needs, surge considerations, equipment recommendations, training, transport issues, staffing considerations, decontamination, pharmacy needs, psychosocial needs, infection control, in-hospital triage, and establishment and management of a family information and support center.[12] To the extent feasible, all health care facilities must be prepared to support the needs of children and families for up to 96 hours after a disaster for the full range of services they require: safety and supervision, lodging and shelter, nutrition and hydration (including infant formula and electrolyte solutions), hygiene and sanitation, and mental health and medical care.

3.4.4.5 Child Maltreatment

Young children are at high risk for physical or sexual abuse, particularly when they are unaccompanied.[23] Offers from well-meaning individuals to provide shelter and food may be considered, but not without screening of the potential guardians. This may be difficult in the aftermath of a disaster, especially if local social services agencies are not optimally functioning. The best advice is to rely on relief agencies to provide for the immediate survival needs of unaccompanied children and adolescents, recognizing that even in disaster shelters administered by responsible, well-established relief agencies, child abuse can and will occur. The National Resource Center for Child Protective Services has established a curriculum for relief agencies to train personnel in the danger of child abuse and to provide effective strategies to help in preventing it.[24] A few simple guidelines will help in preventing child maltreatment in the disaster shelter: know children's whereabouts, keep families together, maintain regular routines, report improper activities, keep a watchful eye, and use a buddy system.

3.4.5 Pediatrics, First Responders, and First Receivers

It is important that health care providers recognize their own feelings in treating children during disasters. Sick or injured children may be helpless and need assistance from adult providers. Despite the most heroic efforts, there will be failures; some children will die. Health care providers want to know they did their best to avoid making mistakes. To help meet these goals, as health responders, we must learn all we can about caring for infants, children, and adolescents in disasters. We must practice our skills often through regular disaster exercises that include pediatric patients. We must discuss our performance afterward with our treatment partners and our medical supervisors or experts in disaster care. As first receivers, children may not show any outward sign of distress or urgency. The silent child must be assumed in danger until proven otherwise. Finally, we must obtain professional help if it is needed in the aftermath of a disaster.

3.5 WOMEN'S HEALTH IN DISASTERS

Women and children account for 75% of displaced persons after a disaster. In part because of their social roles in both predisaster and postdisaster society, and in part because of their unique biological characteristics, women often exhibit poorer mental and physical health outcomes than men in the aftermath of disaster.[25] In addition to the general physical, psychosocial, and access issues that populations face after a disaster, women are subjected to additional hardships. Biologically, women require more regular and intensive sexual and reproductive health services than men.

Traditionally, women have less access to resources that are essential in disaster preparedness, mitigation, and rehabilitation than their male counterparts. They are overrepresented in employment fields such as agriculture, self-employment, and the informal economy, which are most likely to be affected by complex disasters. Women are also primarily responsible for domestic duties such as child care and care for the elderly or disabled; unlike men, they are usually unable to migrate in search of work and are often left alone to head the household.[26] Furthermore, altered home and societal conditions after a disaster can lead to increased stress, feelings of powerlessness, mental health problems, destruction of social networks, and overall instability. These effects are likely to increase individual, family, and community vulnerability to violence.[27]

Given the distinct needs of women in disasters, their participation in community disaster prevention or recovery plans is crucial. Women may contribute their unique experiences and help illuminate the unique vulnerabilities and capacities of the community. Because of their social and economic roles, women bring a different dimension to disaster planning and response and should be intimately involved in the implementation of preparedness, mitigation, and recovery plans.

Lodging and shelter: Often overlooked are the specific lodging needs of women and children after a disaster. Thought must be given to the location of the shelter and the amount of safety and privacy it provides. Does the location of water and food sources or latrines put women at risk? Are there separate restroom facilities for men and women? Do women feel comfortable and secure in their location, or do safety concerns lead to increased stress and anxiety?

Women should feel comfortable bathing, changing clothes, breastfeeding, and otherwise caring for themselves and their families. In certain areas of the world, cultural norms about acceptable behavior for women may contribute to health complications in shelter environments. During the 1998 floods in Bangladesh, for example, shelters did not provide sufficient privacy for females to properly wash or dry their menstrual rags, leading to an increase in urinary tract infections and perineal rashes.[28] Women need to be involved in the planning and design of shelters and temporary living establishments in order to help anticipate such issues before they arise.

Sanitation, pharmaceuticals, and hygiene supplies: In the aftermath of a disaster, access to health care services and supplies is often limited. This poses specific health issues for women. Sanitary supplies (tampons and sanitary napkins) and other supplies related to women's health (including contraceptives) are often unavailable or in limited quantities. Depending on the societal norm, women may be too ashamed or embarrassed to ask for supplies.

Limited access to sanitation may also prompt women to eat and drink less frequently to avoid finding a safe and private place for defecation and urination, which can lead to urinary tract infections and gastrointestinal ailments. A limited water supply also affects women's ability to bathe frequently, which poses additional health risks, particularly during menstruation.

Pregnancy management and health testing: Pregnant women make up a unique subset of the disaster-affected population. Because of their physical and emotional condition, pregnant women may be unable to evacuate or otherwise move around as quickly as other members of the population. They additionally face greater societal marginalization and are particularly susceptible to the psychosocial effects of the loss of family and community networks.

Sheltering options are of primary concern, because a stable place to live provides a sense of security and improved conditions for birthing. Shelters should offer adequate sustenance and nutritional supplements for pregnant women, as their dietary needs differ from those of the general population. This is also true for lactating women, who are unable to properly breastfeed their infants if undernourished and subject to extreme anxiety. Antenatal and postnatal health services and protection should be made available to both pregnant and lactating women to ensure the health of mother and child. Unfortunately, this is rarely the case in postdisaster sheltering environments.[29]

It is important to remember that half of all pregnancies are unplanned. Women may not be aware that they are pregnant; furthermore, disruption of access to care after a disaster may impede access to contraceptives and other reproductive health supplies, increasing the risk of unwanted or unplanned pregnancy. As the first 8 weeks of pregnancy are essential for organogenesis, it is very important to ensure access to testing options and health care information in the aftermath of disaster.

Physical and sexual assault: There are few evidence-based studies that compare violence levels before and after a disaster. However, anecdotal evidence and a few small, systematic studies suggest that physical and sexual assault are highly prevalent following disasters. Studies in the Philippines after the Mt Pinatubo eruption, Nicaragua after Hurricane Mitch, and the United States after the Loma Prieta earthquake have shown increases in domestic violence.[27] It is theorized that women living in a violent relationship before the disaster may experience elevated levels of violence after the disaster as a result of the loss of social support systems that previously afforded some measure of protection. Displaced women and children also are at increased risk of physical and sexual violence, as they may be exploited while trying to meet their basic needs. Reports from eastern Congo and Guinea have shown that displaced women and children have been coerced into sex in exchange for food or shelter.[27]

Health services must include care for survivors of sexual assault and rape. This includes services such as mental health resources, treatment of physical injury, pregnancy prevention options, testing and treatment for sexually transmitted infections, and HIV testing and postexposure prophylaxis. Health care workers should be trained to identify victims of physical and sexual abuse and to provide the appropriate care to these women in a private and sensitive manner.

Psychological impact: Unusual situations such as complex emergencies or disasters are powerful stressors. Disasters not only can introduce new psychosocial stressors but may also magnify previous ones. As discussed in Section 3.8 of this manual, psychological responses to disaster often include guilt, fear, stress, sleep disturbances, and shock. However, not all members of society are affected equally. Various studies have indicated that women and girls are more likely than men and boys to suffer adverse psychological effects.[28] While the exact reasons are unclear, this is perhaps due to the increased familial burden placed on women in the postdisaster setting. It may also be due to an increase in physical, sexual, or emotional violence; a loss of protective shelter; increased disadvantage to productive and economic means; or the effects of physical or emotional losses.[29] Regardless of the reason, it is clear that women have unique mental and behavioral health needs in the aftermath of a disaster, a fact that should be considered in preevent and postevent planning.

3.6 PEOPLE WITH CHRONIC ILLNESS IN DISASTERS

Chronic diseases are the leading causes of death and disability in the United States. Today, about 135 million Americans are living with chronic illnesses, which account for 70% of all deaths and one-third of potential years of life lost prior to age 65 years. Traditionally, preparation for disasters has focused not on the needs of survivors with preexisting chronic medical conditions, but rather on acute injuries, environmental exposures, and infectious diseases. Population-based studies evaluating the indirect mortality (that is, the mortality not directly caused by the event itself, but by the consequences of it, such as lack of access to care) of the general population after large-scale disasters have demonstrated that those with chronic medical conditions, along with women and children, are disproportionately affected. Given that approximately 80% of adults 65 years or older have at least one chronic medical condition and about 50% have at least two chronic conditions, this quickly growing segment of the US population is particularly vulnerable in a disaster.[30]

Populations affected by disasters may carry a large and measurable burden of disabilities and chronic diseases, especially heart disease, cancer, stroke, diabetes, and chronic respiratory disorders.[31,32] Chronic illnesses may be exacerbated by physical, psychosocial, and environmental factors that result from a disaster. These include extreme temperatures, lack of food or water, physical or emotional trauma, and disruptions in the health system. Elderly men and women, many of whom have multiple chronic conditions and comorbidities being treated with multiple medications, are particularly at risk. Similarly vulnerable are ischemic stroke survivors taking anticoagulants, people whose diabetes is controlled by insulin, heart attack survivors taking clot-preventing medications, people with severe lung disease receiving home oxygen therapy, people with hereditary blood disorders, and people receiving hemodialysis for kidney failure. The need to treat chronic conditions is especially magnified when there are catastrophic disruptions of the medical infrastructure, including pharmacies, when access to medical care and medications is severely compromised or totally cut off, and when large-scale evacuations of the population occur.

3.6.1 Medical and Health Record Access

In a disaster or public health emergency, a most basic requirement for people with chronic medical conditions is access to their medications. On September 11, 2001, many frail older adults and persons with disabilities living near the World Trade Center were confined to their high-rise apartments without supplies, electricity, or a mechanism to refill their prescription medications.[30] Hurricane Katrina, on the other hand, forced many residents to evacuate their homes to less familiar surroundings. Approximately one-half of Katrina evacuees lacked medications at the time of displacement.[33] Moreover, most were not able to access their medical records in a timely fashion. The lack of medical records exacerbated difficulties of health care providers in helping individuals reacquire medications or durable medical equipment.[34]

In a disaster, people may arrive at shelters without vital medications, health care information, or records. Under conditions of profound stress, people also may not be able to recall vital health-related information. To help alleviate these challenges, individuals with chronic diseases should be encouraged to wear some form of medical alert identification and carry essential medical information on their person at all times. It is reasonable and prudent for people with chronic medical conditions to maintain an emergency reserve of their prescription medications. People with chronic medical conditions should carry on their person a current list of their prescription medications, which includes indications, doses, and the prescriber's and dispensing pharmacist's contact information.

Individuals with chronic diseases should be educated on disaster preparation. They also must be familiar with strategies for ensuring the availability of adequate dietary, sheltering, and treatment options to protect their health and well-being in various disaster situations. They should discuss medication refill options with a physician or other health care professional to ensure that they have an adequate supply of prescription medications in the event of a disaster or public health emergency.

3.6.2   Medical Care Access

Lack of access to routine health care is a contributing cause to morbidity and mortality after disasters. In addition, indirect effects (eg, loss of electricity) can lead to exposure to extreme heat or cold or interruption of supplemental oxygen supplies. Many people living with chronic diseases rely on routine health care services to maintain their quality of life and live independently. Public education materials, including public service announcements in affected areas, should remind people of actions to ensure that their chronic diseases remain stable and adverse health outcomes are prevented throughout a disaster.

Response efforts must address the needs for durable medical equipment, medical devices, and their associated power requirements. Various outpatient medical services require continuation during a disaster to maintain quality of life (eg, hemodialysis, radiation treatments, chemotherapy, and rehabilitation services). Public and private insurance programs limit the amount of prescription drugs people can order at one time. This restriction therefore limits individuals who may need to fill prescriptions immediately after an emergency. Any disruption of these services can be detrimental to health.

3.6.3   Planning Considerations

Local disaster plans need to address populations that are likely to have chronic medical conditions and to require medical supplies or equipment.[35-37] They need to address evacuation and emergency treatment, as well as strategies to ensure continuity of care to individuals with chronic diseases. Disaster preparation must ensure the availability of medical resources to control chronic diseases and prevent acute events and complications. Guidelines should address triage, clinical evaluation, essential medication supply, emergency medical services (EMS) support, and access to specialty care (to include hemodialysis and ventilator support). A list of essential medications consistent with the predicted burden of chronic diseases should be developed and used in planning for provision of long-term maintenance medications during disasters. Local preparation for the prevention and management of acute exacerbations of chronic diseases should be guided by the following:

➤ Predisaster rates of adverse health outcomes and the chronic disease burden in the community

➤ Awareness of the immediate needs of people with chronic diseases (including a plan for providing essential medications)

➤ Knowledge of the baseline and surge capacity of local and regional health systems to treat and manage chronic diseases

➤ The capacity and capability of the local and regional health systems to rebuild the basic infrastructure needed to support care after a large-scale disaster or public health emergency

3.7 PEOPLE WITH FUNCTIONAL AND ACCESS NEEDS IN DISASTERS

Hurricane Katrina reinforced the stark reality that a large segment of the US population may not be able to successfully plan for and respond to a disaster or public health emergency with resources typically accessible to the general population. The current population is diverse, aging, and focused on maintaining independence as long as possible. Increased consideration needs to be given to people who may be able to function independently under normal situations, but who may need assistance in an emergency situation. In addition to coping with any personal losses or injuries that they may have suffered, people with disabilities who experience a tragic or traumatic event may be deprived of vital connections to attendants, service or guide animals, neighbors, local business owners, and even family members. Many may no longer be able to follow their accustomed routines.

Various public- and private-sector agencies and organizations are working to ensure that the functional and access needs of people are adequately addressed before an emergency. According to the National Organization on Disability (http://www.nod.org), nearly 15% of Americans over 5 years of age have at least one disability.[38] This comprises almost 41 million people who have some sensory, physical, mental, self-care, or employment disability requiring personal care equipment, mobility aids, adaptive feeding devices, service animals, specially equipped vehicles, and/or powered medical equipment.

During a disaster, evacuation of these populations will be challenging, as will decontamination of disabled individuals and their equipment. Some individuals will not understand instructions during a crises, and others may not be capable of following them. For various reasons (including privacy, maintaining independence, fear of bias, and various other social and cultural reasons), people with disabilities, people with health conditions causing limitations, and other at-risk groups may choose not to identify their needs for assistance.

3.7.1 Definitions

Consensus definitions for the terms *special needs*, *functional needs*, and *medical-special needs* continue to evolve. The National Response Framework (NRF; http://www.fema.gov/emergency/nrf) contains a definition of *special needs* to help emergency managers and planners understand the diverse population that has functional and access needs during disasters. The NRF definition of special needs seeks to establish a flexible framework that addresses a broad set of common function-based needs irrespective of specific diagnosis, status, or label (eg, children, elderly, transportation disadvantaged). In other words, this function-based definition reflects the capabilities of the individual, not the condition or label. It is prudent that disaster planners align their language with the NRF definition to enhance intergovernmental communication during an incident.

The definition of *special needs populations* as it appears in the NRF is as follows:

Populations whose members may have additional needs before, during, and after an incident in functional areas, including but not limited to: maintaining independence, communication, transportation, supervision, and medical care. Individuals in need of additional response assistance may include those who have disabilities; who live in institutionalized settings; who are elderly; who are children; who are from diverse cultures; who have limited English proficiency or are non-English speaking; or who are transportation disadvantaged.

➤ *Maintaining independence:* Individuals requiring support to be independent in daily activities may lose this support during an emergency or a disaster. Such support may include consumable medical supplies (eg, diapers, formula, bandages, ostomy supplies), durable medical equipment (eg, wheelchairs, walkers, scooters), service animals, and/or attendants or caregivers. Supplying needed support to these individuals will enable them to maintain their predisaster level of independence.

➤ *Communication:* Individuals who have limitations that interfere with the receipt of and response to information will need that information provided in forms they can understand and use. They may not be able to hear oral announcements, see directional signs, or understand how to get assistance because of hearing, vision, speech, cognitive, or intellectual limitations, and/or limited English language proficiency.

➤ *Transportation:* Individuals who cannot drive or who do not have a vehicle may require transportation support for successful evacuation. This support may include accessible vehicles (eg, lift-equipped vehicles or vehicles suitable for transporting individuals who use oxygen) or information about how and where to access mass transportation during an evacuation.

➤ *Supervision:* Before, during, and after an emergency individuals may lose the support of caregivers, family, or friends or may be unable to cope in a new environment (particularly if they have dementia, Alzheimer's disease, or psychiatric conditions such as schizophrenia or intense anxiety). If separated from their caregivers, young children may be unable to identify themselves, and when in danger, they may lack the cognitive ability to assess the situation and react appropriately.

> *Medical care:* Individuals who are not self-sufficient or who do not have adequate support from caregivers, family, or friends may need assistance with managing unstable, terminal, or contagious conditions that require observation and ongoing treatment; managing intravenous therapy, tube feeding, and vital signs; receiving dialysis, oxygen, and suction administration; managing wounds; and operating power-dependent equipment to sustain life. These individuals require support of trained medical professionals.

Some people with functional and access needs will not require special assistance during an emergency because they are able to care for themselves. Individuals in need of additional response assistance may include those who have disabilities; who live in institutionalized settings; who are elderly; who are children; who are from diverse cultures; who have limited English language proficiency; who are non–English speaking; or who are transportation disadvantaged. Therefore, while some 20% of the total population has a disability, the national planning average used by emergency management offices is notably lower. Accurate planning requires that local authorities have a solid understanding of community demographics.

3.7.2   Communication Challenges

In a disaster or public health emergency, communications should be accessible for people with limited English language proficiency and to members of diverse cultures. This is especially true for people with disabilities, many of whom are unemployed, socially isolated, or in other ways less connected to society than nondisabled people. Individuals who are deaf, deaf-blind, or hard of hearing cannot hear radio, television, sirens, or other audible alerts. Similarly, individuals who are blind or who have low vision may not be aware of visual cues, such as flashing lights and scrolling emergency information on television. Many individuals with cognitive impairment live independently and experience confusion and anxiety, even in minor emergencies. Emergency plans should not rely on a single source of general notification for the community; multiple methods are necessary.

Emergency communications involve two closely interrelated aspects: delivery mechanisms and content messaging. Individuals with disabilities should be informed about realistic expectations of service during and after an emergency, even while demonstrating a serious commitment to their functional needs. Such information can result in a more cooperative relationship with local authorities and enhance their appreciation of the concerns of people with disabilities. Warning methods should be developed to ensure that all citizens have the information necessary to make sound decisions and take appropriate, responsible action. Using a combination of methods will be more effective than relying on one method alone. These might include the use of telephone calls, auto-dialed TTY (teletypewriter) messages, text messaging, e-mails, Braille, audio recording, large-font messaging, and even direct door-to-door contact with preregistered individuals. Additional consideration should be given to the use of open captioning on local television stations, as well as lower-tech options such as dispatching qualified sign-language interpreters to assist in broadcasting emergency information provided to the media.

The medium used to reach people may change at different points in the disaster timeline. Today, the population can receive alerts via relay services or calls placed over the Internet as well as via text messaging, e-mails, social networking Web sites (eg, Twitter, Facebook, MySpace), videophone calls, or online video conferencing programs such as Skype.

3.7.3 Evacuation Challenges

Individuals with functional and access needs will face a variety of challenges in evacuations, depending on the nature of the emergency. People with a mobility disability may need assistance leaving a building without a working elevator. Individuals who are blind or who have limited vision may no longer be able to independently use traditional orientation and navigation methods. An individual who is deaf may be trapped somewhere unable to communicate with anyone because the only communication device relies on voice. Procedures should be in place to ensure that people with disabilities can evacuate the physical area in a variety of conditions with or without assistance.

Community evacuation plans must ensure that people with health-related limitations, including those who have mobility, vision, hearing, or cognitive disabilities, mental illness, or other disabilities, can safely self-evacuate or be evacuated by others. Some communities are instituting voluntary, confidential registries of persons with disabilities who may need individualized evacuation assistance or notification. Whether or not a registry is used, plans should address accessible transportation needs for people who use wheelchairs, scooters, or other mobility aids, as well as people who are blind or who have low vision. It is important to provide accessible modes of transportation to help evacuate people with disabilities during an emergency. For instance, some communities have used lift-equipped school or transit buses during floods to evacuate people who use wheelchairs.

Evacuation of entire communities typically takes place over a longer period of time than facility evacuations. Community evacuations can be even more traumatizing because people are leaving their homes, businesses, and possessions behind. Community evacuation plans should be designed to allow the necessary time, consideration, and assistance for people with disabilities to be adequately notified of evacuation plans. People with disabilities must be able to bring with them special equipment (eg, wheelchairs, dialysis machines, ventilators) and service or guide animals. In some communities, these concerns have led to the creation of staggered evacuation orders with notification of large care facilities ahead of the general population.

Unfortunately, it is often too late at the time of a disaster to educate people, already confused and alarmed by a crisis, about how to escape or to how to help individuals with disabilities. It is critical to ensure that emergency managers have effective evacuation plans and procedures in place for people with disabilities prior to the event. Plans must address strategies for communicating disaster instructions to all ages and populations in a crisis and under unfavorable circumstances, such as the loss of power. As part of disaster preparedness, it is important to conduct regular drills so that residents and employees are familiar with these plans. Disaster drills should pay adequate attention to the functional and access needs of all people, not just those in wheelchairs and with other mobility impairments, but also those with visual, hearing, or cognitive impairments.

3.7.4   Sheltering Considerations

When disasters occur, people are often provided safe refuge in local temporary shelters. Some may be located in schools, office buildings, tents, or other areas. Historically, great attention has been paid to ensuring that these shelters are well stocked with basic necessities such as food, water, and blankets. Many of these shelters may not be accessible to people with disabilities. Even if individuals using a wheelchair can get to the shelter, they may find no accessible entrance, accessible toilet, or accessible shelter area. Many shelters also have a no-pets policy, and some mistakenly apply this policy to exclude service animals. In accordance with Title II of the Americans with Disabilities Act (ADA), general-population shelters should offer individuals with disabilities the same benefits provided to those without disabilities. These benefits include safety, comfort, food, medical care, and the support of family and friends. Disability civil rights laws require physical accessibility of shelter facilities, effective communication using multiple methods, full access to emergency services, and reasonable modification of programs where needed.[21,22,38]

Disaster plans should identify accessible ADA-compliant shelters, which must meet minimal accessibility standards. In addition, the level of medical oversight to be provided must be determined well in advance of an emergency. Whether there will be different classes of shelters (eg, medically managed or designated for functional needs) must be established in the planning phase. Making these determinations ahead of time will help ensure that the needs of those with disabilities utilizing the shelter system will be properly identified and addressed. More information is available from the US Department of Justice's "ADA Checklist for Emergency Shelters" (http://www .ada.gov/pcatoolkit/chap7shelterchk.htm). The checklist can help emergency managers determine whether a building could be used as a shelter and, if so, what barriers must be rectified.

Shelter plans should outline how to obtain resources such as durable medical equipment (ie, wheelchairs, walkers, canes, personal hygiene supplies, skilled staff). Infants and children will need items such as diapers, formula, baby food, and toys. Individuals who require medications, such as certain types of insulin that require constant refrigeration, may find that many shelters do not provide refrigerators or ice-packed coolers. An elderly individual who functions without assistance in his or her home may be confused and in need of assistance in the shelter environment. A person with a cognitive or psychiatric problem may need direction with the change in daily routine. Individuals who use life support systems and other medical devices that rely on electricity to function may not have access to a generator or other source of electricity within a shelter. People who are deaf or hard of hearing may not have access to audible information routinely made available to people in the temporary shelters. Individuals who are blind or who have low vision will not be able to use printed notices, advisories, or other written information.

Individuals who require minimal support or assistance should not be directed to a shelter that provides a greater level of support services than they need. General-population shelters should make appropriate accommodations for individuals with special needs. These accommodations may include physical accessibility, modifications to facilities, pictogram signage and sign-language interpreters, and volunteers to help elderly and/or other individuals who need minimal assistance with activities of daily living. Historically, volunteer organizations (such as the American Red Cross) manage general-population shelter services after a disaster. However, because no jurisdiction can depend on one source to supply all personnel and resources necessary, emergency managers should draw from the skills and resources within special needs planning networks. Whereas moving populations into shelters is generally contraindicated during infectious disease outbreaks and pandemics (instead, sheltering in place is optimal), the responsibilities to maintain resources for populations within their homes with essential food, medications, information, and other supplies will severely challenge the rescue and relief system.

Medical shelters are designed for people whose frailty, mobility, and functional and/or medical needs make them particularly vulnerable and at risk in disaster situations. These shelters are designed for individuals who have preexisting conditions resulting in medical impairments and who have been able to maintain activities of daily living in a home environment before the disaster or emergency situation. Medical shelters are intended to provide a safe environment for those requiring limited medical assistance or surveillance due to a preexisting health problem. They are intended as temporary facilities to provide housing and specialized or supervised care to individuals whose physical or mental health needs exceed the level of care provided by the American Red Cross in disaster shelters but is not severe enough to require hospitalization. Examples of services that can be provided in medical shelters include the following:

➤ Foley catheter maintenance

➤ Diabetes care

➤ Medication management

➤ Blood pressure monitoring

➤ Ostomy care

➤ Stable oxygen and nebulizer therapy

3.7.5   Health Care Considerations

A large-scale disaster or public health emergency may adversely affect the availability of the human services routinely used by individuals with functional and access needs. A number of critical activities and programs delivering human services could be adversely affected by damage to, or excessive demand placed on, key components of the human services resource infrastructure. Potentially affected activities in human services include transportation, child care, child support, developmental disabilities services, foster care, refugee programs, homeless shelters, social services programs, and aging services. Medicare/Medicaid benefits may not be immediately available if affected areas are evacuated, mail service is interrupted, or persons who live in the community are relocated to an institutional setting.

Individuals needing acute medical care should be taken to medical shelters or hospitals. Consideration should be given to a mechanism for transferring people to the appropriate location, taking into account the transportation and sheltering needs of their caregiver and/or family members. Emergency plans should identify personnel and pharmaceuticals available in the jurisdiction to support a surge in the number of individuals needing ongoing medical support. Medical resources available within non-governmental organizations (NGOs) and the private sector should not be overlooked. Trained professionals who have experience working with special needs populations should be identified as part of the planning process to offer health services, including mental health services and services for children.

Disasters may cause psychological distress by forcing individuals with disabilities to confront the limitations imposed by their disabilities on a more or less continuous basis, or it may cause them to relive traumatic experiences from their past. The needs of individuals with disabilities should be considered, too, when they leave a shelter or are otherwise allowed to return to their home. If a ramp has been destroyed, an individual with a mobility impairment will be unable to get into and out of the house. Temporary housing also may be needed that is physically accessible, with appropriate communication devices, such as TTYs, to ensure that individuals with communication disabilities can communicate with family, friends, and health professionals.

Functional and Access Needs Registries

Many communities are developing registries for people meeting specified criteria to voluntarily list themselves, making local emergency authorities aware of their location and specialized support needs. Such registries identify individuals within a community who would be particularly vulnerable in disasters or other serious emergencies. Enrollment provides vital information for the local EMS and other responders by identifying geographic locations and clusters of vulnerable individuals. Emergency planners use this information to plan for transportation, evacuation, sheltering, and health care needs.

It is important to recognize that no matter how comprehensive a registry may be, not all people with functional and access needs will register. Some people may not wish to identify themselves as having a health-related problem. Others may not view their condition as creating a special need. Still others may not be aware of the registry or think to register until after an event occurs. Therefore, any registry should be considered only a guide in an emergency, not a definitive or exhaustive list. With any registry, it is important that policies and procedures are in place to ensure that the registry is voluntary, guarantees confidentiality, and can be updated periodically.

3.8 MENTAL AND BEHAVIORAL HEALTH IN DISASTERS

In times of crisis, communities seek assistance and aid from myriad resources, organized within traditional agencies and social institutions. Such resources may include emergency response personnel, health care institutions and professionals, community mental health organizations, places of worship and faith-based organizations, schools, and voluntary organizations, as well as neighbors and families. Whether the resources of a particular community will be adequate to meet demand is a function of the quality of local and state leadership, the quality of preevent planning, and the quantity and productivity of people in each organization who have the training and commitment to deliver needed care.

"Needed care" includes meeting community expectations for delivery of ongoing services to persons with acute and chronic illnesses, while also addressing the surge in demand for medical and psychosocial care created by a disaster or public health emergency. Although acute stress disorder and posttraumatic stress disorder (PTSD) receive the most publicity after disasters, a majority of persons, including those experiencing somatic symptoms below the threshold for a diagnosable psychiatric disorder, will be sustained by a system of care that includes family and community resources, as well as coordinated primary care and psychiatric, psychological, psychosocial, and behavioral services where they are most effective.[39-44]

A great deal has been learned from crises (such as war) that apply to all large-scale disasters. Interest in these problems is now growing as their frequency and effect among trauma-affected populations have become more apparent. Those populations in need of psychosocial and mental health support represent several overlapping subpopulations of people, including those:

➤ With disabling psychiatric illnesses

➤ With severe psychological reactions to trauma

➤ Who have significant problems but may be able to cope and adapt once security and order are restored (this last subgroup generally represents the majority of the population who have witnessed brutality or sudden and violent loss and will do well with interventions by well-trained volunteers in psychological first aid [as described in Section 3.8.4.2]).

Disasters and Mental Health

While some individuals have a biologic propensity for mental illness, it is important to recognize that everyone who experiences a major disaster will have some type of psychological, psychosocial, and/or behavioral response to the event. This is normal and expected and should be reflected in all emergency planning documents.

Communities, and the support they receive from the outside, must be able to address all subpopulations of care. With the destruction of health care facilities for mental health, outside resources must be able to remedicate and restabilize individuals who require and have lost or been separated from medications to control their psychiatric illnesses.[45]

3.8.1   Planning Goals and Priorities

A fundamental task facing communities is the development of cross-organizational, public-private partnerships that serve a community-wide psychosocial preparedness program. Achievement of this goal requires (1) designation of a leader who is integral to the community, city, county, or regional incident command structure and who is accountable for overseeing the evolving community psychosocial preparedness program; (2) communication and coordination among leaders of the respective public and private organizations that compose the local and regional resources for response; and (3) a plan that is supported by key members of those organizations and that addresses the ability of community care resources to serve the public, including education on psychological and behavioral coping strategies. The leader must be firmly linked to the local and regional incident command structure, as well as being a respected professional who understands and has overseen a comprehensive inventory of clinical, public health, and community psychosocial and behavioral response resources.

Mental health and other response personnel need to provide for the safety, security, and survival (eg, food and shelter) of affected individuals and populations; ensure people are informed of disaster response and recovery efforts; facilitate communications with family, friends, and community; and reduce ongoing hazards. A critical first step in reducing the mental health impact of a disaster is an effective risk communication plan. A spokesperson should be identified who is credible and trusted and who can provide accurate and timely assessments of what is and what is not known. To reduce population fear and anxiety, rumors should be anticipated and debunked as quickly as possible.

Disaster plans should identify locations where people may obtain care for psychosocial needs and screening and referral systems that should be implemented. Family assistance centers or point-of-distribution sites, for example, should offer screening and referral for psychosocial and behavioral disorders in the immediate aftermath of a disaster. Disaster plans also must address specific cultural needs and responses of ethnic minorities, as well as of vulnerable individuals, such as children, the frail elderly, and people with disabilities.

Key Planning Elements to Address Psychosocial Effects of Disasters and Other Mass Trauma Events[39]

➤ Basic resources including food, shelter, communication, transportation, information, guidance, and medical services

➤ Interventions and programs to promote individual and community resilience and prevent adverse psychological effects

➤ Surveillance for psychological consequences, including distress responses, behavior changes, and psychiatric illness, and markers of individual and community functioning before, during, and after a disaster or public health emergency

➤ Screening of psychological symptoms at the individual level

Key Planning Elements to Address Psychosocial Effects of Disasters and Other Mass Trauma Events[39] (continued)

➤ Treatment for acute and long-term effects of trauma

➤ Response for longer-term general human service needs that contribute to psychological functioning (eg, housing, financial assistance when the event creates job loss)

➤ Risk communication and dissemination of information to the public, media, political leaders, and service providers

➤ Training of service providers (in medical, public health, emergency, and mental health systems) to respond to a traumatic event and to protect themselves against psychological harm

➤ Capacity to handle a large increase in demand for services to address psychological consequences in a disaster or public health emergency

➤ Case-finding ability to locate individuals who have not utilized mental health services but need them, including underserved, marginalized, and unrecognized groups of people (eg, undocumented immigrants, homebound individuals) and others with unidentified needs

3.8.2   Stress and Psychological Trauma

In addition to the substantial effect that disasters can have on physical health, they place significant stress and psychological trauma on responders and affected populations. Experiencing a disaster can be one of the most difficult events a person can endure, and it can have both short- and long-term effects. As shown in Figure 3-1, disasters can induce a range of normal responses, including a sense of apprehension, worry, edginess, and difficulty concentrating on anything other than the source of the threat; rational and irrational attempts to remove, or escape from, the threat; and altruistic behaviors intended to ameliorate the situation.

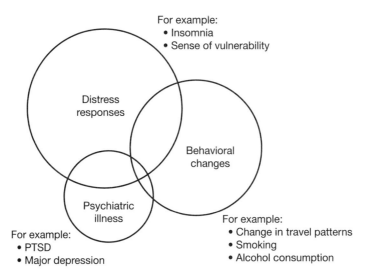

FIGURE 3-1

Psychological Consequences of Disasters and Other Mass Trauma Events[39]

In general, an abnormal response that impairs daily life may occur when symptoms are greater in duration or intensity, when symptoms result in avoidance of certain situations or objects, and if certain patterns of symptoms occur and persist. However, for most people with somatic or psychological symptoms of distress it is reasonable, in the immediate postincident phase, to expect normal recovery. Common emotional and behavioral responses include the following:

➤ Fear

➤ Helplessness

➤ Worry

➤ Anger

➤ Confusion

➤ Difficulty concentrating

➤ Fatigue

➤ Tension

➤ Changes in sleep patterns

➤ Loss of appetite

➤ Stress

It is possible to experience many of these symptoms at the same time. Most people who develop these symptoms will be able to return to normal functioning within a few weeks. Individuals may not be able to make sense out of what happened, which is normal. There is no one way to feel after a tragic event, and people should not think that there is something wrong with them for feeling a certain way or if they respond differently than others. They may wish to talk about the events that occurred and how they are feeling, or they may remain mute, not having the resources within to express their loss or grief. All require a supportive environment. However, people should not feel as though they have to talk about the event if they do not want to.

3.8.3   Mental Health Disorders and Syndromes Associated with Disasters

While many people will recover on their own over time, various syndromes and diagnoses may occur in those who fail to cope rapidly with the trauma and the resulting new realities caused by the incident. A brief understanding of the symptom complexes that make up these disorders will assist emergency response personnel in making appropriate referrals. The management of acute stress and other psychological and behavioral reactions generally aims to foster resiliency, prevent chronic emotional problems, and minimize long-term deterioration in quality of life after the traumatic exposure.

Acute stress disorder: Acute stress disorder comprises a broad set of symptoms, including dissociative symptoms (such as a sense of numbing, detachment, derealization, depersonalization, dissociate amnesia, or absence of emotional responsiveness), persistent reexperiencing of the event, avoidance of stimuli that recall the traumatic event, symptoms of increased arousal, and impairment of normal functioning. Acute stress disorder is characterized by the presence of dissociate anxiety, hyperarousal, avoidance, and reexperiencing symptoms lasting 2 to 4 weeks and occurring within 1 month of the event. Acute stress disorder has most of the same symptoms as PTSD; the length of time that symptoms persist is the prime differentiation. Individuals manifesting this symptom complex require referral to a qualified mental health or primary care professional.

Brief psychotic disorder: Individuals may briefly experience an inability to distinguish what is real from what is not real. Symptoms may include hallucinations, delusions, disorganized memory or speech, disorientation, or confusion. Symptoms may resolve spontaneously, but treatment with psychotherapy, medication, or hospitalization is often indicated.

Chronic or complicated grief: Individuals who have lost loved ones normally will experience an intense period of grief lasting several weeks to months. When the acute grief process persists for more than a few weeks or months, the individual is at risk for complicated grief reaction. While this syndrome will not be noted by initial emergency responders, those caring for survivors after the initial emergency response should be aware of this phenomenon and be prepared to refer people for appropriate mental health evaluation and treatment.

Depression: Depression is a fairly common pathologic response for some people affected by catastrophic events. Symptoms must persist for at least 2 weeks for a

"SAD-A-FACES" Depression Symptom Screening Tool*	
Sleep	Insomnia or hypersomnia
Appetite	Increase, decrease, or weight change
Dysphoria	Sadness/irritability
Anhedonia	Lack of interest/pleasure/sex drive
Fatigue	Decreased energy
Agitation	Psychomotor agitation or slowing
Concentration	Reduced ability to focus
Esteem	Decreased self-esteem or increase in feelings of guilt
Suicide	Feelings that life is not worth living or having an active plan or means to kill oneself

*This is an example of an assessment tool that can be used by caregivers to screen for the possibility of this depression. A minimum of five of these symptoms must be present within a 2-week period to consider the diagnosis.

Source: Montano.[46]

diagnosis of depression to be made. These symptoms include depressed mood and anhedonia.

Generalized anxiety disorder: Individuals may experience persistent and severe anxiety and worry that is global and debilitating. Physical symptoms may be present, and the disorder is frequently associated with both depression and substance abuse. If the symptoms persist, referral to and treatment by a qualified mental health provider or primary care physician is indicated.

Panic attacks: Individuals may experience a time-limited period of extreme anxiety with a host of physical symptoms. A panic attack is a sudden episode of intense fear that develops for no apparent reason and triggers severe physical reactions. Panic attacks usually occur without warning and can occur at any time. Physical associated symptoms include a sense of impending doom, palpitations, shortness of breath, sweating, trembling, chills and hot flashes, nausea, headache, chest pain and tightness in the throat, dizziness or faintness, difficulty swallowing, and abdominal pain. Symptoms may resolve over time or require pharmacotherapy and/or psychotherapy if they persist.

Panic disorder: Individuals with this disorder experience recurrent panic attacks that cause a change of behavior or cognition. This disorder generally requires referral and treatment by a qualified mental health professional or primary care provider.

PTSD: This disorder represents a disabling maladaptive response of at least 1-month duration to a traumatic event. Symptoms fall into three categories: avoidance and emotional numbing; reexperiencing or recurrent flashbacks; and a state of hyperarousal. The following is a screening tool for PTSD and refers to symptoms experienced for at least 1 month:

➤ Do you avoid being reminded of the traumatic experience by avoiding certain places, people, or activities?

➤ Have you lost interest in activities that previously were enjoyable or important?

➤ Have you felt more isolated or distant from other people?

➤ Have you found it hard to have love or affection for other people?

➤ Have you felt that there is no point in planning for the future?

➤ Do you have more trouble than you did before falling asleep or staying asleep?

➤ Do you become jumpy or easily startled by ordinary noises or movement?

Four or more positive responses is strongly indicative of PTSD requiring further evaluation and potential treatment by a qualified professional. Fewer than four positive responses still may be indicative of subsyndromal PTSD and the need for further evaluation. Treatment options for PTSD include antidepressants (selective serotonin reuptake inhibitors) in combination with psychotherapy and teaching individuals grounding and relaxation techniques.

Substance abuse disorder: Individuals who experience traumatic events often may experience an increase in the use of alcohol and other psychoactive drugs. Men are typically more at risk of attempting to cope with a traumatic event through substance abuse. Abuse may be defined as recurrent use in situations that may be physically dangerous, such as driving; use of the involved substance causing a failure to fulfill normal major role obligations and responsibilities; or use of a substance that causes recurrent legal problems. A rapid screen called the CAGE questionnaire can be used to screen for alcohol abuse:

➤ *C*ut down—have you recently thought about cutting down on your drinking?

➤ *A*nnoyed—have you ever been annoyed by criticism of your drinking?

➤ *G*uilt—have you ever felt guilty about your drinking?

➤ *E*ye opener—do you ever have a drink in the morning?

More than one positive response should alert a health professional that the individual might be having a problem with alcohol abuse.

Suicide risk: All people who are suspected of having depression must be assessed for risk of suicide. Individuals most at risk of attempting suicide are young females; people with borderline personality disorder, a history of impulsive behavior, or disrupted intimate relationships; and people with a history of suicide attempts. Individuals most at risk of succeeding in a suicide attempt include older white males, people living alone, people dealing with the recent loss of a loved one, people with chronic health problems, substance abusers, and people with prior attempts at suicide.

3.8.4   Mental Health Considerations for Adults

The psychological effects of any disaster is an important consideration during the recovery phase. Providing for the mental health needs of affected individuals, their families, and emergency response workers is an essential function of crisis management. Feelings of anxiety, sadness, grief, and anger are normal reactions to any disaster event. If the event is a result of an intentional or terrorist act, these normal reactions can be exacerbated. The impact on mental health may extend well beyond those who directly experienced the disaster, perhaps significantly involving those who witnessed events via television or other media. The latter was common among relatives living outside of Haiti after the 2010 earthquake, who were unaware of what was happening to their family members at home.[47-49]

Restoration of mental health after a disaster may be a prolonged process. Clinical management is best when an individual is diagnosed and treated soon after the event. Early intervention can minimize long-term negative psychological outcomes. Appropriate counseling may reduce health risks, work absenteeism, and chronic disease exacerbations attributed to stress and other behavioral and emotional reactions to the event. Treatment may consist of a combination of pharmacologic and nonpharmacologic interventions, which may include group, family, and individual therapy, cognitive behavioral therapy, and other nonpharmacologic interventions. With appropriate treatment, including emphasis on the normal recovery process (talking to others, getting rest and respite, and returning to normal routines), recovery may be facilitated.

3.8.4.1   *Psychological Triage*

Through the use of valid and reliable clinical assessment methods, mental health personnel will assess survivors; identify vulnerable, at-risk individuals and groups; and provide referral or emergency hospitalizations when indicated. Psychological triage must be structured, using a team approach, to identify persons at risk and to reassure persons with normal responses.[42] Triage processes will be designed to identify people:

➤ With acute stress disorder or other clinically significant symptoms stemming from the trauma

➤ Who are bereaved

➤ Who are at risk of suicide

➤ Who have preexisting psychiatric disorders, including substance dependence, affective disorders, and substance-induced mood or anxiety disorders

➤ Who require medical or surgical attention

➤ Whose exposure is particularly intense or of long duration

3.8.4.2 Psychological First Aid (PFA)

Psychological first aid (PFA) refers to simple psychological interventions that enlist the trauma victim's innate coping abilities to facilitate the natural healing process.[50-53] These interventions are intended to provide comfort and reassurance to individuals and ultimately provide them with a sense of empowerment and safety. Despite the profound psychological effect that mass casualty incidents may have on affected populations, simple and thoughtful interventions can often limit and ultimately reverse psychiatric symptoms. PFA is considered the intervention of choice in the immediate aftermath of a disaster. More than 50% of American Red Cross volunteers in the United States are trained in PFA.

Basic strategies to reduce psychological distress include orientation to disaster and recovery efforts, reduction of physiologic arousal, mobilization of support for those who are most distressed, facilitation of reunion with loved ones and keeping families together, providing education about available resources and coping strategies, and using effective risk communication techniques. Key components of this therapeutic stratagem include the following:

➤ Protecting affected people from any further actual or perceived harm; assurance needs to be provided so people feel they are no longer alone and that others will be available to provide support and assistance.

➤ Caring for basic survival needs such as food, shelter, and clothing; this includes providing people with a safe and quiet environment that fosters a sense of physical and emotional safety.

➤ Supporting reality-based practical tasks; often helping individuals develop step-by-step action plans to deal with the physical crisis at hand will help them develop a sense of empowerment and safety, and allowing them to collaborate with caregivers furthers this effort.

➤ Validating people's feelings and thoughts by supportive listening.

➤ Normalizing stress reactions and containing agitation and arousal by informing people that their emotional reactions are normal and are to be anticipated; this includes educating people that these reactions will often resolve by themselves in a short time.

➤ Reinforcing coping skills by discussing with people how they responded to stressful situations in the past and helping them to recruit emotional resources to deal with the current situation.

➤ Keeping families together and providing social support as available.

➤ Being aware of the effect that the incident may have on the entire family.

➤ Providing information and education in a calm, supportive, and honest manner.

➤ Orienting and referring people to other available support services.

3.8.4.3 Outreach and Information Dissemination

After disasters and public health emergences, opportunities will be provided in many venues for survivors and other affected people to come together to heal emotionally. Established community structures and communications vehicles will be utilized to provide information and support. Public health officials will take important steps to promote postcrisis recovery for all affected persons. This can be accomplished by:

> **Psychological First Aid**
>
> PFA is an intervention tool, not treatment. To the trained volunteer, the PFA process may indicate individuals who require further evaluation and treatment by mental health professionals.

➤ Providing memorials and opportunities to grieve

➤ Celebrating heroes and acknowledging survivors and fatalities

➤ Recognizing anniversaries of the event

➤ Creating opportunities for engaging all affected individuals and populations in the physical and emotional healing process

➤ Improving local preparedness for future disasters

Some of the best resources for helping the community recover from a traumatic event are local organizations and institutions in the community, including the American Red Cross, the faith community, social service organizations, and schools. These types of local organizations can reach all populations in the community, including those that are most vulnerable to trauma.

3.8.4.4 Technical Assistance, Consultation, and Training

Organizations, leaders, responders, and caregivers will be supported via dissemination of knowledge, consultation, and training, so that they can improve their capacity to support the reestablishment of community structure, foster personal and community recovery and resilience, and safeguard community health. Under federal emergency support function (ESF) 8, the Department of Health and Human Services (HHS) is designated as the lead agency for provision of health and medical services supplementing state and local resources. The Substance Abuse and Mental Health Services Administration has responsibility for mental health care under federal ESF 8, including assistance in assessment of mental health needs, provision of disaster mental health training materials, and coordinating local, state, and federal mental health response programs.

3.8.4.5 Treatment

Pharmacologic treatment: When a person's psychological symptoms appear severe, unremitting, and unresponsive to applied medical and psychological first aid, medical and psychiatric professionals must be consulted to provide further care. The use of medications to manage psychiatric symptoms in the acute setting can be effective and appropriate. Prescribed medications should be limited to a few days' supply, and appropriate follow-up must be arranged. For anxiety, short courses of benzodiazepine anxiolytics should be considered. For persistent or severe insomnia, hypnotics can be prescribed. Antipsychotics should be reserved for extreme agitation or cognitive disorganization and administered only in a controlled setting if available. Antidepressants are not appropriate for the acute setting. The World Health Organization (WHO) advises that medications used should be available at the local level, especially if they are to be continued under the supervision of trained health and mental health professionals.[54]

Crisis intervention: Crisis intervention refers to a more sophisticated level of mental health intervention. While all affected individuals will experience a variety of emotional responses to a critical incident, most will resolve spontaneously in a short period of time or with just supportive PFA. For individuals whose symptomatology is more complex, persistent, and pervasive, it is important for caregivers to assess the person's potential for self-harm or harm to others. Caregivers should recruit the assistance of others including security, emergency medicine, and psychiatric health providers as needed and as available.

Critical incident stress debriefing: This modality is no longer recommended, because research does not demonstrate any consistent benefit, while it potentially causes psychological harm in some individuals.[44,55-60] Controlled studies do not support the use of group critical incident stress debriefing as a therapeutic intervention for treatment of acute stress disorder or for the prevention of PTSD.

3.8.4.6 Implications for the Emergency Response Workforce

Emergency responders are susceptible to the same psychological reactions as other people. Although some might have more conditioning to traumatic events, the exposure to mass trauma may exceed past experiences, especially when responders become casualties. Of particular concern are acute and posttraumatic stress disorders. To address the psychosocial needs of deployed personnel, emergency response organizations sponsor group meetings in the immediate period after a disaster to provide opportunities for responders to tell their stories, which is a part of personal PFA for maintaining healthy behavior. Talking with others who have experienced similar events helps the healing process.

Responders should be monitored for dissociative symptoms of acute stress disorder as well as for impairment of functioning. Responders who exhibit such symptoms and impaired functioning should be referred for psychiatric care by professionals trained in cognitive-behavioral and pharmacologic therapies. While operational "debriefing" sessions might afford an opportunity for identifying such individuals, supervisors must also be trained to recognize those colleagues in distress. Implementation of these principles requires that an occupational health component of psychosocial response planning be focused on the needs of responders. This cannot be left to volunteers, who are not mental health professionals, no matter how well-intentioned or empathic.

Because responders may experience a wide range of stress reactions, emergency response organizations often provide predeployment training on stress management, such as PFA. The training helps responders recognize common reactions, identify stress-related symptoms, and implement coping skills.

3.8.5 Mental Health Considerations for Children and Adolescents

Children compose a special subset of the population affected by traumatic events. The psychological effects of a disaster can be attributed to the nature of the disaster itself, the level of exposure to the event (direct, indirect), the extent to which children and those around them are affected personally, and individual characteristics of each child. Children also are affected not only by their own reaction to the trauma of the event but by the emotions and behaviors exhibited by parents and others. Because children depend on adults for their emotional and psychological needs, any effects of trauma on adults can exacerbate the psychological effect on children or first be appreciated in the child's behavior.

Responders must be aware that children will not exhibit the same behaviors as adults in response to the event and often will not be capable of verbally expressing their emotions.[61] Behaviors indicative of the potential need to intervene include regressive behaviors such as whining, clinging, fighting, irritability, feeding problems, and bedtime and sleep problems. Other children may exhibit their emotional pain by attempting to be excessively good or compliant.

➤ The response of younger children is characterized by changes in mood and behavior and by anxiety. Younger children may exhibit regressive behaviors, increased temper tantrums, and symptoms of clinginess and difficulty with separation or sleep. Even infants whose lives have been disrupted by a disaster manifest symptoms of crying and irritability, separation anxiety, and a hyperactive startle response.

➤ School-age children may exhibit depression, anger, and despair. Their anxiety may be exacerbated by unrealistic fears for parents, families, and friends. They also may develop problems at school or somatization symptoms, typically with complaints of headache or abdominal pain.

➤ Adolescents differ from adults in their psychological response because they are in a period of development characterized by complex physical, psychological, and social transitions. They are especially vulnerable to the development of major psychiatric disorders such as depression. Of significant importance is the likelihood of engaging in risk-taking behaviors such as drug abuse or sexual relationships. Adolescents also are particularly vulnerable to impulsive behaviors including drug or alcohol use and suicide. In addition, adolescents may try to hide their feelings or symptoms for fear of being perceived as abnormal. It is imperative that these symptoms not be minimized or overlooked because adjustment reactions left unrecognized and untreated can lead to lifelong behavioral and emotional problems.

Responders should not be afraid to talk to children in a clear, honest, empathic, and accurate manner, allowing the child to take the lead in the discussion. Children should not be coerced to talk but should be allowed to talk about their feelings. It may be prudent to limit the child's exposure to repeated media coverage of the event. As soon as possible, children should be provided access to and encouraged to participate in normal activities such as play and school. Assisting parents in their emotional responses to the event will often help their children adjust in a healthy fashion. A child's developmental stage characterizes his or her response to a disaster and is responsible for the wide degree of variability in adjustment to traumatic events. This means that therapeutic interventions should be developmentally appropriate.

3.9 SUMMARY

While the health system seeks to prevent and control injuries and disease in all populations affected by a disaster, particular attention is directed to those with functional and access needs. Such populations include, those who are physically or mentally disabled (blind, deaf, hard-of-hearing, or having cognitive disorders or mobility limitations), those with limited English language skills or who are non–English speaking, those who are geographically or culturally isolated, those who are medically or chemically dependent, the homeless, the frail elderly, pregnant women, and children.

In a disaster or public health emergency, traditional response and recovery operations may not be able to meet all the resulting human needs, in either the short or long term. Addressing the great diversity of special health concerns, language and cultural barriers, and other life circumstances presents multiple challenges for disaster response and recovery systems. People with functional and access needs must be identified and have valid emergency care plans in place, including plans for managing day-to-day problems related to the specific illness or disability, as well as plans for managing health-related needs in the event of a disaster or public health emergency.

Postdisaster mental and behavioral problems can affect all ages and populations, including disaster response personnel. Problems can be wide-ranging, from mild stress responses to more serious PTSD and major depression. Although acute stress disorder and PTSD receive the most publicity after disasters, the majority of affected persons, including those referred to as the "well but worried," have somatic symptoms below the threshold of a diagnosable psychiatric disorder. Ideally, all affected populations will be supported by a coordinated system of family and community health resources, as well as local primary care and psychological services.

REFERENCES

1. Ralston M, Hazinski MF, Zaritsky AL, Schexnayder SM, Kleinman ME, eds. *Pediatric Advanced Life Support—PALS Provider Manual.* Dallas, TX: American Heart Association; 2006.

2. Dieckmann RA, ed. *Pediatric Education for Prehospital Professionals.* 2nd edition. Elk Grove Village, IL: American Academy of Pediatrics; 2006.

3. Gausche-Hill M, Fuchs S, Yamamoto L, eds. *APLS—The Pediatric Emergency Medicine Resource.* 4th ed. Elk Grove Village, IL, and Dallas, TX: American Academy of Pediatrics and American College of Emergency Physicians; 2004 (revised 2006).

4. Emergency Nurses Association. *ENPC—Emergency Nursing Pediatric Course Provider Manual,* 3rd ed. Des Plaines, IL: Emergency Nurses Association; 2004.

5. Mejia R, Fields A, Greenwald BM, Stein F, eds. *Pediatric Fundamental Critical Care Support— PFCCS.* Mount Prospect, IL: Society of Critical Care Medicine; 2008.

6. Salomone JP, Pons PT, McSwain NE, eds. *PHTLS—Prehospital Trauma Life Support.* 6th ed. St Louis, MO: Mosby Elsevier; 2007.

7. American College of Surgeons Committee on Trauma. *Advanced Trauma Life Support® for Doctors (ATLS®) Student Course Manual.* 8th ed. Chicago, IL: American College of Surgeons; 2008.

8. Society of Trauma Nurses. *ATCN®—Advanced Trauma Care for Nurses®.* 2008 ed. Lexington, KY: Society of Trauma Nurses; 2008.

9. Emergency Nurses Association. *Trauma Nursing Core Course: Provider Manual.* 6th ed. Des Plaines, IL: Emergency Nurses Association; 2007.

10. Foltin GL, Schonfeld DJ, Shannon MW, eds. *Pediatric Terrorism and Disaster Preparedness: A Resource for Pediatricians.* AHRQ publication 06(07)-0056. Rockville, MD: AHRQ; October 2006. http://www.ahrq.gov/research/pedprep/. Accessed April 11, 2011.

11. Foltin G, Tunik M, Treiber M, Cooper A, eds. *Pediatric Disaster Preparedness: A Resource for Planning, Management, and Provision of Out-of-Hospital Emergency Care.* Washington, DC: EMSC National Resource Center; 2008. http://www.cpem.org. Accessed April 11, 2011.

12. Pediatric Task Force, Centers for Bioterrorism Preparedness Planning, New York City Department of Health and Mental Hygiene; Arquilla B, Foltin G, Uraneck K, eds. *Children in Disasters: Hospital Guidelines for Pediatrics in Disasters.* 3rd ed. New York, NY: New York City Department of Health and Mental Hygiene; 2008. http://www.nyc.gov/html/doh/downloads/pdf// bhpp/hepp-peds-childrenindisasters-010709.pdf. Accessed April 11, 2011.

13. *Pediatric Tabletop Exercise Toolkit for Hospitals;* 2nd ed. New York, NY: New York City Department of Health and Mental Hygiene; 2008. http://www.nyc.gov/html/doh/downloads/word/ bhpp/hepp-peds-tabletoptoolkit-010709.doc. Accessed April 11, 2011.

14. Garrett AL, Redlener I, eds. *Pediatric Emergency Preparedness for Natural Disasters, Terrorism, and Public Health Emergencies: National Consensus Conference, 2009 Update.* New York, NY: Columbia University Mailman School of Public Health National Center for Disaster Preparedness; 2009. http://www.ncdp.mailman.columbia.edu/files/peds_consensus.pdf. Accessed April 11, 2011.

15. The Sphere Project. *The Sphere Project: Humanitarian Charter and Minimum Standards for Disaster Response.* Geneva, Switzerland: The Sphere Project, 2011. http://www.sphereproject.org/. Accessed April 11, 2011.

16. Pape JW, Rouzier V, Ford H, Joseph P, Warren WD, Fitzgerald DW. The GHESKIO field hospital and clinics after the earthquake in Haiti: Dispatch 3 from Port-au-Prince. *NEJM.* 2010;362:e34.

17. Black K, Barnett P, Wolfe R, Young S. Are methods used to estimate weight in children accurate? *Emerg Med.* 2002;14:160-165.

18. Foltin G, Tunik M, Curran J, et al. Pediatric nerve agent poisoning: medical and operational considerations for emergency medical services in a large American city. *Pediatr Emerg Care.* 2006;22:239-244.

19. American College of Surgeons Committee on Trauma, American College of Emergency Physicians, National Association of EMS Physicians, Pediatric Equipment Guidelines Committee- Emergency Medical Services for Children (EMSC) Partnership for Children Stakeholder Group, American Academy of Pediatrics. Policy statement—equipment for ambulances. *Pediatrics.*

2009;124:e166-e171. http://aappolicy.aappublications.org/cgi/reprint/pediatrics;124/1/e166.pdf. Accessed April 11, 2011.

20. American Academy of Pediatrics Committee on Pediatric Emergency Medicine, American College of Emergency Physicians Pediatric Committee, Emergency Nurses Association Pediatric Committee. Joint policy statement—guidelines for care of children in the emergency department. Pediatrics. 2009;124:1233–1243. http://aappolicy.aappublications.org/cgi/reprint/pediatrics;124/4/1233.pdf. Accessed April 11, 2011.

21. Federal Emergency Management Agency (FEMA), Office for Civil Rights and Civil Liberties, Department of Homeland Security. *Interim Emergency Management Planning Guide for Special Needs Populations*. Comprehensive Preparedness Guide (CPG) 301. Version 1.0. Washington, DC: FEMA; 2008. http://serve.mt.gov/wp-content/uploads/2010/10/CPG-301.pdf. Accessed April 7, 2011.

22. Federal Emergency Management Agency (FEMA). *Guidance on Planning for Integration of Functional Needs Support Services in General Population Shelters*. Washington, DC: FEMA; 2010. http://www.fema.gov/pdf/about/odic/fnss_guidance.pdf. Accessed April 7, 2011.

23. Curtis T, Miller BC, Berry EH. Changes in reports and incidence of child abuse following natural disasters. *Child Abuse Neglect*. 2000;24:1151-1162.

24. Stone A. *Preventing Child Abuse and Neglect in Disaster Emergency Shelters*. PowerPoint Presentation, Participant Handbook, and Trainer's Guide. Albuquerque, NM: National Resource Center for Child Protective Services, 2006. http://www.nrccps.org/documents/2006/ppt/Shelter_Preventing_Child_Abuse___Neglect_final_Nov_2006.ppt. http://www.nrccps.org/documents/2006/pdf/Shelter_Participant_Handboo_final_Mar_2007.pdf; and http://www.nrccps.org/documents/2006/pdf/s_Guide_fina_Nov_2006.pdf. Accessed April 11, 2011.

25. *Gender, Women, and Health: Gender and Disaster*. World Health Organization Regional Office for Southeast Asia; January 2009. http://www.searo.who.int/en/Section13/Section390_8282.htm. Accessed April 11, 2011.

26. *Gender and Natural Disasters*. Pan America Health Organization, Regional Office of the World Health Organization. http://www.paho.org/english/dpm/gpp/gh/genderdisasters.PDF. Accessed April 11, 2011.

27. *Violence and Disasters*. Geneva, Switzerland: World Health Organization Department of Injuries and Violence Prevention; 2005. http://www.who.int/violence_injury_prevention/publications/violence/violence_disasters.pdf. Accessed April 7, 2011.

28. *Gender and Health in Disasters*. Geneva, Switzerland: World Health Organization Department of Gender and Women's Health; 2002. http://www.who.int/gender/other_health/en/genderdisasters.pdf. Accessed April 11, 2001.

29. Weist R, Mocellin J, Motsisi DT. *The Needs of Women in Disasters and Emergencies*. Winnepeg, Manitoba, Canada: University of Manitoba Disaster Research Institute; 2001. http://www.radixonline.org/resources/women-in-disaster-emergency.pdf. Accessed April 11, 2011.

30. Aldrich N, Benson WF. Disaster preparedness and the chronic disease needs of vulnerable older adults. *Prev Chronic Dis* [serial online]. 2008;5:1–7. http://www.cdc.gov/pcd/issues/2008/jan/07_0135.htm. Accessed April 7, 2011.

31. Mokdad AH, Mensah GA, Posner SF, Reed E, Simoes EJ, Engelgau MM; Chronic Diseases and Vulnerable Populations in Natural Disasters Working Group. When chronic conditions become acute: prevention and control of chronic diseases and adverse health outcomes during natural disasters. *Prev Chronic Dis*. 2005;2:special issue. http://www.cdc.gov/pcd/issues/2005/nov/pdf/05_0201.pdf. Accessed April 7, 2011.

32. Miller C, Arquilla B. Chronic diseases and natural hazards: impact of disasters on diabetic, renal, and cardiac patients. *Prehosp Disaster Med*. 2008;23:185–194. http://pdm.medicine.wisc.edu/Volume_23/issue_2/miller.pdf. Accessed April 11, 2011.

33. Greenough GP, Lappi MD, Hsu EB, et al. Burden of disease and health status among Hurricane-Katrina-displaced persons in shelters: a population-based cluster sample. *Ann Emerg Med*. 2008;51:426-432.

34. Tam VC, Knowles SR, Cornish PL, Fine N, Marchesano R, Etchells EE. Frequency, type and clinical importance of medical history errors at admission to hospital: a systemic review. *CMAJ.* 2005;173:510-515.

35. Brodie M, Weltzien E, Altman D, Blendon RJ, Benson JM. Experiences of Hurricane Katrina evacuees in Houston shelters: implications for future planning. *Am J Public Health.* 2006;96:1402-1408.

36. Hurricane Katrina Community Advisory Group, Kessler RC. Hurricane Katrina's impact on the care of survivors with chronic medical conditions. *J Gen Intern Med.* 2007;22:1225-1230.

37. Arrieta MI, Foreman RD, Crook ED, Icenogle ML. Providing continuity of care for chronic disease in the aftermath of Katrina: from field experience to policy recommendations. *Disaster Med Public Health Prep.* 2009;3:174-182.

38. National Organization on Disability. *Functional Needs of People With Disabilities: A Guide for Emergency Managers, Planners, and Responders.* Washington, DC: National Organization on Disability; 2009. http://nod.org/assets/downloads/Guide-Emergency-Planners.pdf. Accessed April 7, 2011.

39. Butler A, Panzer A, Goldfrank L, eds. *Preparing for the Psychological Consequences of Terrorism: A Public Health Strategy.* Washington, DC: National Academies Press; 2003.

40. Inter-Agency Standing Committee (IASC) Reference Group for Mental Health and Psychosocial Support in Emergency Settings. *Mental Health and Psychosocial Support in Humanitarian Emergencies: What Should Humanitarian Health Actors Know?* Geneva, Switzerland: IASC; 2010. http://www.who.int/mental_health/emergencies/what_humanitarian_ health_actors_should_know.pdf. Accessed April 11, 2011.

41. World Health Organization and World Organization of Family Doctors (WONCA). *Integrating Mental Health Into Primary Care: A Global Perspective.* Geneva, Switzerland: WHO Press; 2008. http://www.who.int/mental_health/policy/Mental%20health%20+%20primary%20care-%20final%20 low-res%20140908.pdf. Accessed April 11, 2011.

42. Burkle FM, Chatterjee P, Bass J, Bolton P. Guidelines for the psycho-social and mental health assessment and management of displaced populations in humanitarian crises. In: *The Johns Hopkins and Red Cross Red Crescent Public Health Guide in Emergencies.* 2nd ed. Geneva, Switzerland: International Federation of Red Cross and Red Crescent Societies; 2008. http://www. jhsph.edu/bin/s/c/Forward.pdf. Accessed April 11, 2011.

43. Inter-Agency Standing Committee (IASC). *IASC Guidelines on Mental Health and Psychosocial Support in Emergency Settings.* Geneva, Switzerland: IASC; 2007. http://www .who.int/mental_health/emergencies/guidelines_iasc_mental_health_psychosocial_june_2007.pdf. Accessed April 11, 2010.

44. National Institute of Mental Health. Mental Health and Mass Violence: Evidence-Based Early Psychological Intervention for Victims/Survivors of Mass Violence. A Workshop to Reach Consensus on Best Practices. NIH publication 02-5138. Washington, DC: National Institute of Mental Health; 2002. http://www.nimh.nih.gov/health/publications/massviolence.pdf Accessed April 11, 2011.

45. Burkle FM Jr, Bass J, Bolton P. Becoming responsible in a "socially seismic" environment: mental health as a marker of community recovery. *Disaster Med Public Health Prep.* 2008;2:73-74.

46. Montano CB. Recognition of depression in a primary care setting. *J Clin Psychiatry.* 1994;55(1 suppl):18-34.

47. Safran MA, Chorba T, Schreber M, Archer WR, Cookson ST. Concepts in disaster medicine: evaluating mental health after the 2010 Haitian earthquake. *Disaster Med Public Health Prep.* 2011;5:154-157. http://www.dmphp.org/cgi/content/abstract/dmp.2011.31v1. Accessed April 11, 2011.

48. National Association of School Psychologists (NASP). *Helping Students Cope with the Haitian Earthquake: Guidance for School Mental Health Professionals.* Washington, DC: NASP; 2010. http://www.nasponline.org/resources/crisis_safety/Supporting_Students_Affected_by_Haitian_ Earthquake_School_Mental_Health_ProfessionalsFINAL.pdf.

49. Stige SH, Sveaass N. Living in exile when disaster strikes at home. *Torture*. 2010;20:76–91.

50. Everly GS, Jr., Flynn BW. Principles and practical procedures for acute psychological first aid training for personnel without mental health experience. *International J Emerg Mental Health*. 2006;8:93-100.

51. Parker CL, Everly GS, Jr., Barnett DJ, Links JM. Establishing evidence-informed core intervention competencies in psychological first aid for public health personnel. *International J Emerg Mental Health*. 2006;8:83-92.

52. American Red Cross. *Psychological First Aid: Helping People in Times of Stress*. Washington, DC: American Red Cross; 2006.

53. Brymer M, Jacobs A, Layne C, et al. *Psychological First Aid: Field Operations Guide*. 2nd edition. Los Angeles: National Child Traumatic Stress Network, National Center for PTSD; 2006.

54. van Ommeren M, Barbui C, de Jong K, et al. If you could only choose five psychotropic medicines: updating the interagency emergency health kit. *PLoS Med*. 2011;8:e1001030. http://www.plosmedicine.org/article/info:doi/10.1371/journal.pmed.1001030. Accessed April 11, 2011.

55. Litz BT, Gray MJ, Bryant RA, Adler AB. Early intervention for trauma: current status and future directions. *Clinical Psychology: Science and Practice*. 2002;9:112-34.

56. McNally R, Bryant R, Ehlers A. Does early psychological intervention promote recovery from posttraumatic stress? *Psychological Science in the Public Interest*. 2003;4:45-79.

57. Bisson, JI. Single-session early psychological interventions following traumatic events. *Clin Psychol Rev*. 2003;23:481-499.

58. Bisson JI, Shepherd JP, Joy D, Probert R, Newcombe RC. Early cognitive-behavioral therapy for post-traumatic stress symptoms after physical injury. Randomized controlled trial. *Br J Psychiatry*. 2004;184:63-69.

59. National Disaster Mental Health Work Group. Appendix B: position statement and guidance for MRC units on psychological debriefing. In: *Psychological First Aid Field Operations Guide*. 2nd edition. Medical Reserve Corps, National Child Traumatic Stress Network, National Center for PTSD. 2006. http://www.medicalreservecorps.gov/file/mrc_resources/MRC_PFA.doc. Accessed April 11.

60. National Center for PTSD. *Types of Debriefing Following Disasters*. Washington, DC: National Center for PTSD; 2010. http://www.ptsd.va.gov/professional/pages/debriefing-after-disasters.asp. Accessed April 11, 2011.

61. American Academy of Pediatrics. Psychosocial implications of disaster or terrorism on children: a guide for pediatricians. *Pediatrics*. 2005;116:787-795.

CHAPTER FOUR

Workforce Readiness and Disaster Deployment

CHAPTER CHAIR

Jim Lyznicki, MS, MPH

CONTRIBUTING AUTHORS

Sandra Vyhlidal, MSN, RN

Allen Cherson, DO

Michael J. Reilly, DrPH, MPH

Raymond E. Swienton, MD

4.1 PURPOSE

This chapter provides an overview of personal preparedness and protection issues that health professionals and others should consider when deciding to engage directly in disaster response and relief operations. Important issues include the need for pre-event preparation and planning, ongoing disaster education and training, and knowledge of risk reduction and coping strategies to protect personal health, safety, and well-being.

4.2 LEARNING OBJECTIVES

After completing this chapter, readers should be able to:

➤ Discuss predeployment considerations for participation in disaster response, including team activation and mobilization, risk awareness and mitigation, education, training, and personal fitness for duty.

➤ Describe workforce protection measures in a disaster, including the purpose and types of personal protective equipment and decontamination.

Learning objectives for this chapter are competency-based, as delineated in Appendix B.

4.3 BACKGROUND

The process of systematically activating and mobilizing reserved resources into action is known as *deployment*. Deployment is a means of responding to an overwhelming influx of people in need with quick-responding, trained, and competent professionals, paraprofessionals, and support staff during an emergency or disaster. Along with staffing, deployment also involves the distribution of needed equipment and supplies.

In a disaster, health professionals and other personnel must recognize and appreciate the potential risks and disruptions that are part of disaster operations. Disaster response and recovery operations can be physically and emotionally challenging. Hours can be long, under difficult work conditions. Burnout can come easily if careful attention is not given to pacing oneself, having sufficient time to relax, and minimizing stress. In addition to possessing specific knowledge and skills related to disaster management, responders must possess the fitness to respond and the ability to maintain that fitness once deployed. Sleeping, eating, personal time, and recreation patterns will likely be erratic and affect job performance. Persons may experience stress related to protecting their own safety and well-being, as well as that of others. Additional stress may be related to the care of casualties, the management of mass fatalities, concern for the safety of family members and other loved ones, and unique situational restrictions and limitations encountered at the disaster scene.

Prevention, preparedness, and wellness strategies are essential to help all potential responders develop the strength, resilience, and coping skills to deal with disaster-related health challenges. Much has been learned about the importance of protective factors as simple as immunizations, exercise, good nutrition, adequate rest, healthy human interactions, and support from peers. Personal disaster planning and training can help build resilience by empowering people to deal with serious health emergencies. Personal preparedness for disasters and public health emergencies is covered in greater detail in the Core Disaster Life Support® (CDLS®) course (v3.0) and supporting course manual.

4.4 PREDEPLOYMENT PREPARATION AND PLANNING

All responders have a responsibility to be prepared to perform their duties and to assess whether they are healthy enough to respond effectively. Depending on the event, there may be a large number of serious casualties, who may require ful conditions. Responders must decide whether they can perform their assigned role in less than optimal circumstances and environments. Response personnel who are under medical care for acute and chronic problems should discuss their conditions with a physician or other health professional in advance of any disaster deployment.

Predeployment Questions to Consider

Potential responders should consider the following questions before seeking or accepting a deployment offer:

➤ Can you find extended care for dependent family members (children and adults)?

➤ Can your employer afford your absence?

➤ Do you have any physical limitations that may impair your performance in a particular environment? For example, if you have difficulty ambulating, you may wish to be somewhat discriminating in volunteering for a deployment that will entail considerable movement over uneven terrain, or working in a field facility.

➤ Have you recently had surgery, or have a temporary medical condition that will impair your ability to be deployed or perform your duties at a particular deployment site?

➤ Are you taking prescribed medication that may hamper your abilities to perform your duties in a deployment environment?

➤ If your prescribed medications do not affect your duties, do you have sufficient medications to last for your total deployment?

➤ Are you aware of any issue that may prevent completion of your deployment?

➤ Are you able to share a sleeping environment/room with three or more associates?

➤ Do you have special dietary requirements?

➤ If required, can you work 12-hour or greater shifts for several days?

➤ Are there special requirements at home that need your attention?

➤ Are there seriously ill relatives in the immediate family?

➤ Do you have a plan outlining the way your personal family affairs will be handled during your absence?

4.4.1 Volunteerism and Team Membership

In a disaster or public health emergency, people of all ages and backgrounds will volunteer their services to help people in need. In 2009, more than 63 million Americans volunteered to help communities with an estimated dollar value contribution of nearly $169 billion; this was the largest single-year increase in volunteer numbers since 2003. This increase was led by women between the ages of 45 and 54 years, married individuals, those employed (especially full-time workers), and individuals with high school diplomas or college degrees.[1]

Following recent disasters and terrorist events, considerable national effort has been devoted to increasing the number of volunteer health professionals who are ready, willing, and able to assist in response efforts. Several organized response systems have been developed to provide emergency response teams. Examples include Disaster Medical Assistance Teams (DMATs), the Medical Reserve Corps, and the American Red Cross and numerous other nongovernmental relief organizations (eg, Doctors Without Borders, Project Hope). Individuals who are interested in becoming members of an organized volunteer disaster team must plan ahead to get the requisite education, training, and clearances to participate in response operations.

The Emergency System for Advance Registration of Volunteer Health Professionals

The Emergency System for Advance Registration of Volunteer Health Professionals (ESAR-VHP) is a federal program to support the establishment of state-based processes for the preregistration of volunteer health professionals who can serve at a moment's notice (within their state or across state lines) to provide needed help during a disaster or public health emergency. By registering through this program, a volunteer's identity, license, credentials, accreditation, and hospital privileges are verified in advance, saving valuable time in emergency response operations. Formerly under the Health Resources and Services Administration, ESAR-VHP is now administered by the Department of Health and Human Services (HHS) Office of the Assistant Secretary for Preparedness and Response (ASPR). The ASPR assists each state and territory in establishing a standardized volunteer registration program.

More information about ESAR-VHP is available at http://www.phe.gov/esarvhp/pages/about.aspx.

Occasionally, individuals may self-deploy spontaneously with no affiliation to any responding organization. Such action may add confusion to an already chaotic situation, as well as put these individuals at risk for becoming casualties themselves. These independent people are often underutilized or even turned away because of the lengthy process of assignment approval. Advance membership in a disaster team allows the deploying organization to verify professional credentials, complete personal background checks, and assess individual competencies and skills before a disaster occurs. Members are also provided disaster training related to preparedness, response, and recovery. This training facilitates better matching of skills with work assignments. All these activities speed the process of activation, deployment, and demobilization (returning from assignment). It also enhances volunteer satisfaction as well as success of the mission.

4.4.2 Maintaining Deployment Readiness Status

Prior to deployment, responders must ensure that personal matters are attended to while they are away and that they have made arrangements for the needs of their families and others who rely on them for financial and/or emotional support. It is essential that responders carefully address their own individual situations. This involves taking a close look at personal responsibilities, financial obligations, schooling, ongoing special projects, and clinical workloads that may be adversely affected by a prolonged absence. Employed volunteers should have an agreement with employers on how their sudden absence from the job will be accommodated. Topics to be discussed include (1) approval for 24- to 48-hour leave notification, (2) "backfill" for managing workload during the leave time frame, and (3) agreement on pay (eg, receiving regular pay, using paid time off, or receiving no pay). These issues should be given careful consideration before accepting or volunteering for a deployment.

The disaster responder needs a system in place to take care of personal affairs. Planning should include making arrangements for paying monthly bills and caring for young or elderly relatives, arranging alternative delivery methods for mail and newspapers, arranging for care of pets, listing preferred repairmen, listing credit card numbers with associated contact numbers, canceling or rescheduling business and personal appointments, making sets of house and car keys available to others, showing someone the location of utility (water/gas/electricity) shutoff valves, providing copies of driver's license and passport to trusted individuals, and notifying family and friends of deployment dates. Responders should have a plan for communicating with others during the deployment period. This includes notifying friends and family of the preferred means and modes of communication, such as mobile telephone, e-mail, or other methods. A list of e-mail addresses, telephone numbers, and postal addresses should be in the possession of the volunteer at the time of deployment. If dependent children or adults are involved, disaster volunteers must clarify how their activities and commitments will be maintained during their absence.

Predeployment Planning Considerations

In a major catastrophe, responders should prepare to be self-sufficient and live under potentially austere conditions, with minimal resources and support infrastructure. Careful consideration should be given to the following:

➤ There will be a general lack of privacy and little opportunity for recreation during nonduty hours.

➤ Lodging arrangements could be tents or hastily constructed buildings.

➤ Showers, if available, could be communal or even more rustic.

➤ Opportunities to communicate may be limited initially. Cellular telephones and computers may not be operable.

➤ Receipt of mail or packages via expedited postal or other services may not be possible or be delayed.

➤ Laundry services may be severely limited.

(continued)

> ➤ Religious services and assistance may be limited to nondenominational chaplains.

> ➤ Local health facilities may be damaged severely with shortages of medical supplies, requiring responder to carry a first aid kit for his or her own protection.

> ➤ Sufficient food should be packed for the length of stay.

> ➤ Personal protective equipment (PPE) that is appropriate for the anticipated environment should be packed. This includes preparation for endemic insects and animals.

Readiness for deployment also includes getting legal personal affairs in order. Several legal documents need to be addressed before deployment:

➤ The Power of Attorney for Health Care (POA-HC) is a written document that allows another competent adult (spouse, relative, good friend) the legal power to act on a person's behalf when that person is not able to make his or her own health care decisions.

➤ Supporting the POA-HC is the "Living Will" or "Declaration." In this document, the individual clarifies personal wishes about the treatment desired at the end of life when he or she is unable to give direction or make decisions. State statutes generally provide for the Living Will to take effect when the individual has a terminal condition or is in a persistent vegetative state. It is important that the Living Will be shared with the POA-HC representative because the POA-HC is obligated to follow the wishes expressed in the Living Will and must have an understanding of the wishes and intent.

➤ The Power of Attorney for Finance (POA-F) gives another the power to make financial transactions on behalf of an individual. Setting up a POA-F allows the designated person to conduct business in the name of the deployed, such as banking transactions and selling or buying property. The duration of authority can be temporary (eg, during deployment) or permanent. Some people do not realize there are two different POA documents, one for health care and one for finances. They are not the same.

➤ A will ensures that the estate is distributed according to the person's wishes after death. Without a will, the state makes those decisions and may impose a fee for representation. It is important to understand that, even if one has a will, state laws may override personal wishes. Therefore, it may be beneficial to work with a lawyer to develop this document.

Standard POA and will forms can be obtained from state legislative Web sites, state bar associations, hospital representatives, and some retail stores. Depending on state statutes, most documents can be activated by having the individual's signature notarized or witnessed by two non–family members. Using an attorney is always beneficial in assisting with clarifying state statutes and completing the appropriate forms.

With all these documents, it is important to keep original documents in a safe location, such as a safe deposit box. However, if copies of these documents are stored only in a safe deposit box, they will likely not be available when needed. Thus, it is imperative to provide copies of the POA-HC and the Living Will to the designated power of attorney, clergy, personal physicians, and/or hospital. It may also be desirable to provide the POA-F to designated bank officials.

4.4.3 Personal Health and Wellness

Responders must be positive assets to a team and should not disrupt the momentum of a team that is trying very hard to contribute to the favorable resolution of a catastrophic event. Individuals selected for a disaster assignment must be physically and emotionally capable of performing the duties for which they are selected. *Resilience* is the ability to quickly rebound and adapt to physical and psychological stress and is directly related to a person's physical and psychological health. One can become more resilient by adopting healthy lifestyle behaviors, with a focus on diet, exercise, sleep, and hygiene as essential for preventing injuries and disease and ensuring well-being. Becoming resilient involves taking steps to prevent and avoid predictable dangers to personal health and safety.

Chronic diseases such as heart disease, cancer, and diabetes are among the most common and costly medical and public health problems. Cardiovascular diseases such as heart disease and stroke are leading causes of death and disability and are associated with preventable risk factors, notably high blood pressure, high blood cholesterol levels, and obesity. Also included are behavioral and lifestyle risk factors such as unhealthy diets, physical inactivity, and tobacco use. Many other chronic diseases can be prevented or controlled through exercise and a healthy diet. Disease prevention involves:

➤ Eliminating or controlling personal risk factors;

➤ Recognizing early warning signs;

➤ Undergoing early detection screenings; and

➤ Guarding against potential risks in the environment.

Disaster volunteers are responsible for maintaining personal health before and during deployment. Before deployment, they should have a thorough physical examination and health assessment, with documentation of their current immunization status. Predeployment health screening should include assessment of both the type and dose of medications being taken. People with preexisting health conditions should consider wearing an alert bracelet and make sure this information is on a contact card in their wallet or travel documents. Planning measures include maintaining adequate sleep and nutrition, adequate personal medication supplies, and current immunizations.

Sleep: Most disaster workers average 5.4 hours of sleep during deployment and often work 12-hour shifts with no days off. To enhance sleep, workers should consider packing earplugs, blindfolds, favorite books, and/or headphones with favorite music. In addition, workers may be interested in using mental imaging, relaxation techniques, and establishing an exercise routine during deployment.[2]

Nutrition: Assuming the worst conditions, especially for the first few days of deployment, hydration with water is critical. An adequate supply of bottled water should be packed to sustain responder health. Nonperishable food items and nutritional snacks also should be considered. This includes high-protein, high-fiber bars with added vitamins and minerals; peanut butter; crackers; dried fruit; nuts; and other favorite snacks. Deployment is not the time to diet. It is important to maintain food intake for energy and stable health status.

Medications: Ensuring an adequate supply of personal medications requires planning. The disaster area is not the place to expect accommodations for personal medication prescription refills and over-the-counter medications. Responders should have at least an additional 2-week supply of medications on hand at all times. If the volunteer normally participates in a contracted pharmacy coverage plan, the volunteer may need to work collaboratively with the prescribing physician and coverage plan representatives to receive medications in advance. Over-the-counter remedies should include items the individual routinely uses or uses periodically.

Immunizations: Responders should be up to date on vaccines, as appropriate for their age and health condition.[3] Specific additional vaccinations may be necessary (eg, hepatitis A) depending on the area of deployment and conditions prevalent at the time of deployment.[4] Every disaster volunteer should discuss personal immunization status and recommended immunizations with a primary health care professional. Local and state public health departments provide immunization services at minimal cost.

4.4.4   Personal Equipment and Packing

Disaster volunteers must prepare for deployment by identifying essential basic supplies. First and foremost is having required personal identification readily available at all times (eg, driver's license, passport, photo identification from the disaster response organization, and current professional license). Clothing and other items need to match the weather conditions in the disaster area. Responders should monitor weather forecasts for the affected region. This can be done through the National Weather Service website (http://www.weather.gov) to determine current and projected weather conditions. Responders also should monitor other sites, such as Centers for Disease Control and Prevention (CDC; http://www.cdc.gov) and World Health Organization (WHO; http://www.who.int) for health guidance and alerts. When monitoring news reports, it is important to be aware that initial reports from an incident are often incomplete and based on limited information.

A prepacked bag or suitcase (ie, "go-kit") should be ready to take at a moment's notice.[5,6] It should not be assumed that an individual will remember to pack all essential items in the potentially hectic hours preceding deployment, nor can it be assumed that items can be purchased on arrival at an assigned destination. If it is not feasible to prepack personal items in a suitcase or bag, a packing list should be prepared. The following suggestions might be helpful.

➤ Pack light; volunteers need to carry their own luggage from place to place.

➤ Protect items from moisture and insects (eg, use plastic ziplock bags; package like items together).

➤ Use a suitcase or bag that can fit under a cot.

➤ Pack a "fanny pack" or money belt to contain personal identification papers, money, cellular phone, and contact phone numbers.

➤ Take a backpack to carry drinking water, food and snacks, PPE, hand hygiene products, personal medications, flashlight, and other essential supplies when in the field.

➤ Pack sturdy, practical, comfortable, protective shoes with extra socks (this is not the time to break in new shoes).

➤ Include professional equipment (eg, stethoscope).

➤ Standardize batteries, whenever possible, to reduce the need to carry multiple types.

4.4.5   Professional Credentials and Equipment

Success in meeting a disaster response request is based on volunteer readiness at short notice. To accomplish this, several steps can be taken before actual deployment. The volunteer should be personally prepared to provide documents that validate health care competencies. Such documents may include a professional state practice license and training verification (eg, completion of basic and advanced life support training), professional specialty certifications, and other relevant clinical competencies.[7]

Often the response organization will inform volunteers of recommended personal medical equipment or specialized tools to include with packing. Some organizations issue equipment to volunteers. Unless otherwise stated, the responder is responsible for properly using, caring for, and protecting any loaned equipment against damage. Responders should ensure that received equipment is functional before accepting it and should report any loss, theft, damage, destruction, or misuse of equipment to the assigned supervisor. When returning assigned equipment, the volunteer may be liable monetarily if negligent in performing, maintaining, and securing items. It is important that incident command (usually the logistics section chief) be aware of and updated on all equipment that is being taken or transported for field or deployment use. Equipment considerations include storage requirements, electrical support (battery vs. continuous power), up-to-date safety inspections, and compliance with transportation guidelines.

4.4.6   Predeployment Education and Training

As part of an organized team, volunteer responders need to complete education and training requirements prior to deployment. Once deployed, responders should be receptive to "just-in-time" training to acquire additional knowledge and skills specific to the assignment. Readiness training is available in various didactic and electronic formats through the Federal Emergency Management Agency (FEMA) Emergency Management Institute (http://training.fema.gov/), the National Disaster Life Support program (http://www.ndlsf.org), and other entities to help ensure that all levels of government, private-sector, and nongovernmental personnel know how to work together seamlessly to prepare for, respond to, and recover from the effects of any disaster event, regardless of type, size, or complexity. The level of training indicated for various response personnel depends on their expected roles and functions in a disaster and the likelihood that they will be involved with emergency operations.

In a mass casualty situation, multiple health professions and disciplines may be required to provide emergency care and assistance. In 2005, after Hurricane Katrina, local clinicians and hospitals were the sole source of medical care to the devastated region until the arrival of federal disaster medical assistance teams (DMATs) and were then integrated into the federal response. Knowledge of how to respond to disasters, and how to coordinate that response with other agencies and organizations involved, is essential.[8] It is also essential that health responders have some basic knowledge of the following:

➤ The National Incident Management System (NIMS), including its application to the planning, coordination, and execution of disaster responses

➤ The primary importance of safety in disaster response, including the use of PPE, decontamination, and scene security measures

➤ The need for resourcefulness when the usual medical supplies, personnel, communication, and transportation are not available

➤ Triage principles to maximize survival benefit when limited resources preclude comprehensive care for all of those affected

➤ Strategies to provide effective clinical and public health care in austere settings with limited resources; this includes the ability to adapt or modify skills, attitudes, and behaviors to save the most lives possible

➤ Physical and mental health needs of survivors, including persons with special needs; family and friends of the missing, injured, or dead; the "worried well"; and responders

➤ The importance of teamwork in disaster preparedness, response, and recovery, including the importance of good leadership and good followership during times of crisis

➤ The need to stay calm and keep one's wits when there is maximal chaos and confusion

In 2006, the NIMS Implementation Plan for Hospitals and Healthcare established a list of objectives that were deemed necessary for health care facilities to become NIMS compliant (and thus eligible for federal disaster preparedness funding). Key objectives included incorporation of NIMS components into existing health care facility disaster plans and the identification of appropriate staff for completion of the following independent study courses offered by FEMA:

➤ IS-100.HC: Introduction to the Incident Command System (ICS) for Healthcare/ Hospitals

➤ IS-200.HC: Applying ICS to Healthcare Organizations

➤ IS-700a: NIMS: An Introduction

➤ IS-800b: National Response Framework: An Introduction

The selection of courses is determined by a person's level of responsibility during an incident and the field of work (see http://www.fema.gov/emergency/nims/NIMSTrainingCourses).

4.4.7   Legal Issues for Volunteer Health Responders

Health professionals should be aware of challenges that exist in current government policies with regard to medical liability, standards of care, and license reciprocity to enable them to participate as volunteers in disaster response. Verification of a provider's license and credentials has legal implications both for health care volunteers and for hospitals using their services. Volunteers must consider their legal rights for reemployment after demobilization. A benefit of being deployed by the federal government is the guarantee of reemployment. Volunteers who decide independently and spontaneously to volunteer for a disaster cannot expect this reemployment right unless the employer agrees. Clarification of reemployment should be discussed before deployment. These issues are discussed in more detail in the CDLS® and Advanced Disaster Life Support™ (ADLS®) courses (v3.0) and supporting course manuals.

4.4.7.1   Professional Liability

The risk of civil and criminal liability during disasters is a primary concern of health responders. Health care professionals may be liable for negligent or intentional acts that cause harm to a patient. Immunity from civil liability may be available through:

➤ Governmental sovereign immunity (if the worker or volunteer is a government employee or agent)

➤ Federal and state volunteer protection acts

➤ Good Samaritan statutes

➤ State emergency health powers statutes

➤ Mutual aid compacts

The protections and regulations available to health care professionals vary greatly by state and often depend on the health care professional's method of deployment or status as a volunteer or employee. Legal and regulatory barriers and inconsistencies among states can make it difficult for health care professionals to practice during disasters. Unless a volunteer is deployed through the federal response system or state-approved Emergency Management Assistance Compacts (EMACs), licensure, liability protection, workers' compensation, and the right to reemployment may become issues.[5]

Most state licensing boards have developed quicker licensure recognition processes for disaster events. However, apprehension can arise in the state impacted by the disaster because of inability to function due to the effects of the disaster. Practicing without a license, even during an emergency, can expose an unlicensed individual to civil liability (in which one is held responsible for actions resulting in injuries or losses to others) or criminal changes. Some protection (ie, immunity or indemnification) from civil suits is provided by federal and some state laws for individuals in registries or members of disaster response organizations. It should be remembered that spontaneous, self-deploying responders who have no affiliation with any government or nonprofit organization are unlikely to receive liability protection or injury benefits and are strongly encouraged to join response organizations before a disaster.

While the commonly held Good Samaritan doctrine is designed to encourage people to stop and render aid to those in need, each state recognizes the duties and potential liabilities under this doctrine somewhat differently. It is important to note that, in most states, prior knowledge of an event (ie, being activated, being "dispatched," being told that there is help needed at a particular location) disallows the Good Samaritan laws or governing regulation protection for the response worker. This law may provide protection by providing immunity for liability for ordinary negligence in very defined circumstances and conditions. There is no immunity available for acts that may give rise to criminal liability. The level of protection may be limited depending on the specific state statute.

Some professionals carry liability insurance. It is important for those individuals to determine whether their insurance will cover practice during disasters. It is also critical to understand how such personal protection interacts with insurance provided by sponsoring organizations.

4.4.7.2   Scope of Practice

Disaster situations often involve mobilization of large numbers of health personnel from many states, raising questions about their legal scope of practice in jurisdictions where they are not licensed. While many states provide for licensure reciprocity, volunteer health professionals may not be authorized to provide services outside their scope of practice, even if similarly licensed practitioners in the states would be permitted to provide the services. Some states have amended health care practice acts permitting various health professions to define disaster response as normative within scopes of practice.

Every volunteer should know the limits of his or her position, authority, and expertise. Responders are expected to perform within their scope of practice and with the specific skills in which they were trained. If intubation was not within the scope of practice before deployment, then intubation is not an acceptable practice during deployment. It is important that clear guidance on operational guidelines and clinical policy and procedures be well defined. For example, when many different emergency medical services (EMS) crews from multiple agencies or regions are utilized, it is commonplace that each crew operates by the policy and procedures from its site of origin. Otherwise, the differences in training and education, skills performance, and equipment access would have to be overcome on a just-in-time basis, which raises patient safety and medical control oversight concerns.

Many states have adopted interstate mutual aid agreements, such as EMACs, which allow for volunteer health professionals licensed in one state to practice in another during a declared disaster. Similarly, the Uniform Emergency Volunteer Health

Practitioners Act provides licensure reciprocity for volunteer health professionals who are registered with systems (eg, ESAR-VHP) capable of confirming that persons are licensed and in good standing.[9]

4.5 PERSONAL RISK AWARENESS AND MITIGATION

In deployed environments, responders are at increased risk for injury and illness. To protect themselves, responders need to wear eye, hand, and face protection as appropriate and as directed by the incident command safety officer or his or her designee. This includes safety glasses or goggles, work boots, and leather gloves for physical labor; rubber or latex gloves for handling blood or body fluids; surgical masks; hard hat; earplugs; and N-95 respirators (or other respirator approved by the National Institute for Occupational Safety and Health [NIOSH] for those who are trained and fit-tested). Sandals and sneakers should not be worn. Hardhats should be worn if there is any danger of falling debris; life vests should be used for activities that could result in deep water exposure. Response personnel should drink plenty of fluids regardless of their assigned activity (and not wait until thirsty), avoid very cold drinks or drinks containing alcohol or high sugar content, wear appropriate clothing, and apply sunscreen.

If a responder is injured while deployed, appropriate incident reports need to be completed. All treatments and hospitalizations should be recorded carefully even if care is started in the field or deployed environment. It is strongly recommended that the injured responder also obtain copies of all supporting documentation. Coordination of care with the responder's regular primary care or specialty physicians is important as soon as possible or circumstances allow.

Field hygiene: Response personnel should clean their hands frequently. It is critical to mitigate contamination of the eyes, nose, and mouth, the key portals for pathogen entry. When water and soap are available, infectious and soiled material should be removed as frequently as possible. Waterless, alcohol-based sanitizers may be used when soap and water are not available and when hands are not visibly soiled. An adequate supply of alcohol-based hand sanitizer (carried in a fanny pack or field backpack) is essential. Responders should not be surprised if deployment base camps require hand hygiene before entering the mess tent.

Another hygiene practice that warrants attention is bathing. Responders should always use their own soap; liquid soap is preferred, as bar soap is difficult to air dry. In addition, shower shoes should be worn to protect feet from contact with infectious disease agents and other potential hazards.

Field shelters: Responders need to be aware of the sheltering facilities and conditions at the deployment site. Valuables should be locked in a suitcase or bag; important items should be carried in a fanny pack or money belt. To assist in providing a safe environment, responders should keep their cot or bed area clean and neat. Suitcases and bags should be placed under the cot or bed. Responders should be sensitive to other response personnel who are working different shifts. Some volunteers will be sleeping while others are working, so it is important to be mindful of noise levels.

Injury risks: The risk of injury during and after a disaster is high. Travel may be treacherous due to absent or damaged roads and difficult terrain (eg, mountains, deserts). Hazards such as electrocution from downed power lines and exposed wiring, and structural damage to buildings and roads, pose potential risks. Responders should assume all power lines are "hot" unless qualified personnel confirm otherwise. Other potential hazards include standing water from water system breaks, natural gas leaks, airborne smoke and dust, hazardous materials such as leaking fuels, and exposure to microbes from damaged sewer lines.

Insect bites and stings: Insect-borne diseases (eg, malaria, dengue) may be endemic in the area. Insect bites can be prevented by the following measures:

➤ Using insect repellent that contains one of the following active ingredients: DEET (*N,N*-diethyl-meta-toluamide), picaridin (KBR 3023), oil of lemon eucalyptus (active ingredient is *p*-menthane 3,8-diol or PMD), or IR3535 (3-[*N*-butyl-*N*-acetyl]-aminopropionic acid).

➤ Wearing lightweight long-sleeved shirts, long pants, and a hat outdoors. For greater protection, clothing also may be sprayed with repellent containing permethrin or another Environmental Protection Agency (EPA)–registered repellent (note: permethrin should not be used on skin.)

➤ Remaining indoors in a screened area or using insect repellent frequently on uncovered skin during the peak biting period for malaria (dusk and dawn) and dengue (any time of day).

➤ Sleeping in beds covered by a bed net (preferably treated with permethrin), if not sleeping in an air-conditioned or well-screened room.

➤ Spraying rooms with products effective against flying insects, such as products containing pyrethroids.

Animal bites: Direct contact with animals can spread diseases like rabies or cause serious injury. Even animals that look like healthy pets can have rabies or other diseases. Displaced animals may exhibit dangerous behaviors as they may be scared and hungry. If a person is bitten or scratched by an animal, the wound should be washed well with soap and clean water and then referred for medical attention right away for possible rabies vaccination. If available, a povidone-iodine solution (such as Betadine) can be used to cover the wound after thorough cleansing.

Heat- and cold-related emergencies: People who are not acclimated to hot and humid climates may be at risk for heat-related illnesses such as heat stress, heat exhaustion, or even heat stroke. Because access to medical care may be limited, it is important to prevent heat-related illness while working in high-risk situations. When working in the heat, responders should monitor their condition as well as that of their coworkers. Heat-related illness can cause a person to become confused or lose consciousness. Responders need to pace themselves with activities, know the warning signs and symptoms, and seek medical attention if symptoms of heat exhaustion or heat stroke are observed. Responders also should avoid prolonged exposure to cold temperatures, know the warning signs and symptoms of hypothermia and frostbite, wear appropriate clothing, and seek emergency care if signs and symptoms of hypothermia or frostbite develop.

Exposure to blood and body fluids: Responders should take the following precautions to minimize exposure to infectious disease agents:

➤ Protect the face from splashes of body fluids and fecal material by using a plastic face shield or a combination of eye protection and surgical mask. In extreme situations, a cloth tied over the nose and mouth can be used to block splashes.

➤ Protect hands from direct contact with body fluids and from injuries that break the skin by using a combination of a cut-proof inner layer glove and a latex (or similar) outer layer. Wash hands with soap and water or with an alcohol-based hand cleaner immediately after glove removal.

4.6 WORKFORCE ACTIVATION AND MOBILIZATION

Registered volunteers will receive a request for service and be expected to reply quickly (usually in less than 8 hours) based on availability during a disaster. Notification for needed services will often occur by preestablished communication methods agreed on between the volunteer and the deploying organization, such as text messaging, e-mail, personal cellular phone, business or home telephone, or a combination. The notification message (ie, the "alert") seeks a quick reply regarding volunteer availability for a set time frame (usually 1 or 2 weeks). The message typically includes an overview of the disaster, setting of the needed health care services (eg, mobile hospital, emergency department, temporary prehospital shelter), and anticipated location (ie, city and state).

In most instances, volunteers will have less than 24 hours to indicate their availability. Once a person has agreed to serve, he or she can expect to receive deployment orders within the next few hours. A usual time frame for mobilization (relocating from home base to area of need) is within 24 to 48 hours after confirmation of activation. Deployment orders typically include the following:

➤ Confirmed dates

➤ Time frame

➤ Destination

➤ Job assignment

➤ Contact person with phone number

➤ Reporting time with directions

➤ Attire preference with recommended clothing needs

➤ Lodging, travel, and transportation arrangements

Travel may include preestablished airline electronic tickets, contact information for an individual to make airline reservations, or specific driving arrangements. The responder should anticipate mobilization to include reporting to a central location (eg, base camp) and then being assigned to a service site (eg, mobile hospital, temporary shelter). If the volunteer is expected to drive to a destination, obtaining directional map information (eg, http://www.mapquest.com or http://www.maps.google.com) or a global positioning system device before departing is a great asset in making the journey safer and less stressful.

On arrival at the deployment location, responders must check in with deployment support staff or other designated personnel to verify arrival. Responders will then check in with the disaster supervisor for orientation. After orientation, responders will obtain equipment that is required to perform assigned duties. As directed, responders will report to a specified workstation and assume job responsibilities. During the orientation or initial debriefing, lodging and meal accommodations will be clarified. During deployment, responders are accountable to demonstrate full and consistent compliance with all predeployment policies and check-in procedures.

4.7   WORKFORCE PROTECTION

The goal of disaster response is to save lives safely, which may involve responders putting their own safety at risk. As discussed in Chapter 1, many types of potential hazards and dangers need to be considered before a disaster scene is entered. If the precise cause of an incident is not immediately apparent, or if there is suspicion that something is unusual, responders should take necessary precautions to minimize risk to themselves and others. Even if real-time identification of the precise cause is possible, responder safety remains paramount.

Personal Protection

Protecting yourself from becoming a casualty is the number 1 priority. Report any recognized or suspected hazard to appropriate authorities. Do not enter any disaster scene or take any action until authorities determine it is safe.

Multiple safety issues and challenges may arise during the management of disasters. The hazards for rescue personnel are significant. In many disasters, the majority of nonlethal injuries presenting to hospitals occur after the initial impact. These include blunt and penetrating traumatic injuries, electrical shocks, burns, smoke inhalation, and toxic fume exposures. Downed power lines are commonly encountered after natural disasters and pose a particularly dangerous hazard during night operations or when flooding is present. They may be less visible during a flood, and flooding can also limit access to pathways that would avoid them. Natural or propane gas leaks are also a significant hazard, and the risk of fire and explosion warrants careful handling by trained rescue personnel. Law enforcement and hospital security personnel must have a well-coordinated plan for maintaining access and egress routes approaching and surrounding the disaster scene.

Triage, treatment, and evacuation of casualties become secondary considerations if scene conditions do not permit intervention without endangering rescuers. The immediate scene may be too dangerous to allow any responders in to provide care. In a disaster, first responders and affected individuals must act quickly to protect themselves as they help trapped and injured persons. Under these conditions, personal health and safety must remain a primary concern. In some circumstances, emergency evacuation of response personnel from a disaster scene may be necessary because of:

➤ Temperature extremes

➤ Precipitation

➤ Changes in wind direction

➤ Smoke and fire hazards

➤ Potential violent situations

➤ Potential structure collapse

➤ Uncontrolled release of hazardous materials

➤ Presence of secondary devices

All responders need to be aware of their surroundings with an eye for things that seem unusual or out of place and thus may indicate a potential problem. This is part of surveillance, whether for law enforcement or public health. In any disaster, response personnel must recognize and appreciate the potential risks and disruptions that are part of response operations. Safety and security in a disaster are dynamic, ever changing as the situation unfolds. Vigilance is paramount.

Risk reduction measures are implemented to lower the possibility of exposure to actual or potential hazards. For disaster responders, this involves engineering controls, administrative controls, PPE, and decontamination. Engineering controls (eg, shutdown of heating and air conditioning systems, sprinkler systems, negative–air pressure rooms in hospitals) are used to remove a hazard at the scene, to remove reliance on human behavior, or to place a barrier between responders and the hazard. Well-designed engineering controls can be highly effective in protecting responders. When engineering solutions are not feasible, administrative controls offer methods to reduce exposure. Administrative controls (eg, respiratory protection programs, disaster plans, standard operating procedures) are policies, procedures, and practices that minimize the exposure of responders and affected populations to hazardous conditions. They are considered less effective than engineering controls in that they do not usually eliminate the hazard and they rely on human behavior. Rather, they lessen the duration and frequency of exposure to the situation. The least effective controls are PPE and decontamination, as responders are still present in a potentially hazardous environment.

4.7.1 Disaster Scene Exclusion Zones

Disaster scenes involving the release of hazardous substances or materials are managed by means of a three-zone system of perimeter isolation. The purpose of delineating these three zones, which are mapped out in 360° surrounding the site of the release, is to contain and confine the contamination to a specific geographic area. These three exclusion zones are called the hot, warm, and cold zones.

The *hot zone* is the area where the site of the release occurred and where most of the contamination is located. All work activities within the hot zone are exclusively performed by members of a hazardous materials (HAZMAT) response team who are specially trained and equipped to work in this environment. Response activities that will be performed in the hot zone include identifying the agent if it is unknown, stopping the spread of the release (usually by finding and sealing, patching, or overpacking the container releasing the hazardous substance), and rescuing casualties.

The *warm zone* is the location where workers enter and leave the contaminated hot zone, before entering the contamination-free cold zone. The warm zone has a special location designated as the decontamination corridor, where decontamination of response team members and contaminated victims will take place. All decontamination activities take place within the warm zone, and all contaminated runoff from decontamination remains within the warm zone.

The *cold zone* is the contamination-free area. Far enough from the site of the release and upwind of any vapor plume hazards, the cold zone is where casualty collection, triage, treatment, and transportation of casualties coordinated by EMS will take place and where other responders and incident command elements will be located.

Hospitals and other health care facilities that receive casualties from the disaster scene will consider the activation of protocols and procedures to minimize exposure of staff, patients, and others in the facility to potentially hazardous materials.[10] A decontamination zone should be established outside the facility and a postdecontamination zone within the facility. Four potential groups may arrive at the decontamination zone: (1) exposed casualties without other injuries and who require decontamination; (2) exposed casualties with other injuries and who require decontamination; (3) casualties requiring verification of decontamination elsewhere; and (4) worried, yet previously unexposed, people.

Recommendations in this section are for informational purposes only. Federal guidance should be consulted for more detailed information on personal protection, worker safety, and specialized training requirements for dealing with HAZMAT incidents in hospitals and other health care facilities.[10,11] Additionally, 29 CFR 1910.120 contains the federal regulations concerning Hazardous Waste Operations and Emergency Response (HAZWOPER) with which first responders and first receivers must comply in responding to or receiving casualties from a HAZMAT incident.[12]

4.7.2   Selection and Use of PPE

Before entering any disaster scene, it is important that responders protect themselves through the selection and use of appropriate PPE.[10-13] Each responder must be aware of commonly used PPE and must know where to seek expert HAZMAT advice regarding selection and proper use of specific PPE when situational awareness and hazard assessments warrant protective actions. One of the early determinations by the safety officer should be the level of PPE needed by persons entering the hot zone, people staffing the decontamination area, and even security personnel dealing with the members of the public approaching treatment facilities. PPE is intended to minimize contact with contaminated persons, objects, and environments. This includes protecting the skin, mouth, eyes, nose, lungs, and other body parts vulnerable to vapor or liquid exposure and penetration. PPE provides a hazard barrier that allows function in a hazardous area and must be used properly during all phases of response. Casualty care may have to wait until proper PPE is available.

PPE includes two components: (1) respiratory protection, and (2) protective garments and barriers. For health responders, this may require more than gloves, gowns, and masks, including helmets, air-purifying respirators, work gloves, self-contained breathing apparatus (SCBA), steel-toed shoes, and reflective clothing.

The component of any PPE that is most useful is *respiratory protection*. Responders should be instructed to remove respiratory protection last when dealing with nondecontaminated patients, to reduce the likelihood of inhaled material. For the purposes of responding to or receiving casualties from most disasters, there are two types of respiratory protection: air-purifying respirators and supplied air devices.

Air-purifying respirators (APRs) are defined under 29 CFR 1910.134(b) of the Respiratory Protection Standard as "a respirator with an air-purifying filter, cartridge, or canister that removes specific air contaminants by passing ambient air through the air-purifying element." Typically these are either gas mask–type respirators or mechanically "powered" APRs (or PAPRs). APRs filter contaminants from breathing air through cartridges or filters, resulting in inhaled air that has been purified. For APRs to be used in a toxic environment, the hazardous agent must be known, as must the concentration of the agent in the work area. The concentration of any hazardous material must not exceed a level considered to be immediately dangerous to life or health (IDLH). An IDLH atmosphere is defined by the Occupational Safety and Health Administration (OSHA) as "an atmosphere that poses an immediate threat to life, would cause irreversible adverse health effects, or would impair an individual's ability to escape from a dangerous atmosphere." If the concentration of any hazardous agent exceeds the IDLH level, an APR does not provide sufficient protection. Further, responders using APRs breathe filtered air; thus, APRs are not acceptable in oxygen-deficient environments (that is, environments with oxygen concentrations less than room air). Under these two conditions, responders must use supplied air devices.

Supplied air refers to one of two types of respiratory protection devices, the SCBA or the supplied airline respirator. Both devices provide a full-face mask through which a responder breathes clean, contaminant-free air, supplied through a back cylinder (SCBA) or a hose that runs from a generator or large breathing air tank in a clean environment. Supplied air devices are required in environments in which the hazardous material is unknown, oxygen is deficient, or IDLH.

Protective clothing refers to the garments that are worn by first responders or first receivers when performing tasks such as decontamination. Such clothing is rated on the basis of the time it would take for a hazardous chemical to penetrate the garment; the longer the time, the more protective the suit. The highest level of protective clothing is a fully encapsulating vapor-tight suit. The second highest level is a fully or partially encapsulating suit that is resistant to liquid chemicals. The third level of protective clothing is a hooded coverall typically constructed with a laminated or plasticized Tyvek®-type material. This is designed to keep a worker's clothes clean but is not protective against liquid chemicals or vapors. The lowest level of protection is simply a laboratory apron or other uniform-type clothing that provides no chemical protection. Protective clothing is typically combined with a corresponding level of respiratory protection to meet EPA-recommended levels of PPE (A, B, C and D, as explained in the following section).[10,11]

4.7.2.1   PPE Levels

OSHA has adopted the EPA levels of PPE, which are discussed in detail in Appendix B of 29 CFR 1910.120.[11,12] A brief summary is provided in this section. Each level is a combination of chemical protective clothing and respiratory protection. Proper selection of the appropriate level of protection will depend on the unique circumstances of the event and the mission assigned.

Level A PPE should be worn when the highest level of respiratory, skin, eye, and mucous membrane protection is needed. It involves:

➤ Positive-pressure, full-face-piece SCBA, or positive-pressure-supplied air respirator with escape SCBA (NIOSH approved)

➤ Totally encapsulating chemical-protective suit

➤ Gloves, outer, chemical-resistant

➤ Gloves, inner, chemical-resistant

➤ Boots, outer, chemical-resistant, steel toe and shank

➤ Disposable protective suit, gloves, and boots (depending on suit construction, may be worn over totally encapsulating suit)

Level B PPE should be selected when the highest level of respiratory protection is needed, but a lesser level of skin and eye protection is sufficient. Level B is the minimum level recommended on initial site entries until the hazards have been identified and defined by monitoring, sampling, and other reliable methods of analysis, and equipment corresponding with those findings has been provided. Level B requires either supplied air or SCBA but lacks the full encapsulation. Level B protection involves:

➤ Positive-pressure, full-face SCBA, or positive-pressure-supplied air respirator with escape SCBA (NIOSH approved)

➤ Hooded chemical-resistant clothing (overalls and long-sleeved jacket; coveralls; one- or two-piece chemical-splash suit; disposable chemical-resistant overalls)

➤ Gloves, outer, chemical-resistant

➤ Gloves, inner, chemical-resistant

➤ Boots, outer, chemical-resistant, steel toe and shank

Level C protection should be selected when the type of airborne substance is known, the concentration has been measured, criteria for using air-purifying respirators are met, and skin and eye exposure are unlikely. Periodic monitoring of the air must be performed. Level C protection involves:

➤ Full-face or half-mask APRs (NIOSH approved)

➤ Hooded chemical-resistant clothing (overalls; two-piece chemical-splash suit; disposable chemical-resistant overalls)

➤ Gloves, outer, chemical-resistant

➤ Gloves, inner, chemical-resistant

Level D PPE is universal precautions as practiced in any health care facility. It should not be used on any site where respiratory or skin hazards exist. it involves:

➤ Coveralls

➤ Boots/shoes, chemical-resistant steel toe and shank

The selection of PPE may vary depending on the threat analysis or known hazards. The appropriate level of PPE to be used at the scene will be determined by local response experts, such as HAZMAT personnel. Important considerations include the following:

➤ Is there an immediate danger to life or health?

➤ What agent was released?

➤ How was the agent released (eg, gas, liquid, particles)?

➤ Is the release site confined?

➤ What is the responders' proximity to the release site?

➤ What are their expected roles and job duties during the event?

It is important to adhere to routine safety precautions, policies, and procedures at all times. Respirators approved by NIOSH should be worn whenever there is risk of exposure to airborne and dust-borne contaminants (see http://www.cdc.gov/niosh/npptl/topics/respirators/disp_part/RespSource.html).

4.7.2.2 PPE Challenges

When working in PPE in a hazardous or potentially hazardous environment, it can be technically difficult to perform some clinical procedures successfully. Such procedures include, the use of autoinjectors for nerve agent antidote administration, chest decompression by means of a needle thoracentesis, and advanced

---

Universal Precautions

Actions taken to assist casualties may increase risk of exposure to blood and body secretions, thereby increasing risk of exposure to human immunodeficiency, hepatitis B, and hepatitis C viruses. These viruses can pass from an infected individual to a rescuer through broken skin or mucous membranes such as the eyes, nose, or mouth, or from open wounds. Risk of exposure can be reduced by following universal precautions to the extent possible, particularly by wearing protective equipment such as face masks, eye shields, and gloves for any invasive procedure or contact with blood and other body fluids. With proper precautions, the risk of contracting these viruses through blood and body secretions is low.

airway management. The PPE necessary to operate in a hazardous contaminated environment can significantly impede the ability of health care personnel to use their basic senses:

➤ Touch may be impaired by gloves.

➤ Smell may be impaired by the type of respiratory protection being used (eg, powered and nonpowered APRs, SCBA).

➤ Hearing may be impaired by the type of respiratory protection, the necessity for hearing protection, and loud noises in the immediate environment. Any type of respiratory protection may present communication challenges.

➤ Sight may be limited if visual fields are narrowed by the type of airway protection being used by the responder.

If lifesaving care cannot be administered in the level of PPE required at the scene, it is recommended that injured persons be provided whatever supportive measures are available and then be rapidly decontaminated and moved to a clean area for further medical evaluation and treatment. It is critical that clinical responders practice performing medical procedures while wearing appropriate PPE under various disaster situations. The selection and use of PPE is discussed in more detail in the ADLS®course (v 3.0) and supporting course manual.

4.8   CASUALTY DECONTAMINATION

Decontamination is generally performed by trained and appropriately equipped personnel to reduce a person's exposure to hazardous materials and minimize the chance of secondary contamination of responders, health care providers, and others. It involves the process of removing or deactivating harmful contaminants such as chemical agents and radioactive materials from external body surfaces. The decision to decontaminate should be made early, even if it is based on incomplete information. Once the decision is made to proceed, it should be assumed that every exposed individual is contaminated until proven otherwise. In some instances, such as after nerve agent or cyanide exposure, antidote administration must proceed simultaneously with or prior to decontamination by health care providers in PPE.

Decontamination should be considered in all explosive events, any hazardous materials release or exposure, or when individuals may have been exposed to radioactive materials. If casualties can be adequately and reliably screened for contaminants (ie, by use of a Geiger counter for radiation), then decontamination is not necessary. If contaminated casualties, or casualties whose status regarding contamination is unknown, arrive at a health care facility, they should not be allowed to enter the facility until they have been properly decontaminated.

4.8.1   Types of Decontamination

Decontamination is a primary objective for initial casualty care. It consists of two types, dry and wet:

Dry decontamination essentially consists of removal of clothing and/or debris. In many instances, the *removal of clothing* may eliminate up to 90% of contamination.

Wet decontamination consists of washing in a shower or wiping down the casualties with a soap-and-water solution or some form of moistened cloth. Showering with tepid water and a liquid soap with good surfactant properties is the preferred method for removing hazardous substances from skin and hair. Water alone is good, soap and water are better. Bleach solutions should be avoided for human decontamination but are useful for equipment decontamination.

During a mass casualty event, it is often asked who will prioritize individuals for decontamination. This question may have different answers depending on available resources and whether decontamination is taking place on-scene by first responders or at a health care facility by first receivers. Emergency treatment before decontamination is usually not advised, because the performance of invasive procedures could introduce contamination into a person's body and if emergency or life-saving interventions must be performed before decontamination, the individual may not survive the 5- to 10-minute decontamination process. Each agency and facility should have its own specific protocols for determining what, if any, treatment would be provided before decontamination.

A simple way to describe the process of mass decontamination is wet, strip, flush, and cover. First, individuals are wetted down while wearing their clothes to trap particulates or other debris and prevent these contaminants from becoming airborne. Next, individuals are asked to remove all their clothing and place it into a labeled plastic bag, which will be stored in a secure location for evidence preservation, decontamination, or destruction at a later date. Individuals are then flushed for a minimum of 5 minutes with the decontamination solution of choice (usually soap and water). Finally, individuals are dried off, covered with a privacy garment, and moved to a location for further medical assessment. The method of decontamination is generally standard for the general public after all chemical disasters with few exceptions.

All individuals who are decontaminated require temporary clothing and blankets appropriate for the climate and the person's age and size. Once decontamination is completed, they should be screened to determine the need for further medical and mental health care. Those who do not require definitive treatment can be moved to a separate area for observation and monitoring for delayed symptoms. Those requiring medical attention should be triaged and transported to the appropriate care area. Decontamination issues and challenges are discussed in greater detail in the ADLS® course (v 3.0) and supporting course manual.

4.8.2 Special Decontamination Considerations

Nonambulatory casualties: These casualties will require special procedures when they are moved through a mass decontamination process. Facilities using tents may have a dedicated lane for these individuals, whereby they are placed onto a slideboard and are moved through the decontamination process on a conveyor system. If the agency or facility does not have a dedicated nonambulatory lane, the nonambulatory person can be moved through on a stretcher or wheelchair as long as the device does not introduce contamination into the clean area and the person is moved to allow decontamination of the areas touching the wheelchair or stretcher. Additional staff will be required to facilitate this process.

Children: Decontamination personnel must be cognizant of unique challenges in decontaminating children in general and children with special health care needs in particular. Family members may not cooperate with instructions by decontamination personnel, either because they do not understand the instructions or because their family would be separated. Children are at increased risk of hypothermia, fear, and psychological consequences from the decontamination process, as well as embarrassment from disrobing. Pediatric decontamination also can be resource intensive, as two to three people may be needed to decontaminate a child. Whether to use decontamination procedures for asymptomatic children after a known or suspected exposure is often a decision that must be made before the agent has been identified.

Current mass casualty decontamination procedures designed for adults carry further challenges. Children have a higher surface area and a more difficult time with temperature regulation; decontamination with room-temperature or colder water can lead to dangerous hypothermia. Although hypothermia may be a risk, it is less risky than not decontaminating a child. Young children may be unable to understand the concepts of decontamination and will be unable to comprehend why they must be separated from their family and asked to strip down with strangers. Finally, response personnel should ensure that clothing is available for children after decontamination. This includes diapers for infants.

Many shower systems are not suitable for children, who require systems that use warm water and are high-volume but low-pressure. Shower decontamination units designed for young children and infants must be able to accommodate an adult (parent or caretaker) as well as the child. Specific questions to be addressed for pediatric decontamination are as follows:

➤ Is the water pressure appropriate? Will it injure a child?

➤ Is the water temperature acceptable? If water is not warm it may cause hypothermia.

➤ Can the process handle the nonambulatory child, as well as infants, toddlers, and children with special health care needs?

➤ Does the method and equipment used allow decontamination of a child with a parent or caregiver?

➤ Will children follow instructions?

➤ Have mental health concerns been addressed?

➤ What are the long-term effects of such decisions?

Like nonambulatory patients, children will require more time to decontaminate and additional staff to assist them through the decontamination process. The following should be considered when decontaminating children:

➤ Keep children with their families or a caregiver whenever possible.

➤ Have the child go through the decontamination tent with the parent, and allow more time to ensure that both the parent and child have been washed for a minimum of 5 minutes.

➤ Be conscious of the increased risk of hypothermia in the pediatric population.

➤ Take steps to ensure that decontamination water is heated when possible and that blankets and heaters are used in the postdecontamination area.

➤ Attempt (when possible) to have dry pediatric-specific garments (eg, gowns, diapers) available in various sizes for use at the decontamination location.

Individuals with functional and access needs: Individuals may have difficulty being processed through decontamination lines for a variety of reasons. If communication is a problem, decontamination areas should have signs depicting what should be done at each location or personnel available to guide a visually impaired person through the decontamination process. Individuals with assistive devices (eg, wheelchairs, walking sticks, walkers) should not be allowed to travel through the decontamination process with these aids. Hearing aids, prosthetics, and other medical devices should be sealed in a plastic bag with the person's name and left with his or her belongings. When the immediate crisis is under control, these devices can potentially be decontaminated and returned to the individual.

4.9 WORKFORCE DEMOBILIZATION AND DEPLOYMENT-RELATED STRESS

Demobilization orders come from incident command. Demobilization is a planned process involving the organized transition of functions or cessation of services and a dismantling of equipment and site-based resources. It is not an emergency evacuation (which is the unplanned but immediate need to evacuate personnel from an area or scene because of serious threats to responder health, safety, and security). Demobilization is the process of "standing down" and disbanding resources when emergency response needs have been met. As disaster operations shift from response to recovery, demobilization efforts will focus on the return of all resources (ie, personnel, equipment, supplies) to their original locations.

At the completion of deployment, response personnel complete unfinished reports; brief their replacements, subordinates, and supervisors; return incident-issued equipment or supplies; and complete any additional documents requested by their supervisors (eg, travel voucher, time and attendance verification, and performance evaluation [if applicable]). Responders may be requested to participate in a debriefing ("hot wash") to discuss the strengths, weaknesses, and opportunities for improvement related to operational responses. Findings of the debriefing are captured in a report called the *after-action review*. Demobilized responders will receive information on travel arrangements (eg, designated airline, departure time, transportation arrangements). On arrival home, responders must notify their home unit or organization of their return.

Although disaster work can be rewarding, it can be stressful when loss of life, serious injuries, missing and separated families, and other traumatic situations are encountered. Symptoms of stress are often normal and generally temporary, but stress can be dangerous to physical and emotional well-being. Occasionally, some empathic disaster workers internally absorb the traumatic stress of disaster survivors. The relief worker may feel inadequate in meeting the overwhelming needs of disaster victims. The buildup of stress over time may lead to a state of exhaustion and difficulty in functioning, commonly known as compassion fatigue or, in some cases, posttraumatic fatigue syndrome.[14,15] After returning home, responders need to keep in mind that:

➤ Everyone who experiences a disaster is affected by the situation.

➤ It is normal to feel sadness, grief, and anger about what happened and what was seen.

➤ It is natural to feel anxious about personal safety and the safety of one's family.

➤ Acknowledging personal feelings will help an individual move forward more quickly.

➤ Focusing on one's contributions, strengths, and abilities can help in healing if an individual is troubled by the experience.

➤ Everyone has different needs and different ways of coping. This is normal.

➤ It is healthy to reach out for and accept help if needed.

Mental and behavioral health issues are discussed in much greater detail in Chapter 3, "Population Health and Mental Health in Disasters."

4.10 SUMMARY

In any disaster, health professionals and other response personnel must recognize and appreciate the potential risks and disruptions that are part of disaster operations. Damage caused by natural and human-caused disasters creates myriad health and safety risks for affected populations and emergency responders. Depending on the event, there may be a large number of serious casualties, which may require search, rescue, and support operations under potentially hazardous and stressful conditions. Without proper precautions, additional casualties may result from secondary hazards such as structural collapse, excessive heat, motor vehicle crashes, downed power lines, ruptured gas mains, release of hazardous materials by fires or explosions, and infectious disease outbreaks.

All responders have a responsibility to be prepared to perform their duties and to assess whether they are healthy enough to respond effectively. In addition to possessing specific knowledge and skills related to disaster management, emergency responders must possess the fitness to respond and ability to maintain that fitness once deployed. They must decide whether they can function in less than optimal circumstances and environments.

Before entering any disaster scene, it is important that responders protect themselves through the use of appropriate PPE. The appropriate level of protection depends on the unique situation. PPE is intended to minimize contact with contaminated persons, objects, and environments. It protects those body parts that are vulnerable to exposure and penetration: the skin, the mouth, the eyes, the nose, and the respiratory tract.

Disaster response and recovery operations can be physically and emotionally challenging. Responders may experience stress related to protecting their own safety and well-being, as well as that of others. Additional stress may be related to the care of casualties, the management of mass fatalities, and the unique situational restrictions and limitations encountered at the disaster scene. In addition to the substantial effects that disasters can have on physical health, they place significant stress and psychological trauma on responders. Experiencing a disaster can be one of the most difficult events a person can endure, and it can have both short- and long-term effects. Most people who experience a disaster, whether as a casualty or as a responder, will have some type of psychological, physical, and/or emotional response to the event.

REFERENCES

1. Corporation for National and Community Service, Office of Research and Policy Development. *Volunteering in America 2010: National, State and City Information*. http://www.nationalservice.gov. Accessed March 25, 2011.

2. Jenkins J, Frederisksen K, Stone R, Tang N. Strategies to improve sleep during extended search and rescue operations. *Prehosp Emergency Care*. 2007;11:230-233.

3. Centers for Disease Control and Prevention (CDC). Recommended adult immunization schedule—United States, 2010. *Morbid Mortal Wkly Rep (MMWR)*. 2010;59:1-4. http://www.cdc.gov/mmwr/PDF/wk/mm5901-Immunization.pdf. Accessed March 25, 2011.

4. Centers for Disease Control and Prevention. *Traveler's Health Web Site*. http://www.nc.cdc.gov/travel/. Accessed March 25, 2011.

5. Office of the Civilian Volunteer Medical Reserve Corps. *Preparing for a Federal Deployment*. Ft Lauderdale, FL: QuickSeries Publishing; 2010.

6. Seligman PJ, Cunningham B. USPHS deployment readiness. In: Carmona RH, Darling RG, Knoben JE, Michael JM. *Public Health Emergency Preparedness & Response: Principles and Practice*. Washington, DC: Public Health Service Commissioned Officers Foundation for the Advancement of Public Health; 2010.

7. Coyle G, Sapnas K, Ward-Presson K. Dealing with disaster. *Nurs Manage*. 2007;38:24-29.

8. James JJ, Benjamin GC, Burkle FM Jr, Gebbie KM, Kelen G, Subbarao I. Disaster medicine and public health preparedness: a discipline for all health professionals. *Disaster Med Public Health Prep*. 2010;4:102-107.

9. Hodge, JG , Pepe RP, Henning, WH. Voluntarism in the wake of hurricane Katrina: The Uniform Emergency Volunteer Health Practitioners Act. *Disaster Med Public Health Prep*. 2007;1:44-50.

10. Occupational Safety and Health Administration (OSHA). *Best Practices for Hospital-Based First Receivers of Victims From Mass Casualty Incidents Involving the Release of Hazardous Substances*. Washington, DC: OSHA; 2005. http://www.osha.gov/dts/osta/bestpractices/firstreceivers_hospital.pdf. Accessed March 25, 2011.

11. US Department of Health and Human Services (HHS), Centers for Disease Control and Prevention. *Guidance on Emergency Responder Personal Protective Equipment (PPE) for Response to CBRN Terrorism Incidents*. Washington, DC:DHHS; 2008. http://www.cdc.gov/niosh/docs/2008-132/pdfs/2008-132.pdf. Accessed March 25, 2011.

12. Occupational Safety and Health Administration. *29 Code of Federal Regulations (CFR) 1910 Occupational Safety and Health Standards*. Applicable OSHA standards include 29 CFR 1910.120 – HAZWOPER; 29 CFR 1910.132 – Personal Protective Equipment – General Requirements; 29 CFR 1910.133 – Eye and Face Protection; 29 CFR 1910.134 – Respiratory Protection. http://www.wbdg .org/ccb/OSHA/29cfr1910.pdf. Accessed March 25, 2011.

13. Institute of Medicine. *Preparing for an Influenza Pandemic: Personal Protective Equipment for Healthcare Workers*. Washington, DC: National Academies Press; 2008.

14. Frank D, Korioth S. Measuring compassion fatigue in public health nurses providing assistance to hurricane victims. *Southern Online J Nurs Res*. 2006;7:1-13. http://www.snrs.org/publications/ SOJNR_articles/iss04vol07.pdf. Accessed March 25, 2011.

15. Figley C. Compassion fatigue as secondary traumatic stress: an overview. In Figley C, ed. *Compassion Fatigue: Coping with Secondary Traumatic Stress Disorder*. New York: Bruner/ Mazel;1995.

CHAPTER FIVE

Mass Casualty and Fatality Management

CHAPTER CHAIR

Arthur Cooper, MD, MS

CONTRIBUTING AUTHORS

Steven Parrillo, DO

Seth C. Jones, BS, NR – Paramedic

J. Marc Liu, MD, MPH

Jim Lyznicki, MS, MPH

Raymond E. Swienton, MD

5.1 PURPOSE

This chapter describes the basic principles and practices of mass casualty management, including mass casualty triage and mass casualty assessment, as well as mass fatality management. The focus is to orient first responders and first receivers to the rapid clinical decision making and prioritization necessitated by the altered care environment that results when large numbers of casualties require urgent treatment. Applying a rational approach to casualty sorting and assessment that supports timely identification and intervention is vital in recognizing those casualties with the best chance of survival. Basic concepts in mass fatality management are also addressed. Professional action and ethical decision making during casualty management are additionally reinforced.

5.2 LEARNING OBJECTIVES

After completing this chapter, readers should be able to:

➤ Describe the rationale, elements, and actions for performing mass casualty triage, utilizing standardized triage categories and SALT methodologies and reinforcing the need for information reporting and sharing.

➤ Discuss an all-hazards, scalable casualty management approach, including life-saving interventions, clinical decision making, and casualty transport under potentially hazardous, stressful, and resource-constrained circumstances.

➤ Describe the concepts and principles of mass fatality management for health professionals in a disaster or public health emergency.

➤ Discuss the importance of professionalism and ethics in mass casualty care.

Learning objectives for this chapter are competency-based, as delineated in Appendix B.

5.3 BACKGROUND

When disaster strikes, emergency medical needs at the scene may quickly overwhelm local resources. To save the most lives possible, quick decisions must be made for the efficient use of immediately available resources. In a disaster, the clinical management of casualties may be different than what is typically encountered in nondisaster health care settings. In day-to-day emergencies affecting limited numbers of patients, triage involves the temporary prioritization of medical care delivered in physician offices, clinics, and emergency departments, with the objective to do the greatest good for each individual patient. In large-scale disasters or public health emergencies involving multiple casualties, the objective is different: it is to do the greatest good for the greatest number of possible survivors. It is essential to remember this distinction during any true disaster or public health emergency. Decisions on prioritization of care will affect not just initial treatment and transport, but the entire subsequent course of mass casualty care.

Provision of medical care when the situation suddenly exceeds or overwhelms the available local resources or facilities is the operational definition of a medical disaster. Access to medical resources may be further limited by communication, transportation, and other constraints. Providing medical care in such an altered care environment is different from providing care under normal circumstances. Specifically, the altered care environment demands that resource utilization be a priority in clinical decision making. Thus, it is important to consider not just an individual's requirements but also the effect that the utilization of potentially limited resources may have on other casualties.

As such, the principles and basic skills of mass casualty triage are important for all providers to understand. This is true not only for on-scene first responders, but also for hospital-based first receivers. Understanding mass casualty triage will allow field providers to understand how casualties have been prioritized and hence where to direct their efforts. It will also allow hospital providers to understand how decisions at the scene were made, to interpret reports from the scene, and to manage the "worried well" and "walking wounded," who may converge at the doors of their facilities. It is important to note that disaster casualties are not always transported by emergency medical services (EMS); the more significant the disaster, the less likely that casualties will be transported by a structured EMS system. Individuals transported by themselves or bystanders outside a structured EMS system do not always require minimal care only; they may require limited, if delayed, care, and occasionally even extensive or immediate care. Such casualties can represent significant challenges to hospitals, as they typically arrive early, often in large numbers, before the hospital even learns about the incident—making the hospital and its staff vulnerable to potential contaminants and possible lockdown.

The importance of basic knowledge and skills in disaster casualty assessment also cannot be overstated. Casualty management must include expeditious recognition of the presence of immediately life-threatening situations; this allows emergent life-saving interventions to be performed as necessary. Initial assessment is based on acuity and severity of injury and illness, as well as potential salvageability given the available treatment options. For example, in a disaster situation, first responders and first receivers might initially be able to provide care only for immediately life-threatening problems in the highest-priority casualties; other casualties would need to be monitored for deterioration in clinical status, but at first might be able to receive supportive care only. As resources became available, assessment and therapeutic interventions would be distributed according to the severity of need, balanced with likelihood of survival.

5.4   GENERAL PRINCIPLES OF MASS CASUALTY TRIAGE

The goal of mass casualty triage is to create a formal, reproducible process for sorting casualties, so that (1) those who are treated first will be those among the most seriously ill or injured who have a reasonable possibility of survival and (2) those who are treated last have the least severe illnesses or injuries or are very unlikely to survive, while (3) those who require minimal or no treatment can initially be separated from the others, such that scarce medical resources can first be directed to those with the greatest needs.

Mass casualty triage is a systematic method for organizing casualties at the scene of a mass casualty event. Mass casualty triage decision making encompasses three important considerations when determining an ordered prioritization:

1. The presence of a life-threatening, limb-threatening, or vision-threatening condition

2. The immediately available life-saving and similarly emergent medical and surgical interventions that can be delivered

3. The availability of transportation assets, including their capabilities and capacities, and their timely access to arrival at health care facilities

Because triage balances patient condition with available resources, a casualty with a life-threatening injury will not always be assigned to the highest or most acute triage category. Moreover, once the immediately available interventions are attempted, the triage category may be changed due to a low likelihood of survival resulting from a lack of on-site medical intervention or timely access to available transportation capabilities and capacities. This is the nature of disaster triage. Clearly it necessitates a solid understanding of the dynamic condition of sorting casualties, given the treatment resources and transport assets available during a mass casualty event.

Mass casualty triage must therefore take into account both dynamic changes in the sudden demand of casualties requiring care and significant constraints in the supply of resources needed to provide that care. Disaster triage differs from day-to-day triage in that there are large numbers of casualties to be prioritized (demand), constrained by a scarcity of resources (supply), including an infrastructure that is insufficient to handle the number of casualties. There may be limited equipment available at the scene; transport assets may not be sufficient for the numbers of casualties; and hospital resources may be strained or overwhelmed such that alternative transport destinations may need to be considered. Providers may also be faced with potential dangers to themselves and their patients, such as the possibility of hazardous materials that require decontamination and use of appropriate personal protective equipment (PPE) as well as the possibility of secondary devices or other hazards. Functional and sensory limitations may also be imposed on providers utilizing PPE (for more details, see section 5.6.3). Finally, because of the overwhelming numbers and needs, multiple agencies may find themselves working together to execute an appropriate response. This requires interoperability of command and coordination as well as communication: in other words, a common language and understanding of the steps that need to be taken, and when.

Mass Casualty Triage

Mass casualty triage involves rapid categorization of casualties with potentially severe injuries or illnesses who require immediate medical attention at the scene. In a disaster, health care needs exceed the immediately available resources. Therefore, not all casualties may initially receive full medical care. In a serious mass casualty event, this can be a daunting and difficult challenge.

It is likely that an event that causes multiple casualties will be stressful and upsetting to the casualties, bystanders, and rescuers alike. This will lead to a chaotic scene where people are unlikely to be orderly and patient. Therefore, rescuers will need to rely on a common mass casualty triage method to help them organize and control the chaos of the scene, in an attempt to minimize self-triage of casualties to the closest health care facility. Instead, rescuers will attempt to move individuals from the scene in an organized manner so that the chaos of the scene does not move to the local hospitals. Emphasis is placed on not allowing ambulatory casualties with minor injuries to overwhelm the local hospitals before the more severely injured people can be transported. For example, amid the early "chaos" phase at the scene of an explosion, many will evacuate themselves or others by means of civilian transportation, without receiving any treatment at the scene. In the 1995 Oklahoma City bombing, more than half of the casualties, including some with critical injuries, were transported to the hospital in privately owned vehicles. When people self-evacuate, they are likely to seek care at the nearest hospital. This must be taken into account when distributing casualties via an organized evacuation system.[1]

Triage is a dynamic process. For example, a casualty triaged as immediate at one time might improve considerably or perhaps deteriorate further at a later time. As another example, a victim of a gunshot to a long bone is normally triaged to a trauma center; however, if demand (number of casualties) is high and/or supply (trauma center capacity) is low, that same patient may need to be managed at a local hospital, freeing the trauma center for more complex cases (eg, head, chest, abdomen).

As noted, triage is both dynamic and continuous. *Primary* triage guides initial treatment and transport decisions. *Secondary* triage further prioritizes casualties and medical resources once all initial needs have been determined and categorized and may be followed by *tertiary* triage. As part of secondary and tertiary triage, a medical provider must use clinical judgment to assess the severity of a casualty's condition when compared with available resources. In other words, the way a casualty will be triaged is dependent on the equipment, personnel, and facilities available to the casualty at that time. As such, a casualty who would be quickly treated in a fully equipped hospital might be considered unsalvageable in a remote location where there were very limited medical resources. For example, a head-injured casualty with a weak pulse and agonal breathing would normally receive volume resuscitation and assisted ventilation in the field followed by endotracheal intubation and mechanical ventilation at a trauma hospital. However, in a remote location where venous access and ventilatory support devices, and even hospitals, are scarce, a responder might need to bypass that casualty and move on to another.

In large-scale disasters, patients already hospitalized with illnesses may be able to be transferred from local hospitals to regional tertiary care centers as in normal operations. On the other hand, sick patients may need to be kept at local hospitals (even though in normal conditions those same patients would be transferred) in order to maintain capacity at the regional tertiary care center to manage more critical patients. For the same reason, sick patients may also need to be "back"-transferred from the regional tertiary care center to their local hospitals (the local hospital that is normally the sender now becomes the receiver, while the regional tertiary care center that is normally the receiver now becomes the sender).

In addition, not all disasters result in a distinct incident scene. Population-based triage optimizes the use of limited resources when casualties are dispersed across a large region, such as during an infectious disease outbreak or a flood. The population-based, bioevent-specific, SEIRV triage methodology is introduced in Chapter 9, "Biologic Disasters," while the principles of population-based triage are discussed in the Advanced Disaster Life Support® (ADLS®) course (v3.0) and supporting course manual.

5.4.1   Mass Casualty Triage Systems

Mass casualty triage was first described by Baron Dominique Jean Larrey, the surgeon-in-chief of Napoleon's army. Two hundred years later, many different mass casualty triage systems are used.[2] In the United States in particular, there has been a lack of national standardization in mass casualty triage. Different locales use different systems.

Regardless of which mass casualty triage system is used, it must be simple, accurate, rapid, and reproducible across numerous types of providers and various conditions.

Table 5-1 provides a list of triage systems that are commonly used today. It is important that every potential responder know and practice the triage system used by his or her agency or agencies. Several of these triage systems are compared and contrasted in a summary table provided in Chapter 2 of the ADLS® course manual (v3.0)

TABLE 5-1 Examples of Mass Casualty Triage Systems Used Today

CareFlight[3]
CESIRA
Homebush[4]
JumpSTART[5]
Military triage[6]
Pediatric Triage Tape (PTT)[7]
SALT[8]
Simple Triage and Rapid Treatment (START)[9]
Triage SIEVE[3,10]

Among the multiple triage systems that currently exist—of which very few have been prospectively validated—it is important that a locality, organization, or agency choose a system that addresses three key components: acuity, severity, and salvageability. Mass casualty incidents and disasters frequently cross jurisdictional lines and thus involve responders from multiple local agencies, who may be using different triage tools.

The NDLS™ program and all its courses (CDLS®, BDLS®, and ADLS®) promote SALT (*Sort/Assess/Lifesaving Intervention/Treatment and/or transport*) triage, which was recently developed through a collaborative effort funded by the Centers for Disease Control and Prevention (CDC).[8]

The SALT triage methodology is a national consensus-based mass casualty triage model that was developed by using the best scientific evidence available at the time it was created.[8] It is simple to use and easy to remember. SALT instructs providers to globally *sort* casualties into priority tiers by their ability to follow simple commands, then to individually *assess* casualties within each tier, while applying *lifesaving interventions* and assigning priority for *treatment and/or transport*. SALT is fully compliant with the Model Uniform Core Criteria for Mass Casualty Triage that recently were identified to ensure interoperability and standardization when responding to mass casualty events.[8,11]

Common Triage Methodology

While the operational and clinical implications of using multiple triage systems at the same incident are unknown, it seems reasonable to presume that for operational simplicity, communication interoperability, and clinical efficiency, it is preferable for all responders at a given incident to be using the same triage system; or, at the very least, operate from some common elements (eg, nomenclature of triage categories).

5.4.2 Limitations of Triage Systems

Most currently available mass casualty triage methodologies were designed to be used for victims of traumatic injuries, including explosive and incendiary injuries. They appear less useful for victims of chemical, biologic, radiologic, or nuclear injuries. Moreover, few current triage systems have been tested rigorously. Triage systems may also be limited by language barriers and age, as well as by functional and sensory impairment of the casualties.

5.4.3 Triage Categories

All mass casualty triage systems group casualties into large categories. Many systems use five categories that can be identified by an assigned color and/or label. Commonly used color-coded triage categories include the following (see Table 5-2):

➤ *I*mmediate (red)

➤ *D*elayed (yellow)

➤ *M*inimal (green)

➤ *E*xpectant (gray)

➤ *D*ead (black)

Helping responders easily remember the title and priority order of triage categories is important. *ID-MED* provides an easy-to-remember mnemonic for the sorting of live casualties based on the commonly used triage categories of *i*mmediate, *d*elayed, *m*inimal, *e*xpectant and *d*ead. The use of the acronym ID-MED reminds the responder performing triage assignment of the priority ordering of live casualties as well as of the operational task.

Casualty conditions can change over time, necessitating regular reassessment and potential reclassification to a different triage category. Reassessment should be performed as frequently as the situation allows. The need to quickly consider all the casualty and resource factors makes mass casualty triage a challenging process.

TABLE 5-2 Mass Casualty Triage Categories

Triage Category	Description	Color Code
Immediate	Requires immediate care for a good probability of survival	Red
Delayed	Requires care that can be safely delayed without affecting probability of survival	Yellow
Minimal	Sick or injured but expected to survive with or without care	Green
Expectant	Alive, but with little or no chance of survival given current available resources	Gray
Dead	A fatality with no intrinsic respiratory drive	Black

5.4.3.1   Immediate (Red) Triage Category

"Immediate" casualties are those classified as the highest priority to receive care. These are casualties with a life-threatening condition that requires immediate management in order to survive. With immediate care, such casualties are expected to have a good chance at survival (in contrast with the "expectant" category described below).

Examples of immediate casualties include the following:

➤ A 30-year-old man with a large laceration to his left thigh that has uncontrolled, pulsatile bleeding

➤ A 64-year-old woman who is breathing but has no palpable radial pulse

➤ A 4-year-old girl with a fever and acute respiratory distress

➤ A 34-year-old man who is found wandering around after an explosion and now can tell neither his name or where he is nor follow simple commands

5.4.3.2   Delayed (Yellow) Triage Category

The "delayed" category is used for casualties requiring medical intervention for survival, but who have a condition that is less time sensitive than the immediate group. This group of casualties can wait for care for a short period of time without significantly affecting their probability of survival.

Examples of delayed casualties include the following:

➤ An 18-year-old woman who is having abdominal pain but is alert with normal vital signs

➤ A 5-year-old boy with a laceration and deformity to his right forearm, but who is able to move his right hand while crying, "My arm hurts—I want my mommy!"

5.4.3.3   Minimal (Green) Triage Category

The "minimal" category is used for casualties who have minor injuries or illness and are expected to survive even if they do not receive medical attention. In general, because these casualties have the highest chance of survival, they are cared for after the higher-priority casualties. This casualty group should ideally be managed definitively in a manner that prevents them from overloading a nearby hospital that is vital to the management of more acute-severity casualties. The use of secondary treatment centers, urgent care facilities, and alternative care facilities is a consideration for these medical care needs.

Examples of minimal casualties include the following:

➤ A 37-year-old man with bruises, abrasions, and nonbleeding lacerations

➤ A 12-year-old girl with left lower leg pain, but no deformity, good pulses, and normal vital signs

5.4.3.4   Expectant (Gray) Triage Category

Casualties who are triaged to the "expectant" category are those who are considered to have a low probability of survival with the currently available medical resources.

It is entirely possible that a casualty initially triaged as expectant (gray) might actually be triaged as immediate (red) were there greater availability of resources. In fact, the inability to perform a critical lifesaving intervention because of a resource or skill limitation could well force a casualty triaged as immediate (red) to be triaged as expectant (gray). As previously noted, triage is a dynamic process and reassessment is paramount.

Expectant (gray) casualties should also include those likely to die even if all necessary resources were available to care for them. In a mass casualty setting, such resources are better expended on other casualties with higher chances of survival. Expectant (gray) casualties are therefore placed in the lowest priority for treatment and transport.

However, it is important to remember that casualties assigned to the expectant (gray) category should not simply be ignored. Resuscitation should be attempted as soon as sufficient resources become available. Potentially salvageable casualties in this group should therefore be reassessed along with other casualties as the response progresses. At the same time, those who are truly unsalvageable should be afforded comfort care.

Examples of expectant casualties include the following:

➤ A 16-year-old boy with third-degree full-thickness burns over 80% of the body

➤ A 25-year-old man exposed to a known source of ionizing radiation, who reports vomiting and headache starting approximately 15 minutes after the exposure

➤ A 30-year-old woman with a through-and-through gunshot wound to the head with exposed brain matter

5.4.3.5 Dead (Black) Triage Category

A casualty triaged to this category manifests complete absence of the signs of life (ie, detectable life-sustaining cardiopulmonary function). Attempts at basic life-sustaining interventions may be initiated, but only if sufficient personnel are available; such efforts are highly unlikely to be successful and should never detract from the care of other casualties with higher chances of survival.

Casualties categorized as dead (black) are those who are not breathing after basic airway opening maneuvers are attempted. In children, providers may also attempt to give two rescue breaths, ideally using a bag-valve-mask device. However, if there is still no respiratory effort, they too must be considered dead. When there are not sufficient personnel at a scene to treat all of the casualties, a casualty found to be in respiratory or cardiac arrest must be considered dead, and no attempts at resuscitation should be made. This is in contrast to a scene where there are ample personnel and resources, in which mass casualty triage is not employed, and resuscitation should be attempted. Note that there is a very low probability of survival after blunt traumatic cardiac arrest.[12] Therefore, in a mass casualty situation, devoting resources to a blunt trauma casualty in cardiorespiratory arrest would deprive other casualties of life-sustaining resources.

Application of these triage categories to the types of injuries and illnesses likely to occur in a given disaster should be considered in the context of the type of disaster observed. Table 5-3 lists potential triage category assignments (based on acuity, severity, and salvageability) for injuries likely to be encountered in an explosive or incendiary disaster.

TABLE 5-3   Triage Categories of Common Traumatic Injuries

Immediate (Red): severe, life-threatening injuries that require surgical procedures of moderately short duration; high likelihood of survival:

- Mechanical airway obstruction
- Sucking chest wounds
- Tension pneumothorax
- Maxillofacial wounds with potential airway compromise
- Unstable chest and abdominal wounds
- Incomplete amputations
- Exsanguinating hemorrhage
- Second- or third-degree burns involving 40%-60% of total body surface area (TBSA)

Delayed (Yellow): injuries that can tolerate delay prior to surgical intervention without unduly compromising the likelihood of a successful outcome:

- Stable abdominal wounds with possible visceral injury, but without hemodynamic instability
- Soft tissue wounds requiring debridement
- Maxillofacial wounds without airway compromise
- Traumatic crush injuries without crush syndrome
- Traumatic amputation with controlled bleeding
- Immobilized cervical spine injuries
- Smoke inhalation without respiratory distress
- Vascular injuries with adequate collateral circulation
- Major orthopedic injuries requiring operative manipulation, debridement, and external fixation
- Most eye and central nervous system injuries
- Second- or third-degree burns involving 15%-40% of TBSA

Minimal (Green): injuries that require little more than first aid and should be rapidly directed away from the triage area:

- Superficial wounds
- Closed, uncomplicated fractures
- Auditory blast injury
- Psychiatric or emotional disorders
- First- and second-degree burns involving <15% of TBSA

Expectant (Gray): injuries that require an unjustifiable expenditure of limited resources and should be triaged away, *but not abandoned:*

- Agonal respirations
- Profound shock with multiple injuries
- Unresponsive individuals with penetrating head wounds
- Quadriparetic individuals with probable high spinal cord injuries
- Mutilating explosive wounds involving multiple anatomic sites and organs
- Second- and third-degree burns involving >60% of TBSA

In general, rescuers should provide treatment and/or transport to causalities in the immediate (red) group first, then to those categorized as delayed (yellow), then to those categorized as minimal (green), and finally to those categorized as expectant (gray). In some cases, incident command may direct that the most appropriate use of resources will involve combining different categories of casualties. For example, a single ambulance with one provider and a driver might not be able to transport two immediate (red) casualties at the same time, but it might be able to accommodate an immediate (red) casualty on the stretcher, a delayed (yellow) casualty in the patient compartment jump seat, and a minimal (green) casualty in the passenger seat in the front of the vehicle. Alternatively, resources might become available that make transport of less severely injured casualties first more appropriate. For example, a nontraditional transport vehicle like a bus may arrive on scene. Such a vehicle would likely not be appropriate for the transport of casualties categorized as immediate (red), but might be used to evacuate minimal (green) casualties from the scene, even as more severely injured casualties still await transport. Flexibility will allow for better use of resources.

During the course of a disaster, casualty conditions and provider resources can change, so it is important to reassess casualties as time allows. For instance, casualties may decompensate and require assignment to higher triage categories. Also, as more medical resources become available, casualties initially triaged as expectant (gray) may receive necessary care. Last, given the chaotic circumstances of a mass casualty event, mistakes are likely to occur. Reassessment therefore gives rescuers the chance not only to detect changes in casualty status (and hence triage category) as early as possible, but also to correct any initial triage errors that may inadvertently have been made.

5.4.4   Triage Tags and Casualty Care Documentation

Once a casualty has been assessed, it is important for a rescuer to clearly and concisely communicate his or her findings to other rescue personnel. This is typically done by attaching a triage tag to the casualty that identifies the category to which he or she has been assigned. This will help avoid duplication of effort, since subsequent personnel who have contact with that casualty will immediately know the category to which he or she had previously been assigned. If there are no formal triage tags available, it is completely appropriate to improvise. Individuals can be labeled by using makeshift tags made of ordinary paper or by writing on the individual or his or her bandages with lipstick, felt-tip markers, or other means. No matter which method is used, the tag or label should be securely tied (or written) directly to (or on) the person, not to his or her clothing (which may be removed for decontamination, evaluation, or treatment). Tags should account for the dynamic nature of triage and should allow for a casualty's triage category to be changed if his or her condition changes. Some triage tags also contain areas where detailed information can be written to assist subsequent caregivers; this information can become the foundation of the casualty's "medical record." Some agencies will also use separate geographic areas for casualties with different triage categories and may physically move casualties to the areas that have been designated for their individual triage categories.

It is unreasonable to expect care providers in a mass casualty situation to maintain the same level of recordkeeping that is generated during single patient interactions. Some consideration should be given to how care will be documented and what data will be included. The primary reasons are to ensure that continuity of care is maintained and that necessary treatments are not overlooked because of poor communication and the general chaos of such events. Again, this may be as simple as adding notes to the triage tag, writing directly on the individual, developing specific mass casualty care records for prehospital and/or hospital use, or transmitting some type of electronic record. However, plans must be in place for instances in which an event interferes with routine procedure and does not allow communication to occur as it normally would.

5.5   SALT MASS CASUALTY TRIAGE METHODOLOGY

SALT stands for *Sort–Assess–Lifesaving interventions–Treatment/transport*, which are the key activities that must be completed during the triage process (Figure 5-1). SALT triage is intended to facilitate rapid sorting and assessment of casualties of all ages, injured in any type of event, by first responders at the scene of a disaster, once it is safe to enter. SALT triage is designed to optimize survival and to be easy to teach and to remember.

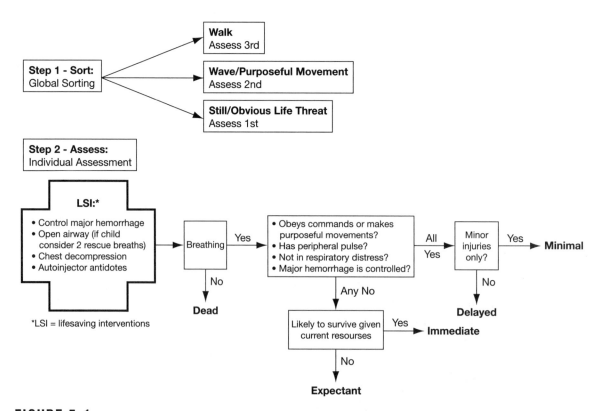

FIGURE 5-1
SALT Mass Casualty Triage

5.5.1 SALT Step 1: Global Sorting

SALT begins with a *global sorting* of casualties, prioritizing them into tiers for individual assessment. In this first step, casualties are asked to *walk* to a designated area. The responder should shout or use a public address system to say "If you need help please move to _____." Those who walk to the designated area are the last priority for individual assessment, because they are the least likely to have a life-threatening condition. Specifically, the ability to walk indicates that they are likely to have the following:

➤ Intact airway, breathing, and circulation (they are unlikely to have severe breathing difficulties or low blood pressure because they are able to walk from the scene)

➤ Intact mental status (because they are able to follow commands)

Those who remain should be asked to *wave* (or follow a command) or be observed for purposeful movement (such as trying to free oneself or self-treat an injury). The responder should shout or use a public address system to say "If you need help, please wave your arm or leg." Those who remain *still* and do not move, and those with obvious life threats (such as major bleeding) are assessed individually first, because they are the most likely to need life-saving interventions. Those who wave are individually assessed next. Those who walked to the designated location are individually assessed last.

It is important to note that the global sorting process will not be perfect. It is an initial attempt to organize numerous casualties, but stable casualties may not follow the direction to move to a designated area, while unstable casualties may be helped or carried by other casualties or bystanders to the designated location. Therefore, all casualties must be individually assessed, even if they are able to walk. It should never be assumed that individuals are minimally injured simply because they have been evacuated by self or others to the designated area. Many possible communication limitations can be encountered during global sorting, which may include noise level, hearing impairment, language barriers, and visual barriers, among numerous others.

5.5.2 SALT Step 2: Individual Assessment

SALT continues with the *individual assessment* of casualties, according to global sorting.

Casualties in the first priority tier (those who could not *walk* to the designated area, did not *wave* or demonstrate similar purposeful movement, and are *still*, or have an obvious life threat) are given rapid life-saving interventions that meet ALL the following criteria:

➤ Can be provided quickly

➤ Can greatly improve a casualty's likelihood of survival

➤ Do not require a care provider to stay with the casualty

➤ Are within the responder's scope of practice

➤ Require only equipment that is immediately available

Lifesaving interventions that meet these criteria include the following:

➤ Opening of the airway with simple basic life support (BLS) maneuvers, including head tilt-chin lift (if trauma is not suspected), modified jaw thrust with spinal motion restriction (if trauma is suspected), or insertion of airway adjuncts (but not advanced airway maneuvers such as endotracheal intubation). In a child, two rescue breaths may also be given, ideally using a bag-valve-mask device, if no breathing is seen

➤ Performing needle decompression if signs of a tension pneumothorax are evident

➤ Control of any major hemorrhage using pressure dressing or arterial tourniquet

➤ Providing autoinjector antidotes to casualties with suspected chemical exposure.

After appropriate lifesaving interventions are performed, casualties should be prioritized for treatment and/or transport by assigning them to one of the five triage categories described above (immediate, delayed, minimal, expectant, or dead):

➤ Casualties who are not breathing even after lifesaving interventions have been attempted should be triaged as *dead* and designated with the color black.

➤ Casualties who are breathing should be assessed for neurologic status and respiratory and circulatory effort (ie, ability to follow commands or make purposeful movements; signs of respiratory distress; uncontrolled hemorrhage; and presence of peripheral pulses).

➤ For those who do not obey commands, OR do not have a peripheral pulse, OR are in respiratory distress, OR have uncontrolled major bleeding, providers should consider whether these individuals are likely to survive given the available resources.

  ➢ If the casualty is judged unlikely to survive, he or she should be triaged as *expectant* and designated with the color gray.

  ➢ If the casualty is judged likely to survive, he or she should be triaged as *immediate* and designated with the color red.

➤ For casualties who do obey commands, AND have palpable radial pulses, AND are not in respiratory distress, AND have no uncontrolled major bleeding, providers should consider whether these individuals' injuries or conditions are minor (ie, they could go untreated without affecting the likelihood of survival or increasing the potential for loss of limb or eyesight).

  ➢ If the casualty is considered to have more serious injuries or conditions, he or she should be triaged as *delayed* and designated with the color yellow.

  ➢ If the casualty is considered to have only minor injuries or conditions, he or she should be triaged as *minimal* and designated with the color green.

Once again, each casualty should be individually assessed as described above, starting with those who during global sorting were still and did not move, followed by those who followed the wave command, and then those who followed the walk command.

5.6 CASUALTY ASSESSMENT

A thorough clinical assessment is the basis for clinical decision making. Once the scene is safe to enter, and as conditions, time, and personnel allow, a more thorough individual assessment consisting of a focused (eg, SAMPLE; see section 5.6.2.1) history and detailed (head-to-toe) physical examination should be completed for each casualty. Medical records and wallet cards with accurate names and addresses, as well as contact information for family members or legal guardians, should be sought while the opportunity to obtain such information still exists. It will be challenging, but nonetheless vitally important, to document the information obtained about each casualty. It should be remembered that casualties may be transported or evacuated to distant health care facilities; thus, the only information that in the end may be available is what first responders are able to collect in the field.

Limitations in diagnostic testing, inaccessible past medical records, and lack of available family members increase the value of well-done and well-documented clinical assessments in the field whenever possible. Additional limitations to obtaining thorough clinical assessments include lack of privacy to expose casualties properly, environmental or weather extremes, and inadequate lighting, among numerous others.

5.6.1 Primary Assessment

During initial assessment, the status of ventilation, oxygenation, and perfusion takes precedence over critical elements of the casualty history and the specific mechanisms and patterns of injury and illness observed in guiding clinical decision making. The initial or primary assessment should be done by standardized methods, such as the guidelines provided by the American College of Surgeons or the American Heart Association, when appropriate. Providers should not take time to obtain casualty history until the functional integrity of the airway, breathing, and circulation has been ensured.

> **Personal Protective Equipment**
>
> No casualty should be examined without some form of PPE being worn by the provider.

A (Airway): Injuries to the airway are rapidly fatal. Hence, prompt assessment for potential airway compromise is the first priority. If the individual can speak, the airway is patent. If respirations are noisy, a partial obstruction is present. If respirations are absent, complete obstruction should be considered, particularly if severe, rocking, "see-saw" chest wall movement is apparent. Initial attempts to establish an airway in trauma include a combined jaw thrust and spinal stabilization maneuver, insertion of an oropharyngeal or nasopharyngeal airway as appropriate, or simply the removal of foreign debris. Individuals unable to protect their own airways should receive a definitive airway either through orotracheal intubation or needle cricothyroidotomy. However, rescue airways may suffice if the equipment or skills for establishing a definitive airway are not available. As stated, measures to establish a patent airway must be instituted simultaneously with measures to stabilize the cervical spine. Rapid extrication from an unstable structure must be weighed against full cervical spine immobilization.

B (Breathing): Airway patency does not ensure adequate ventilation or oxygenation. An injured person may have significant pulmonary injury with or without coexisting airway compromise. For example, a bullet wound might cause tension pneumothorax; blunt trauma might cause flail chest with associated pulmonary contusion; an explosive event might cause barotrauma or systemic air embolism. In individuals with asymmetrically decreased breath sounds, assessment of tracheal position relative to the midline can determine whether there is mediastinal shift, which would indicate a contralateral tension pneumothorax or, rarely, massive hemothorax. The former must be treated immediately by needle thoracostomy, the latter expeditiously by rapid volume resuscitation, followed urgently in both cases with chest tube placement by a qualified provider.

C (Circulation): The first step in addressing circulation is to control all sources of external bleeding. Obvious sources of external hemorrhage should be initially controlled with direct pressure and pressure dressings. The appropriate use of tourniquets is now a necessary clinical skill for all medical providers who may be involved in managing acutely and potentially severely injured patients. Thus, if conventional methods fail to control bleeding, the use of commercially manufactured arterial tourniquets, such as the C-A-T® (Combat-Application-Tourniquet®), and topical hemostatic agents, such as Quikclot® powder (zeolite) or gauze (kaolin) and HemCon® (chitosan), may be considered. The use of arterial tourniquets and topical hemostatic agents has been shown to control life-threatening hemorrhage in the military setting, especially for traumatic amputations caused by improvised explosive devices (IEDs), and their use should be considered for similar types of injuries in civilian trauma as well (see Chapter 6).[13-16] However, the role of neither of these modalities has yet been scientifically validated in the civilian setting.

Once life-threatening hemorrhage has been controlled, the individual's hemodynamic status should be assessed by evaluation of vital signs in conjunction with clinical signs of perfusion: the level of consciousness, skin color and temperature, peripheral pulses, and capillary refill time. Shock, if not due to other causes such as tension pneumothorax or profound hypoxia, must be assumed to be the result of hemorrhage. Cool clammy skin, pallor, and thready pulses characterize hypovolemic shock. In the field setting, efforts should focus initially on control of external hemorrhage. If an individual appears to remain in shock once external hemorrhage has been adequately controlled, immediate, rapid volume resuscitation should be initiated, ideally with an isotonic balanced salt solution. If in a hospital setting, rapid transfusion with appropriate blood components should be considered when the patient's hemodynamic status does not improve quickly.

Recently, the Military Committee on Tactical Combat Casualty Care has made recommendations for the management of trauma patients with hemorrhagic shock. Recommendations in the Seventh Edition of the Pre-Hospital Trauma Life Support (PHTLS) Course indicate that individuals with uncontrolled internal hemorrhage should be resuscitated if they have a change in mental status or if they become unconscious (due to the hemorrhage) and should be resuscitated to an improvement in mental status (corresponding to a systolic blood pressure of approximately 80-90 mm Hg or a mean arterial pressure of 65 mm Hg).[17] These recommendations for hypotensive resuscitation may also be reasonable to follow in the disaster setting to minimize hemorrhage and conserve resources, because clinical and experimental evidence has shown that large fluid boluses and rapid infusions have resulted in increased bleeding and mortality.[18,19]

Once the ABCs have been addressed, the primary assessment should focus on detecting life-threatening concerns, such as unconsciousness or altered mental status, and identifying signs of significant intracranial injuries, neurologic function impairment, serious intrathoracic or intra-abdominal organ system signs, or even toxidromes.

D (Disability): Additional assessment of disability reminds providers to document the baseline neurologic status, which is important because it may impact subsequently on management and prognosis and it can provide rapid early indication of significant intracranial injuries. Examining the pupil size and response, the motor function of the extremities, and the level of consciousness by using the Glasgow Coma Scale (GCS) or its pediatric modification, as appropriate (Table 5-4 and Table 5-5, respectively), can indicate an intracranial mass lesion as well as evaluate mental status. The motor response component of the GCS has the strongest association with severe injury and has been demonstrated to have a 94.6% sensitivity for field triage.[20]

E (Exposure and environment): This cue reminds the provider to visually and palpably screen all external body surfaces of the casualty for evidence of injury. While practical considerations at the scene, such as need for rapid extrication and evacuation, ambient temperature and weather conditions, and many others, may affect one's ability to temporarily disrobe a casualty, the importance of completely exposing the individual cannot be overstated. In conjunction with police, explosive ordnance disposal teams, or other appropriately trained personnel, the casualty should be searched for any weapons, chemical contamination, or forensic evidence. Hypothermia may develop during resuscitation, so measures such as warmed intravenous fluids, warmed blankets, and removal from a cool environment as quickly as feasible are important considerations.

TABLE 5-4   Glasgow Coma Scale (GCS)

Best Eye Opening Response	Best Oral Response	Best Motor Response	Score
		Obeys commands	6
	Oriented	Localizes pain	5
Spontaneous	Confused	Withdraws from pain	4
To voice	Inappropriate words (mumbling)	Flexion to pain	3
To pain	Incomprehensible sounds (moaning)	Extension to pain	2
None	None	None	1

TABLE 5-5   Glasgow Coma Scale (GCS) Pediatric Modification

Best Eye-Opening Response

>1 year of age	<1 year of age
4: Spontaneously	Spontaneously
3: To oral command	To shout
2: To pain	To pain
1: No response	No response

Best Oral Response

>5 years of age	2 to 5 years of age	0 to 23 months of age
5: Oriented and conversive	Appropriate words and phrases	Smiles, coos, cries appropriately
4: Disoriented and conversive	Inappropriate words	Cries
3: Inappropriate words	Cries/screams	Inappropriate crying/screaming
2: Incomprehensible sounds	Grunts	Grunts
1: No response	No response	No response

Best Motor Response

>1 year of age	<1 year of age
6: Follows command	Not applicable
5: Localizes pain	Localizes pain
4: Flexion withdrawal	Flexion withdrawal
3: Flexion abnormal (decorticate)	Flexion abnormal (decorticate)
2: Extension (decerebrate)	Extension (decerebrate)
1: No response	No response

5.6.2   Secondary Assessment

After all immediately life-threatening injuries are identified and treated in the primary assessment, the secondary assessment begins. A consistent and methodical approach to casualty history, and thorough physical examination, are the mainstays of evaluation.

5.6.2.1   Casualty History

Obtaining casualty history is vitally important. It should be recorded if at all possible. One reasonable approach is the "SAMPLE" history advocated by most life support training organizations (*S*ymptoms, *A*llergies, *M*edications, *P*ast illnesses, *L*ast meal, *E*vents and environment). The SAMPLE history can serve to alert the treating health care provider to injury and illness status, as well as potential comorbidities that may affect provision of care. Additional history from eyewitnesses and scene responders, as well as situational reports from incident command, should be sought when time allows.

5.6.2.2 Casualty Physical Examination

The secondary assessment continues with a detailed head-to-toe physical examination. If possible, the individual should be completely disrobed to allow thorough examination to be performed, so as not to miss significant injuries. In field settings, this can be complicated by environmental conditions or similar circumstances. Once the physical examination has been completed, it is essential that casualties be kept warm and that they be covered appropriately to prevent any further deterioration in their conditions.

5.6.3 Implications of Personal Protective Equipment (PPE) for Casualty Management

As noted in Chapter 4, PPE may be needed during the primary encounter with casualties at the scene of a disaster. If hazard assessment at the scene or known contamination or exposure of a casualty requires levels of PPE beyond the usual barrier methods for avoiding blood or bodily fluid contamination that should be utilized during every casualty encounter, it may be difficult to assess the casualty and may be technically challenging to perform clinical interventions. If lifesaving interventions cannot easily be provided because of the level of PPE required at the scene, it is recommended that the casualty be rapidly evaluated by trained personnel then rapidly decontaminated and moved to a clean area for further medical evaluation and treatment. If it is not possible to rapidly decontaminate the casualty, whatever supportive measures are available should be provided to the casualty, as long as they pose no significant risk to scene responders.

It is important for all scene responders and health care providers who use higher levels of PPE to be properly trained and experienced in the limitations and restrictions likely to be encountered. The PPE necessary to operate in a contaminated environment can significantly impede the ability of health care personnel to use their basic senses:

➤ Touch may be impaired by the type of gloves being worn by the responder.

➤ Smell may be impaired by the type of airway protection utilized by the responder (eg, self-contained breathing apparatus, or SCBAs; powered air-purifying respirators, or PAPRs; nonpowered air-purifying respirators, or APRs).

➤ Hearing may be impaired by the type of airway protection utilized by the responder, the necessity for hearing protection, and loud noises in the immediate environment.

➤ Sight may be limited if visual fields are narrowed peripherally or otherwise obscured by the type of airway protection utilized by the responder.

5.7 CASUALTY TRANSPORT AND EVACUATION

Evacuation from a disaster scene involves the evacuation of both casualties and rescue personnel from an acutely hazardous environment or situation. Scene evacuation can become complicated if there is nowhere for casualties to go or if resources to evacuate casualties are severely limited. Some individuals may be able to self-evacuate from the scene under direction from incident command, but many will need either assisted evacuation or medical evacuation. Initial evacuation is a coordinated effort by multiple local agencies, particularly police, fire, and EMS, under the supervision of incident command. Evacuation does not require ambulance transport for all injured or ill people.

Casualties must be prioritized for treatment as well as transport to definitive care. The disposition options for injured and ill people include treatment at and release from the scene, transportation to local hospitals, and transport to secondary hospitals. A top priority is to avoid overwhelming the closest hospitals. Equitable and rational distribution of casualties among available regional facilities reduces the burden on each hospital to a manageable level, potentially even to nondisaster levels. At times, definitive care may be hundreds of miles away. Methods of executing safe and efficient movement of casualties, as well as family and others, may need to be arranged through local, regional, and national resources. This function may require coordination among multiple private vendors, nongovernment relief organizations, and many governmental agencies.

Transport officials should have a good working knowledge of local and regional hospital and transport capabilities to distribute casualties throughout the area. Burn victims, pediatric casualties, those with multisystem trauma, and those with certain injuries requiring hyperbaric therapy should be sent to the appropriate specialty hospital. Stable individuals with minor injuries should be distributed evenly and equitably among medical centers in the region. Institutionalized patients and homebound patients with special health care needs should be known to the regional EMS system in advance, and specific plans should be developed to ensure their timely evacuation. Ideally, balanced casualty distribution will be achieved via a centrally controlled EMS system working with incident command in collaboration with a regional Health Emergency Operations Center (HEOC). Such operations should be planned in advance and exercised both as tabletop drills and as full-field exercises before being executed in an actual disaster situation.

Protecting the overall safety and security of casualties in transit is a difficult undertaking. Transport distances can be considerable, requiring technical support such as short-range (rotary wing; ie, helicopters) and long-range (fixed wing) aircraft in addition to prolonged ground evacuation methods. The use of distant health care facilities places many challenges on the operations of this evacuation. Surge evacuation is the transfer of disaster-affected people seeking health care services to distant facilities. This is necessary when local medical surge capacity and capabilities become grossly exceeded in volume, acuity, or specific service need (eg, hemodialysis, other medical or surgical subspecialty care). Deterioration of clinical health status during prolonged transit is likely. Appropriate observation and monitoring by medical providers, on-board medical equipment, access to emergency care in transit, and routine dosing of essential medications are some of the operational challenges typically encountered. Meeting the basic comfort care needs of casualties (eg, temperature-controlled evacuation vehicles, sufficient on-board food and water, access to toilets/restroom facilities) can also present significant challenges.

5.8 MASS FATALITY MANAGEMENT

The initial focus of any mass casualty event is to provide care and transport to potential survivors. Unfortunately, first responders also may encounter dead casualties, which requires an understanding of the fundamentals of mass fatality management.

The importance of not disrupting the remains of the deceased or displacing their personal belongings or other important nearby items is key. Personal identification, linkage of personal items to the remains, and evidence gathering are some of the important reasons not to disrupt the remains or displace surrounding items, as such disruptions and displacements may delay the identification process. However, it is no less important for responders to know and understand a crucial exception to this rule: when the remains or their effects are blocking access to live casualties, they must be moved. Therefore, while the forensic objective is to cause as little disruption as possible, an area that could contain live casualties should never be avoided because of the presence of remains.

It is also vitally important for all responders to remember that mere exposure to dead casualties generally poses no significant health risk.[21,22] Thus, the hazard assessment in the search and rescue area and at the casualty collection point, not unfounded fears or concerns over the presence of dead bodies in the surrounding area of operations, should guide responders' and receivers' actions.

Once the scene has been cleared of live casualties, including those in the expectant triage category, the focus can shift from casualty management to fatality management. This involves many action steps and organizational procedures, including moving the deceased to morgues, identifying them, determining cause of death, returning personal effects to family members unless retained for forensic purposes, and making final disposition decisions for the bodies. All of this must be done while preserving evidence and maintaining its chain of custody for law enforcement to investigate the cause of the incident. This requires the coordination of efforts from numerous agencies, including EMS, public health, health care, public safety, and morgue personnel. It is important to note that, much like mass casualty management, mass fatality management can involve a geographically defined scene, such as a building collapse, or may involve a more diffuse area, such as would be seen during an infectious disease outbreak.

Depending on available personnel and their skill sets, mass fatality management may take place in parallel with mass casualty management. The local medical examiner (coroner in some jurisdictions) or designee will likely oversee the implementation of the mass fatality plan and typically has the authority under law to do so. This person is responsible for:

➤ Taking charge of dead bodies and human remains associated with the disaster

➤ Identifying and examining remains

➤ Moving the deceased to the morgue(s) (permanent or temporary)

➤ Maintaining custody of the bodies until they are released

➤ Determining cause of death

➤ Returning personal items to family members

➤ Making final disposition decisions for the bodies

➤ Determining and recording cause of death and the circumstances surrounding the death

➤ Issuing death certificates

Mass fatality management is discussed in more detail in the ADLS® course (v3.0) and supporting course manual.

5.8.1   Mass Fatality Event Definition

The definition of a mass fatality incident is similar to that of a mass casualty event. A mass fatality event occurs when the number of deaths exceeds the ability of local jurisdictions to care for them. This may mean that a community alters its typical process for fatality management or needs other agencies or communities to provide additional resources. There is no predefined number of deaths that constitutes a mass fatality event; like a mass casualty event, the definition is based on resource availability.

5.8.2   Field Fatality Management

Field fatality management involves locating, sorting, and removing bodies and body parts as well as personal effects from the scene and securely transporting them to an identification center or temporary morgue where they can be safely preserved. Human remains should always be treated with dignity and respect and kept covered whenever possible, away from public view and scavenging animals. Each body or body part should be tagged. Unless otherwise indicated, the responder should assume that the site is a crime scene. This means that the chain of custody for potential forensic evidence must be maintained at all times. Documentation of how and where remains were found must also be maintained as requested for investigational purposes.

Recovery of human remains begins after a thorough, careful, well-documented review of the scene has been completed. Only after approval by the forensic expert in charge can bodies and body parts be moved to an identification center or temporary morgue. If bodies need to be moved to temporary locations for safety or logistical reasons, these locations should be away from public view and scavenging animals whenever possible.

5.8.3   Morgue Operations

Once a facility has been established, various stations may be set up for the examination of remains. These stations will be used for evaluation of cause of death and collection of evidence related to potential criminal activities that are being investigated surrounding the event. They will also be used to initiate identification of the remains.

When possible, remains are identified by means of documents found with or near the casualty, but definitive identification in this manner may not be possible. In these cases, identification may need to be facilitated by documentation brought to the facility by family members, friends, or other community resources. Confirmation of identification may require the expertise of pathologists, anthropologists, DNA experts, dentists, and mortuary affairs specialists. Successful identification is of great importance because it carries legal, ethical, religious, and financial significance.

Areas will also need to be set up for holding bodies and allowing family members to view and/or visit the remains of their loved ones. This becomes especially important when there is an ongoing criminal investigation and bodies cannot be quickly released to families or funeral homes. Morgue access must be well controlled because crowds are likely to assemble as people search for their loved ones. This means that fatality management plans should include the resources and personnel for providing security. Record keeping and organization of morgue data must be meticulous. Chain of custody procedures must be followed to the letter whenever there is a concern that the incident may have resulted from a crime. This includes managing personal effects of casualties as potential evidence and returning them to family members when appropriate.

Facility management includes the activities necessary to allow the morgue—which may also serve as an identification center, whether temporary or permanent—to function. That would include maintenance of refrigeration, radiology and laboratory facilities, security, and crowd control. Resources for running such facilities may be provided by a response team, such as a National Disaster Medical System (NDMS) Disaster Mortuary Operational Response Team (DMORT). Similar to a Disaster Medical Assistance Team (DMAT), a DMORT may be mobilized if an incident is declared a federal disaster. The DMORT can provide needed personnel and equipment, possibly including a Disaster Portable Morgue Unit (DPMU). However, for small incidents and prior to mobilization of a DMORT, local medical examiners or coroners will need to acquire local resources for responding to potential mass fatality events in their communities.

Bodies must be kept cool to forestall decomposition. Emergency preparedness plans therefore need to identify resources for providing refrigeration. This may involve recruiting refrigerated trucks, or even buildings with refrigerated areas, for temporary storage of bodies. These temporary storage areas require a reliable source of power to maintain operations for the entire time they are being used. Predisaster planning must also consider the long-term implications for those trucks or facilities after the event has concluded, as it may not be considered socially desirable to return them to their original purpose (eg, transport or storage of food products). Recently, DMORTs have tested a commercially available device called a Mortuary Enhanced Remains Cooling System (MERCS). The device is small and portable and can be made operational in 15 minutes.

5.8.4 Provider and Survivor Management

Dealing with dead and expectant casualties is difficult for providers and survivors alike. Appropriate mental and emotional support should be made available as part of the recovery effort. Family Assistance Centers are sites where families and loved ones can gather and be protected from the media and the public. Authorities can meet regularly with the families and update them as needed. It is often at these facilities that families will be notified about the fate of their loved ones. Grief counselors and spiritual advisors should be there to provide support during this process to both survivors and providers.

5.9   CASUALTY REPORTING, IDENTIFICATION, AND TRACKING

All casualties transported to area hospitals, alternate care facilities, or morgues should first be identified at the scene, so they can be accounted for and tracked. Records must indicate all facilities that receive casualties. Mechanisms should be in place to help relatives, neighbors, and emergency management personnel identify persons who are still in danger and need assistance. This includes mechanisms to help reunite families and loved ones after an event, as well as assist efforts to identify missing persons.

5.9.1   Casualty Reporting

Casualty reporting includes a broad range of activities that over the course of an event will become increasingly detailed. In the initial minutes of the response, it may be as simple as reporting the number of casualties to incoming responders and hospitals that are preparing to receive them. Later in the event, the focus may shift to informing family or friends of casualty location and condition. Reporting of disease or injury surveillance findings to public health entities, or potential criminal activities to law enforcement agencies, may also be required. It will also be important to report the general situation to the community at large via media reports citing the number of dead and injured and the current status of the event (eg, all casualties have been moved from the scene to local hospitals).

There will also be concern regarding how to balance individual rights to privacy with the general recovery of the community. This must be done in accordance with applicable standards for protection of personal health information and regulations such as the privacy rules established under the Health Insurance Portability and Accountability Act (HIPAA), which may allow some modification for disasters. This is best addressed through planning that takes into account the needs and desires of the community.

5.9.2   Casualty Identification and Tracking

The importance of identifying individual casualties and tracking their movements cannot be overlooked and must be considered a crucial part of every responder's duties. Efforts to identify and track casualties should begin when they are first individually assessed and assigned to triage categories, including those categorized as expectant and dead. For deceased casualties, tracking will be done as part of mass fatality management. Regardless of the system a community uses to track casualties, time must be taken both to populate that system with basic identifying information and to keep that information with the individual. The quality and depth of the information initially available will likely improve as the casualty moves through the medical system. Moreover, with each level of care, the casualty's condition or available medical resources may improve. This may allow casualties to provide more information about themselves and/or allow medical staff more time to identify the casualty and gather more information. However, it is also possible that a casualty's condition might worsen during the course of care, underscoring the importance of gathering as much information as possible during initial contact with each casualty and keeping that information with him or her.

Depending on the resources of the community and the setting of the event, tracking information can be maintained in a variety of ways, from using a formal electronic system, to writing information on a triage tag, to simply recording information on a piece of tape attached to a casualty's arm. This documentation should include basic patient information, since time and personnel constraints may prevent responders from documenting the detailed information they would collect under normal circumstances. Basic information should include, at a minimum, the individual's name, date of birth, location found, triage category, and destination. A community's formal tracking system may be as simple as having information provided by radio or paper recorded at a dispatch center or as comprehensive as having an electronic system that generates a database of casualty information. Many communities have begun using bar or similarly coded triage tags that provide each casualty with a tracking number. If such a system is used, this number should also be recorded and reported to facilitate casualty tracking. A limited number of complete tracking systems for mass casualty situations have been developed over the years. These all-in-one systems were specifically designed to address the issues of casualty identification, care records, reporting, and tracking.

Regardless of the approach used, all response plans should include a defined system for casualty tracking. All responders should make every attempt to contribute to tracking efforts while performing their duties.[23] Plans should also include contingencies for when common means of communication are not functioning, or loss of power or other necessary infrastructure limits the capacity of systems to operate as planned.

As was seen during the aftermath of Hurricane Katrina, tracking evacuees as well as casualties is vital. Few will forget the huge numbers of children who were separated from their families and the number of days it took to reunite them.[24] Identification and tracking of the remains of nearly 3000 casualties in the aftermath of the events of September 11, 2011, was also an enormous task. In response to the issues that were faced during this process, the State of New York, with the support of a federal grant, developed the Unified Victim Identification System. This system identifies and catalogues DNA from disaster victims in a database that is then used for reporting.

5.10 PROFESSIONALISM AND ETHICS IN MASS CASUALTY CARE

At a disaster scene, adherence to established health practices and professional conduct is paramount. Clinical decision making must always be guided by defined— hence defensible—practices that are based both in science and in customary acts when compared with the moral, ethical, and acceptable practice of medicine, nursing, or allied health professions. Simply stated, would a peer-professional make similar decisions or take similar actions if faced with the same circumstances and situations? This question should be a filter for each disaster-based casualty clinical decision. If the answer is "no," the assistance of like-trained professionals should be sought if at all possible before such decisions or actions are implemented. Professionalism goes beyond just clinical decision making.

Volunteer as well as career responders should follow incident command policies to protect the privacy and confidentiality of disaster victims (eg, taking of photographs, unless authorized for purposes of identification). Responders should not talk to media representatives unless permitted by a supervisor and/or public information officer. If the responder has any questions regarding the release of casualty-related information, the assigned supervisor will provide guidance. All must adhere to local, state, and federal laws at all times.

Professionalism is also about maintaining safety and security at all times. Proper identification of all health personnel is an important safeguard. It is therefore necessary to keep a photo identification badge visible at all times. Responders must adhere to established safety standards and protocols and wear appropriate PPE at all times. They must also maintain situational awareness by staying alert and reporting any hazardous conditions immediately. Responders should also demonstrate cooperation, efficiency, integrity, and accountability with respect to the duties assigned. This includes adhering to the chain of command and following duly authorized instructions. For many in the health professions, large-scale disasters create conflicting obligations. For example, the need to take care of personal responsibilities (eg, the responder's own health status) may sometimes outweigh the obligation to perform professional duties.

Cultural and ethical issues may be potential flash points. Notions of modesty and respect, as well as status, may have to be considered, both to eliminate the potential for conflict and to provide compassionate care for all affected populations. Whenever feasible, decontamination should be done with considerations of modesty taken into account. Mass casualty situations may require bodily exposure and performance of diagnostic and treatment procedures in public settings. For certain subcultures and religious groups, the amount of the human body that may be displayed to those outside the family or to providers of the opposite sex can differ considerably from customary patterns in the industrialized world. Even though the casualty may realize that such exposure is necessary, this can create considerable discomfort. Compassion must therefore be maintained and discretion exercised during all efforts to care for the ill and injured.

Separation of sexes is also important, not only for reasons of modesty, but also for security concerns, particularly prevention of predatory activities. Men and women must therefore be properly separated. In addition, children must be properly protected from potential predatory activities. For these reasons, decontamination lanes should always be separated by sex and include sufficient security to maintain them in that manner.

Challenging ethical dilemmas will be encountered, particularly when authorities make decisions for the distribution of scarce resources and for access to limited health care services. Interventions may be limited both by resource availability and by outcome potential. A large-scale disaster in a heavily populated area could produce hundreds, if not thousands, of casualties, involving traumatic injuries, burns, and other medical problems. Medical systems throughout most of the industrialized world are currently operating at near full capacity. Hospitals and pharmacies generally use just-in-time inventory systems. As a result, supplies of many, if not all, medically necessary pharmaceuticals and equipment will be exhausted early in the response phase to a catastrophic event. This reality will require new thinking and new approaches to the treatment of large numbers of casualties. Triage paradigms in such situations will have to take into account the realities of limited resources for a potentially unlimited number of casualties. The federal and certain state and municipal governments have made some attempts at developing guidelines for ventilator allocation in pandemic influenza.[25]

As noted, difficult decision making is best left to a group process through seeking peer consensus whenever feasible. The effectiveness of group decision making was evident from the experience of the military field hospital that was established by the Israeli Defense Forces in Haiti shortly after the earthquake in Port au Prince in 2010.[26] Changing medical requirements at the scene require that health responders operate with maximum flexibility and versatility regarding triage, treatment, and transport policies and priorities.[27] Ethical dilemmas in mass casualty care are discussed further in the CDLS® and ADLS® courses (v3.0) and supporting course manuals.

5.11 SUMMARY

A mass casualty or mass fatality event occurs when the number of victims overwhelms the resources available to care for them. A similar event may not be considered a mass casualty or mass fatality event in another community because of its different capabilities and capacities. By familiarizing themselves with the basic principles for managing mass casualty and mass fatality events, providers can better respond when such events occur.

The initial goal of mass casualty triage is to sort and assess casualties to identify those with life-threatening injuries and initiate lifesaving treatment as soon as feasible. Once this is done, casualties with less serious injuries can be further assessed and triaged for transportation from the scene on the basis of treatment priority and available resources.

Primary and secondary assessment, ideally performed once the casualty has been evacuated from the scene and simply documented as time and resources allow, follow mass casualty triage. Performing such assessments and related interventions while wearing cumbersome and sensory-limiting PPE, documenting clinical information, and even keeping a triage tag on a given casualty throughout triage, treatment, and transport, are some of the challenges that may be encountered during mass casualty management in large-scale disasters.

Fatalities are an unfortunate reality of the mass casualty response. While most medical responders will not have a formal role in mass fatality management, it is important that all potential responders understand the fundamentals of handling fatalities, including the importance of preserving evidence and identifying remains. Initial fatality management principles also include knowing to move fatalities only if they prevent responders from accessing and attempting to keep personal effects with the deceased to facilitate identification. In addition, a basic understanding of actual health risks posed by dead bodies and how to protect oneself and other responders from these risks is critical.

The importance of casualty reporting, identification, and tracking was seen after the September 11, 2001, disasters and Hurricane Katrina. In both instances, the recovery phase involved numerous people searching for loved ones. In the heat of response, when people need medical attention to save their lives, it is easy to overlook the value of time spent on documentation. Sparing a few seconds or minutes to contribute information to casualty tracking systems, whether they are electronic, paper, or oral, may spare families days of anguish wondering about the fate of their loved ones. Tracking should be considered a responsibility of all providers who may have contact with any casualties throughout the continuum of care (eg, from the field to the hospital to the morgue).

The importance of maintaining professionalism and ethical decision making during mass casualty care is paramount. Clinical decisions based in science, customary practice, and peer-review consensus should guide care during altered care situations. Cultural, ethnic, religious, gender, and age-appropriate sensitivities must be addressed whenever feasible. Professionalism involves adherence to proper personal and group safety and security measures at all times. Challenges will arise during times of disaster, and it is important to comply with, inform, and seek assistance from the proper chain of command.

REFERENCES

1. Hogan DE, Waeckerle JF, Dire DJ, Lillibridge SF. Emergency department impact of the Oklahoma City terrorist bombing. *Ann Emerg Med.* 1999;34:160-167.

2. Jenkins JL, McCarthy ML, Sauer LM, et al. Mass-casualty triage: time for an evidence-based approach. *Prehosp Disaster Med.* Jan-Feb 2008;23(1):3-8.

3. Garner A, Lee A, Harrison K, Schultz CH. Comparative analysis of multiple-casualty incident triage algorithms. *Ann Emerg Med.* Nov 2001;38(5):541-548.

4. Nocera A, Garner A. An Australian mass casualty incident triage system for the future based upon triage mistakes of the past: the Homebush Triage Standard. *Aust N Z J Surg.* Aug 1999;69(8):603-608.

5. Romig L. The JumpSTART Pediatric MCI Triage Tool. January 2, 2008. http://www .jumpstarttriage.com/JumpSTART_and_MCI_Triage.php. Accessed February 10, 2008.

6. Wiseman DB, Ellenbogen R, Shaffrey CI. Triage for the neurosurgeon. *Neurosurg Focus.* Mar 15 2002;12(3):E5.

7. Hodgetts T, Hall J, Maconochie I, Smart C. Paediatric triage tape. *Prehosp Immediate Care.* 1998;2:155-159.

8. Lerner EB, Schwartz RB, Coule PL, et al. Mass casualty triage: an evaluation of the data and development of a proposed national guideline. *Disaster Med Public Health Prep.* 2008;2(suppl 1):S25-S34.

9. Benson M, Koenig KL, Schultz CH. Mass casualty triage: START, then SAVE—a new method of dynamic triage for victims of a catastrophic earthquake. *Prehosp Disaster Med.* Apr-Jun 1996;11(2):117-124.

10. Hines S, Payne A, Edmondson J, Heightman AJ. Bombs under London: the EMS response plan that worked. *JEMS.* Aug 2005;30(8):58-60, 62, 64-57.

11. Lerner EB, Cone DC, Weinstein ES, Schwartz RB, Coule PL, Cronin M, et al. Mass casualty triage: an evaluation of the science and refinement of a national guideline. *Disaster Med Public Health Preparedness.* 2011;5:129-137.

12. Willis CD, Cameron PA, Bernard SA, Fitzgerald M. Cardiopulmonary resuscitation after traumatic cardiac arrest is not always futile. *Injury*. May 2006;37(5):448-454.

13. Beekley AC, Sebesta JA, Blackbourne LH, Members of the 31st Combat Support Hospital Research Group. Prehospital tourniquet use in Operation Iraqi Freedom: effect on hemorrhage control and outcomes. *J Trauma*. 2008;64:S28-S37.

14. Kragh JF, Walters TJ, Baer DG, et al. Practical use of emergency tourniquets to stop bleeding in major limb trauma. *J Trauma*. 2008;64:S38-S50.

15. Kragh JF, Walters TJ, Baer DG, et al. Survival with emergency tourniquet use to stop bleeding in major limb trauma. *Ann Surg*. 2009;249:1-7.

16. McManus JG, Wedmore IS. Modern hemostatic agents for hemorrhage control: a review and discussion of use in current combat operations. *Business Briefing: Emerg Med Review*. 2005. http://www.touchbriefings.com/pdf/1334/ACF444.pdf

17. Salomone JP, Pons PT, McSwain NE, eds. *PHTLS: Prehospital Trauma Life Support*. 6th ed. St Louis, MO: Mosby Elsevier; 2007.

18. Bickell WH, Wall MJ, Pepe PE, et al. Immediate versus delayed fluid resuscitation for hypotensive patients with penetrating torso injuries. *N Engl J Med*. 1994;331:1105-1109.

19. Sondeen JL, Coppes VG, Holcomb JB. Blood pressure at which rebleeding occurs after resuscitation in swine with aortic injury. *J Trauma*. 2003;54(5 suppl):S110-S117.

20. Meredith W, Rutledge R, Hansen AR, et al. Field triage of trauma patients based upon the ability to follow commands: a study in 29,573 injured patients. *J Trauma*. 1995;38:129-135.

21. World Health Organization (WHO). Management of dead bodies in disaster situations. Disaster Manuals and Guidelines Series, No 5. http://www.paho.org/english/dd/ped/DeadBodiesBook.pdf. Accessed June 16, 2010.

22. Centers for Disease Control and Prevention (CDC). Interim Health Recommendations for Workers Who Handle Human Remains After a Disaster. http://emergency.cdc.gov/disasters/handleremains.asp. Accessed June 16, 2010.

23. Recommendations for a National Mass Patient and Evacuee Movement, Regulating, and Tracking System. AHRQ publication AHRQ-09-0039-EF. http://archive.ahrq.gov/prep/natlsystem/. Accessed August 16, 2010.

24. National Center for Missing and Exploited Children. Hurricane Katrina Success Stories. http://www.missingkids.com/missingkids/servlet/PageServlet?LanguageCountry=en_US&PageId=2102. Accessed August 16, 2010.

25. Powell T, Christ KC, Birkhead GS. Allocation of ventilators in a public health disaster. *Disaster Med Public Health Prep*. 2008;2:20-26.

26. Merin O, Ash N, Levy G, Schwaber M, Kreiss Y. The Israeli field hospital in Haiti—ethical dilemmas in early disaster response. *N Engl J Med*. 2010;362:e38. http://www.nejm.org/doi/pdf/10.1056/NEJMp1001693. Accessed March 25, 2011.

27. Kreiss Y, Merin O, Peleg K, et al. Early disaster response in Haiti: the Israeli field hospital experience. *Ann Intern Med*. 2010;153:45-48. http://www.annals.org/content/153/1/45.full.pdf+html. Accessed March 25, 2011.

CHAPTER | SIX

Explosions and Traumatic Disasters

CHAPTER CHAIR

Arthur Cooper, MD, MS

CONTRIBUTING AUTHORS

Alexander Eastman, MD, MPH

Raymond E. Swienton, MD

Michael Wainscott, MD

Daniel B. Fagbuyi, MD

6.1 PURPOSE

This chapter describes principles and practices for the management of explosions and traumatic disasters. It reinforces the general concepts of situational awareness, incident management, workforce protection, and casualty management, which were explained in Chapters 1–5 of this manual. The application of these principles in the context of explosions and traumatic disaster preparedness, mitigation, response, and recovery is described. Casualty management guidance for unique and specific injuries related to traumatic and explosive disasters is provided.

6.2 LEARNING OBJECTIVES

After completing this chapter, readers should be able to:

➤ Discuss the background and epidemiology of explosions and traumatic disasters, including the vulnerability of civilian populations, limited scientific literature basis and case-based examples.

➤ Discuss three primary types of explosions that should be considered in disaster preparedness and response planning.

➤ Describe the four blast-related mechanisms of injury related to explosions and traumatic disasters.

➤ Identify important hazard-specific considerations involved in the preparedness and response to explosions and traumatic disasters.

➤ Discuss clinical decision making relevant to explosions and traumatic disasters, including immediate lifesaving interventions and organ system–specific injury and illness management.

➤ Identify individuals who may be at increased health risk in an explosion or other traumatic disaster.

Learning objectives for this chapter are competency-based, as delineated in Appendix B.

6.3 BACKGROUND

Explosions and traumatic disasters occur commonly throughout the world, attributed to terrorism, conflict-based disasters, industrial mishaps, transportation incidents, and structural collapse, among other causes. The more widespread use of bombs and improvised explosive devices (IEDs) is a concern for health professionals and counterterrorism experts worldwide. To prepare effectively, those who will be tasked with mitigating the consequences of these incidents when they occur must become proficient not only in the mechanics of these incidents, but also in all aspects of the care of people affected by trauma and explosives.

Civilian populations are vulnerable to such disasters; typically common gathering places or highly populated urban areas will be targeted or impacted directly by these events. Because the time available to prepare for such disasters prior to their occurrence is minimal, these types of disasters require quick decisions and fast action on the part of emergency medical providers. Despite widespread concern over biologic and chemical attacks, conventional explosive devices are by far the most commonly used terrorist weapons, accounting for about 75% of all terror events worldwide; firearms are responsible for most of the rest.[1] Bombings and shootings causing multiple civilian casualties are dramatic and gain immediate public attention, accomplishing the terrorist's motive of causing immediate panic much more readily than in the case of an insidious bioweapon attack.

There is a solid scientific basis for the majority of basic and advanced trauma management. The same cannot be said for explosions and traumatic disasters, as much of the published literature is retrospective and anecdotal.[2-6] The nature of such events (which commonly occur without warning, suddenly overwhelming response efforts) limits documentation and data capture. Such events are also not amenable to rigorous scientific design methodologies or experimental modeling. The tragic events of September 11, 2001, have spurred tremendous efforts in disaster training and research, as medical and civic leaders recognize that a mass traumatic event can strike any community on an overwhelming scale at any time. For example, in addition to the 2,752 deaths at "Ground Zero" in New York and the 189 deaths at the Pentagon outside Washington, DC, on that date, New York City area and National Capital Region hospitals treated 1,103 and 106 patients, respectively, hospitalizing 181 and 57 of them, many of them affected with severe burns.[7-14] Moreover, untold numbers continue to suffer psychological sequelae from the attacks, especially posttraumatic stress disorder (PTSD).[15-17]

While there have been several other domestic civilian disasters of a similarly massive scale in the United States prior to September 11, 2001, 6 of them were associated with death tolls exceeding 1000, 4 of which were due to natural disasters. In fact, except for 2001, bomb-related deaths in the United States have been fewer than 50 per year.[18] Even so, the number of criminal bombings in the United States has doubled in the last decade, and the probability of future terrorist attacks on US soil is very likely.[19]

6.4 TYPES OF EXPLOSIONS

There are three general types of explosions: nuclear, mechanical, and the most common type, chemical. A basic understanding of these types of explosions is helpful in determining the mechanisms of injury that may result following explosions.

6.4.1 Nuclear Explosions

The most powerful type of explosion is nuclear. The explosive power from the alteration of atomic and subatomic structures is catastrophic in its destructive impact, with the force to destroy urban centers. The basic science and mechanisms of injury in nuclear explosions is described in Chapter 7, "Nuclear and Radiologic Disasters."

6.4.2 Mechanical Explosions

Mechanical explosions are the result of a physical process, rather than a nuclear or chemical reaction. A boiling liquid expanding vapor explosion (BLEVE) is an example of a mechanical explosion. When an enclosed vessel or container holding a liquid under pressure is exposed to heat sufficient to raise the temperature of the contained liquid above its boiling point, a BLEVE can occur. If the container is damaged, either from corrosion of or damage to the container, and a leak subsequently develops, the resulting sudden drop in pressure causes violent boiling of the remaining liquid, followed by vigorous release of its vapor. This in turn causes a rapid, secondary increase in pressure inside the enclosed vessel, which then explodes, because the vapors accumulate faster than they can decompress via the existing leak. BLEVEs can result in significant explosions and traumatic disasters. Although infrequent, BLEVEs usually occur as industrial or transportation accidents (eg, railroad tank car, tank trailer on an 18-wheeler). Both flammable and nonflammable liquids (eg, water, liquid nitrogen, liquid helium, other refrigerants) stored or transported under pressure can result in BLEVEs. If the liquid is flammable, which is often the case, a large fireball follows as the result of a fuel air explosion (ie, vapor cloud explosion).

6.4.3   Chemical Explosions

Chemical explosions are the most common type of explosions. They result from the rapid chemical conversion of a solid or liquid explosive material into a rapidly expanding gas, with an ensuing energy release. Explosives are arbitrarily considered "high energy" or "low energy," depending upon whether or not the speed of the explosion exceeds the speed of sound (approximately 343.2 m/sec, or 1,126 ft/sec, in dry air, at standard temperature and pressure [STP]).

Low-energy explosives release energy progressively by a rapid combustive process called *deflagration*, defined as the stepwise ignition of flammable solids or liquids in layers, producing an advancing front that moves at *less* than the speed of sound. Examples of common low-energy explosives are petroleum products (such as Molotov cocktails) and black powder ("gun" powder).

High-energy explosives release energy immediately by a sudden explosive process called *detonation*, defined as the instantaneous transformation of solid or liquid material into gases, producing a *blast wave* that moves at *more* than the speed of sound, filling the same volume within a few microseconds, putting the adjacent physical space under extremely high pressure. The highly pressurized gases expand rapidly and compress the surrounding medium (air or water), generating a pressure pulse that is propagated as a radial blast wave in all directions at speeds from 1500 to 9000 m/ sec. Following this, a chaotic *blast wind* occurs as the contiguous air fills the relative vacuum that travels behind the blast wave. Examples of common high-energy explosives are nitroglycerine (a liquid mixture of glycerol with nitric and sulfuric acids); dynamite (a mixture of nitroglycerine and diatomite invented by Alfred Nobel); gel-ignite (a polymer bonded dynamite); 2,4,6-trinitrotoluene (TNT); triacetone triphosphate (TATP); Semtex (a ubiquitous plastic explosive); and ammonium nitrate-fuel oil (ANFO) mixtures. An ideal, or nonreflected, blast wave is depicted in Figure 6-1.[20-21]

The initial, almost instantaneous, rise in pressure gives blast waves associated with high-energy explosives the unique characteristic of *brisance*, or shattering ability. Low-energy explosives do not release energy fast enough to have brisance. The magnitude of the positive phase impulse (PPI) or "peak overpressure" is the primary determinant of the severity of blast injury and is governed by three factors:[21]

1. *The size of the explosive charge:* The larger the charge, the greater the peak overpressure will be and the longer its duration.

2. *The distance from the blast:* The peak overpressure is inversely proportional to the cube of the distance from the blast. Nearby presence of

reflecting or absorbing surfaces, such as walls or other people, will alter the peak pressure.

3. *The surrounding medium (air or water):* Because water is denser than air, blast waves propagate farther underwater, and the positive phase impulse will last longer.

The negative phase impulse (NPI) contributes significantly to the overall blast injuries. The combined effects of PPI and NPI, causing shattering and shearing forces, contribute to the mechanisms of injuries from explosions.

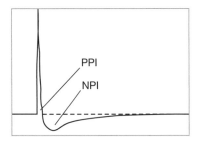

FIGURE 6-1
Idealized blast wave as it passes over a fixed point in space. The X-axis represents elapsed time; the Y-axis represents arbitrary units of pressure. NPI indicates negative phase impulse; PPI indicates positive phase impulse.[21]

It is vital to recognize that when reflected by a solid surface, multiple blast waves are created, and the combined or additive effects may be magnified by many times the amount of the pressure generated by the original incident wave, such that a complex pattern of overpressures is created.[22] Thus, individuals who are between the blast and a wall, or who are in corners, can have injuries several times more severe than what would be expected for a given blast pressure.[23] A recent Israeli study reported an 8% overall mortality rate in open-air terrorist bombings, but a 49% mortality rate in bombings in enclosed spaces. Similarly, the incidence of primary blast injuries in enclosed spaces was twice that seen in open-air bombings. Body armor may protect from penetrating injury, but may also act like a wall around the chest, thus exacerbating any blast effect.[24]

The most common type of industrial accident that results in a explosion and traumatic disaster involves ammonium nitrate fertilizer. The April 16, 1947, disaster in Texas City, Texas, was such an event and is regarded as the worst industrial disaster in US history, killing 581 individuals and maiming 3500 others. The April 19, 1995, bombing of the Alfred P. Murrah Federal Building in Oklahoma City, Oklahoma, which killed 168 people, including 19 children, and injured 853 others, also mainly resulted from the explosion of ammonium nitrate fertilizer and was the deadliest terror attack to occur on American soil prior to September 11, 2001.

The most common devices now utilized by terrorists are enhanced blast weapons and improvised explosive devices (IEDs). These weapons use blast overpressure to exert their effects but can produce casualties through multiple mechanisms including secondary and tertiary effects.[25] IEDs are weapons that can be made of almost any type of explosive and can be concealed in almost any type of container. They are "homemade" devices designed to cause death or injury by using explosives alone, or in combination with metallic objects or toxic substances, and range from simple parcel and pipe bombs to larger backpack and truck bombs. It is the ease with which their components can be obtained and concealed that have made them the weapon of choice for most terrorists worldwide in recent years.[5,26-33]

6.5 MECHANISMS OF BLAST INJURY

Multiple mechanisms of injury are related to blast effects on the human body. Understanding these mechanisms of injury is informed by a basic knowledge of the types of explosions described in the preceding section. Important variables, such as the type of blast material used, location of the blast relative to the casualty, and surrounding medium of the explosion, are all important considerations affecting resulting injury patterns and severity of injuries.

Blast injuries associated with explosions are typically caused by chemical explosions. The blast wave, blast wind, the resulting disruptions in the local environment, and their effects on the human body are the basis for the blast mechanisms of injury. The mechanisms of injuries are described as primary, secondary, tertiary, and quaternary.

6.5.1 Primary Blast Injury

Primary blast injury (PBI) is caused by the blast wave, as described above. As the blast wave itself passes through the body, it causes damage by several different mechanisms. On a molecular level, *spalling* occurs when particles from a denser medium are thrown into a less-dense medium as the pressure wave passes through. In the lungs, for example, particles of liquid spall into the alveolar space, much as water is thrown into the air in an underwater explosion.[34] Blast waves passing through organs containing pockets of gas, such as the ears or the sinuses, cause *implosion* of the air pockets, followed by rebound expansion once the wave has passed. Because air is easily compressible by a passing blast wave while fluid-containing tissues are not, the differential *inertia* associated with these substances allows *shearing* to develop at such air-fluid interfaces, thereby causing the tearing and disruption of adjacent body tissues.

Primary blast injury is essentially a form of barotrauma that is unique to explosions, which causes damage to air-filled organs. These injuries are limited to high-energy explosives and result from the impact of the overpressure wave with body surfaces. Body parts that are gas filled, such as the lungs, gastrointestinal (GI) tract, and middle ear of the auditory system, are most susceptible. The traumatic injuries from primary blast injuries that may occur are listed in Table 6-1. Except for "blast ear," which may result from overpressures as low as 5 pounds per square inch (psi), the presence of the other traumatic injuries requires a live casualty to have been fairly close to the epicenter of the explosive event, as the blast wave dissipates quickly with distance.

TABLE 6-1 Traumatic Injuries from Primary Blast Injuries

Blast ear	Tympanic membrane rupture and middle ear damage
Blast lung	Pulmonary barotrauma
Blast belly	Abdominal hemorrhage and perforation
Blast eye	Globe rupture
Blast brain	Traumatic brain injury without physical signs of head injury

PBIs are certainly not the most common injury caused by explosives, but their true incidence is unknown. PBIs may have a subtle and delayed presentation and may be easily missed in a mass casualty incident or event when providers are faced with multiple casualties with more dramatic and overt injuries. Individuals with a PBI injury may present with no outward sign of trauma or injury. It should be noted again that the wearing of body armor does not necessarily protect personnel from the barotrauma produced by the blast wave.[35] PBIs should be specifically considered in all blast casualties to avoid unnecessary morbidity and mortality. It is also important to remember that in open-air bombings, the incidence of PBI will be less than in enclosed space bombings.

6.5.2   Secondary Blast Injury

Secondary blast injury (SBI) is also caused by the forces associated with the blast wave. SBI results in penetrating or blunt trauma caused by the acceleration of fragments and debris by the blast through or against body surfaces. SBIs may derive from primary bomb elements (ie, fragmentation of the explosive device container and its contents) or secondary elements from the surrounding environment (ie, the powerful blowing of objects in the area of the explosion whose inertia is overcome by the force of the blast). Because they can strike any part of the body, all parts of the body can be affected.

Secondary blast injuries are typically responsible for the majority of casualties resulting from an explosive event. SBIs are the most common type of blast injury in part because the casualties need not be in close proximity to the epicenter of the explosive event, as is the case for PBIs. SBIs were a significant cause of morbidity in the bombing of the Alfred P. Murrah Federal Building in Oklahoma City, Oklahoma, as the building had a glass façade that shattered and was propelled over an area of many city blocks.[36]

Weapons and explosive devices are often designed to increase the likelihood of SBIs. Terrorists often deliberately pack small metal objects, such as nuts, bolts, screws, nails, or ball bearings, around an explosive in an attempt to increase secondary blast injuries. Military shell casings are specifically designed to fragment to achieve a similar goal (the eponymic term "shrapnel" should be discarded, as it refers to a specific type of fragmenting artillery shell used during World War I but no longer used today). Fragment injuries occur in 20% to 40% of blast casualties, with increased incidence in enclosed spaces. At missile speeds of 50 feet per second, skin may be lacerated. At speeds of more than 400 feet per second, body penetration and significant tissue damage are likely.[34]

6.5.3 Tertiary Blast Injury

Tertiary blast injuries (the abbreviation "TBI" is rarely used, to avoid confusion with "traumatic brain injury") occur when the individual is propelled through the air (body displacement) by the blast wind or when a structure collapses with resultant casualties. The momentum imparted by the force of the blast may propel the person against a stationary object, causing injury on impact.[36] With body displacement, typical injury patterns of blunt trauma occur as the body strikes a solid object or the ground. A high-explosive blast wind may propel a 75 kg adult with an acceleration of nearly 15 times the force of gravity. Such an event results in a high incidence of skull fractures, head injuries, and long bone fractures, but because the individual is thrown, any body part can be affected. The types of injuries that could occur from body displacement could also include closed or open head injury, blunt chest and abdominal trauma, impalement injury, or traumatic amputation.

The structural collapse of buildings and other structures may lead to compartment syndromes, as well as crush, entrapment, and blunt force injuries, and are responsible for the high mortality rate.[4] Length of entrapment time has been shown to double mortality in people who cannot be extricated for 24 hours or more, due chiefly to acute renal failure, even though they may reach the hospital alive.[37]

6.5.4 Quaternary Blast Injury

Quaternary blast injuries are described as additional injuries beyond primary, secondary, and tertiary injuries. This group contains several important physical mechanisms of injury including fire, toxic contaminants, dangerous fumes, dust, smoke, and other environmentally -based substances, as well as the associated psychological mechanisms of injury.

Some of the conditions included in quaternary blast injuries are listed in Table 6-2. These associated injuries, and the exacerbation of underlying chronic diseases in blast casualties, adds markedly to the complexity, morbidity, and mortality of blast or explosive events.

TABLE 6-2 Injuries and Illnesses Associated with Quaternary Blast Injury

Burn injuries (flash, partial, and full thickness)
Toxidromes from chemical exposures
Inhalation injury
Respiratory distress from asthma or chronic obstructive pulmonary disease (COPD)
Acute coronary syndrome (ACS) or acute myocardial infarction (AMI)
Hypertensive emergencies
Psychosocial and behavioral emergencies

Another important consideration in this type of blast injury is the intentional inclusion of substances that may cause more injury, illness, or panic. The radiation dispersal device (RDD), or "dirty bomb," is an example of this, and is described in greater detail below and in Chapter 7, "Nuclear and Radiologic Disasters." The purposeful addition of adulterants that result in tissue contamination or systemic illness are referred to as quinary blast injuries in some literature.[38,39]

6.6 SITUATIONAL AWARENESS AND DETECTION

It is important to remain focused on the basic principles of the all-hazards approach to disaster casualty management in the initial response to explosions and traumatic disasters. Specific preparedness planning for areas identified in local or regional hazard vulnerability analyses should be incorporated into the strategic readiness wherever possible. This may include industrial facilities, hazardous materials transportation routes, presence of military installations, and other likely "targeted" areas or events when considering explosions and traumatic disasters. Terrorism, or any individual or group that is motivated to use violence within our communities, places every mass gathering event or well-populated area on a list of concern.

The likelihood of intentional "targeting" of the emergency response community and health facilities (ie, "secondary devices") must be considered during any explosion or traumatic disaster occurrence until appropriate law enforcement agencies have eliminated such threats.

It is worth reviewing the all-hazards approach to hazard assessment at the scene, as reinforced in the DISASTER Paradigm™, which demonstrates the importance of continual observation and careful reinspection of the scene. Practical questions that should be considered by all responders at the scene of a explosion and traumatic disasters are listed in Table 6-3.

TABLE 6-3 Assessing Hazards at the Scene of an Explosion or Traumatic Disaster

Are there downed power lines?

Is there debris and trauma at the scene?

Do you see fire and people with burns?

Are blood and body fluids apparent on the scene?

Do you see any hazardous materials?

Is there smoke or toxic inhalants?

Do you see a structural collapse or a structure that looks like it could collapse?

Are there any reports of possible secondary devices on the scene?

Is there the possibility of exposure to chemical/biologic/radioactive material?

Site safety after an explosive event, structural collapse of an occupied building, or any other cause of large-scale traumatic injuries is challenging. The threat of additional detonations or further collapse is of particular concern. This is demonstrated starkly by the fact that most of the fatalities among rescue personnel on September 11, 2001, occurred when the World Trade Center towers collapsed. While instances of this "second hit" phenomenon have occurred far more frequently in international human conflict zones (Palestinian intifada, asymmetric warfare in Iraq and Afghanistan), it is important to note that such events have also occurred within the United States (Atlanta Olympic and nightclub bombings, school and abortion clinic shootings, in addition to the World Trade Center towers collapse). Despite the urgent needs of injured people, first responders must refrain from entering the disaster scene until it has been declared safe by duly authorized public safety officials. The same rule applies to sites of potential evacuation. Casualties should not be moved to such sites until they, too, have been deemed free of potential hazards. The Jonesboro, Arkansas, mass shooting (1998) is a good example of this. The school-age perpetrators of this massacre activated a fire alarm that forced individuals outside the building where they were well within their line of fire.

As mentioned previously in this chapter, first responders and receivers must also contend with possible contamination of casualties with chemicals or radioactive materials, either in the case of in industrial incident or terrorist event. While industrial mishaps involving toxic chemicals occur with some frequency, there have been no reported incidents to date involving a "dirty bomb." Even so, the threat of such an intentionally contaminated explosive device, or the possibility of explosions at nuclear power plants, mandates early screening for radiological contamination as well as chemical contamination, for which close coordination with both radiation safety officials and industrial hygiene officials is of vital importance. It is important to note that the presence of a hazardous material may not be immediately obvious. Providers must maintain a high index of suspicion and initiate screening for toxic substances after any explosive event thought to be intentional or terrorist related.

6.7   CLINICAL DECISION MAKING

The information obtained through casualty history and the primary and secondary assessments are the basis for determining a differential diagnosis or list of probable injuries or organ systems affected. The possibility of contaminants with chemical, biologic, and radioactive agents should be considered.

Once a patient is transported to a medical treatment facility, a complete physical examination (including a careful otoscopic examination) should be performed. Laboratory and radiologic evaluation should be obtained as indicated to include hemogram, coagulation studies, basic metabolic profile, urinalysis, and standard trauma radiographs, including lateral cervical spine, chest, and pelvic X rays. More advanced imaging such as the Focused Assessment with Sonography for Trauma (FAST) examination, computed tomography (CT) of the head, spine, chest, and abdomen, as well as other diagnostic methods, may be utilized depending upon clinical findings and resource availability.

Table 6-4 shows an overview of explosion-related physical injuries commonly seen in various organ systems.

TABLE 6-4 Overview of Explosion-Related Injuries

System	Injury or Condition
Auditory	Tympanic membrane rupture, ossicular disruption, cochlear damage, foreign body
Eye, Orbit, Face	Perforated globe, foreign body, air embolism, fractures
Respiratory	Blast lung, hemothorax, pneumothorax, pulmonary contusion and hemorrhage, A-V fistulas (source of air embolism), airway epithelial damage, aspiration pneumonitis, sepsis
Digestive	Bowel perforation, hemorrhage, ruptured liver or spleen, sepsis, mesenteric ischemia from air embolism
Circulatory	Cardiac contusion, myocardial infarction from air embolism, shock, vasovagal hypotension, peripheral vascular injury, air embolism–induced injury
CNS Injury	Concussion, closed and open brain injury, stroke, spinal cord injury, air embolism–induced injury
Renal Injury	Renal contusion, laceration, acute renal failure due to rhabdomyolysis, hypotension, and hypovolemia
Extremity Injury	Traumatic amputation, fractures, crush injuries, compartment syndrome, burns, lacerations, acute arterial occlusion, air embolism–induced injury

Source: http://www.bt.cdc.gov/masscasualties/explosions.asp.[40]

6.7.1 Lifesaving Skills

Most casualties with lethal injuries will die immediately. Approximately 10% to 15% of casualties with critical injuries (mainly secondary and tertiary blast injuries) may be saved with appropriate management.[5,41,42] Immediate lifesaving interventions and emergency care for any unstable casualty should not be withheld from any patient regardless of contamination status, provided that appropriate PPE is worn. The fundamental principles and skills of basic life support and advanced life support should be followed in caring for all casualties of explosions and traumatic disasters. Once decontaminated, therefore, all casualties should initially be managed in accordance with Pre-Hospital Trauma Life Support (PHTLS), Advanced Trauma Life Support® (ATLS®), and Advanced Burn Life Support (ABLS), Advanced Trauma Care for Nurses® (ATCN®), and Trauma Nursing Core Course (TNCC) guidelines.[43-47]

6.7.2 Pulmonary Blast Injury

The hallmark of pulmonary trauma from a primary blast injury (PBI) is an injury to the respiratory system, called "blast lung." The enormous pressure differentials generated in explosions tear the delicate alveolar walls and disrupt alveolar capillary interface, leading to multifocal hemorrhage, hemothorax, pneumothorax, traumatic emphysema, or alveolovenous fistulae. Communication between the airways and the pleural space will lead to pneumothorax, which, in an already compromised lung, can cause even more rapid respiratory failure.

The signs and symptoms of pulmonary PBI may include difficulty completing sentences in one breath, rapid shallow respirations, poor chest wall expansion, hemoptysis, decreased breath sounds, or wheezes. Individuals with alveolovenous fistulae may develop hemoptysis or arterial gas embolism. Arterial gas embolism results from passage of gas from the alveoli to the pulmonary venous system, to the left side of the heart, and finally to systemic circulation (see Section 6.7.3). A person with arterial gas embolism will most commonly present with signs and symptoms of stroke with an acute neurological deficit. Individuals may also present with an acute coronary syndrome if air bubbles enter the coronary circulation. Although particulate irritants or worsening of preexisting heart or lung disease may also present with similar symptoms, respiratory insufficiency following an explosion should be first assumed to be caused by a blast injury and should be treated as such. Chest radiograph in these cases will show the characteristic "butterfly" pattern of hilar-based, fluffy infiltrate.

The treatment of pulmonary PBI focuses on correcting the effects of barotrauma and supporting gas exchange. Pulmonary PBI can cause acute respiratory insufficiency within minutes to hours after an explosive event. Those with immediate and severe respiratory distress or massive hemoptysis have less chance of survival, and a definitive airway should be placed. In those with only mild to moderate respiratory distress, oxygenation should be supported by a non-rebreathing mask. Any activity should be minimized, because exertion following a blast has been shown to increase the severity of PBIs.[6,48-51] Casualties with asymmetric breath sounds should be managed with needle thoracostomy (a large-bore angiocatheter, greater than 3.5" in length in an adult and 1.5" in a child to ensure pleural penetration, inserted into the pleural space through the second intercostal space at the midclavicular line) followed by chest tube placement to decompress the pneumothorax. Special care should be taken in the intubated patient with evidence of pulmonary blast injury to avoid hyperventilation and high peak and plateau airway pressures, as these may cause (or worsen) tension pneumothorax or arterial gas embolism. Some providers, therefore, advocate prophylactic placement of bilateral chest tubes in pulmonary PBI before positive pressure ventilation begins.[52,53]

If mechanical ventilation is unavoidable, pressure controlled modes and permissive hypercapnia to facilitate oxygen exchange while keeping airway pressures at less than 35 cm of water are recommended.[54] Refractory hypoxemia has been managed successfully with ventilatory strategies used in acute respiratory distress syndrome, namely pressure controlled inverse ratio ventilation, independent lung ventilation, high frequency jet ventilation, and as a last resort, extracorporeal membrane oxygenation.[49] Deterioration of individuals after positive pressure ventilation following pulmonary blast injury is often attributed to arterial gas embolism.

6.7.3   Arterial Gas Embolism

As mentioned in the previous section, a dreaded complication of pulmonary PBI is the development of arterial gas embolism, which is thought to be responsible for most of the sudden deaths that occur within the first hour after blast exposure. Air emboli result from direct communication between the bronchial tree and disrupted pulmonary vasculature. Air may enter the pulmonary venous system as a result of a positive pressure gradient caused by low venous pressure (as in hypovolemia), increased airway pressure (as in positive pressure ventilation or tension pneumothorax), or both. Importantly, only those with clinical evidence of pulmonary PBI seem to be at risk.

Arterial gas embolism often manifests as rapid decompensation immediately following intubation and positive pressure ventilation. Such a collapse is usually unresponsive to resuscitation.[49] While vascular obstruction from air bubbles may occur anywhere, the most catastrophic are those in the coronary or cerebral circulation. As little as 2 ml of air injected into the cerebral circulation can be fatal. Signs and symptoms correspond to the location of embolic occlusion, including blindness due to air in retinal vessels, focal neurological deficits, loss of consciousness following cerebral obstruction, and chest pain from myocardial ischemia following coronary obstruction. Air emboli to the skin may produce cutis marmorata, a reddish-blue mottling discoloration of the skin. Tongue blanching may also be seen. Arterial gas embolism is likely to be the cause of rapid death solely from PBI in immediate survivors.[49]

Management of suspected air embolism begins with simultaneous placement in the left lateral decubitus and Trendelenburg positions, to sequester air bubbles in the tips of the right and left ventricles, and the administration of supplemental 100% oxygen, which promotes not only short-term oxygenation, but also absorption of arterial bubbles. A primary goal is to keep airway pressure less than intravascular pressure to minimize further risk of arterial air embolism, which is generally the case in the spontaneously breathing patient. In the intubated and ventilated patient, airway pressures should be kept as low as possible while still maintaining adequate oxygenation and ventilation. Overzealous ventilation or high positive inspiratory pressures must be avoided. If it is possible to determine which lung is injured, it should be positioned dependent to the left atrium. Alveolar pressure can thereby be made lower than vascular pressure. If unilateral, the injured lung may be isolated by selective intubation of the uninjured lung. Right mainstem intubation can be reliably accomplished by advancing a normally placed endotracheal tube (ETT) distally until left-sided breath sounds disappear.

Left mainstem intubation may be accomplished with a 92% success rate by turning the individual's head 90 degrees to the right, rotating the ETT 180 degrees, and passing it distally.[49] If cervical spine injury is a concern, an alternate method is to rotate a normally placed ETT 90 degrees counterclockwise before advancing it. If lung isolation and resuscitation are unsuccessful, immediate thoracotomy and hilar clamping may be needed. The definitive treatment for arterial air embolism is hyperbaric oxygen therapy. Nonemergent surgery should be delayed, and regional or local anesthesia is preferred in those needing immediate surgery.

6.7.4 Traumatic Asphyxiation

Traumatic asphyxia occurs when the chest is suddenly and markedly compressed by a heavy object to such a degree that both respirations and venous return to the heart are impeded. The sharp increase in thoracic and superior vena cava pressure and the lack of valves in the vessels result in retrograde flow of blood and transmission of pressure from the right heart into the great veins of the head and neck. Children seem to be more vulnerable to traumatic asphyxiation owing to their relatively more pliable and cartilaginous chest walls.

Traumatic asphyxia is seen following a variety of disasters. Natural disasters (particularly earthquakes) or any event with structural collapse, as seen in the 1981 Kansas City Hyatt Hotel Skywalk collapse, or a crowd surge, such as that seen in various international soccer stadium riots, are likely to be associated with traumatic asphyxia.

Although individuals with traumatic asphyxiation often present quite dramatically, the condition itself is usually relatively benign and self-limiting in those who survive the initial asphyxial insult. Signs and symptoms may include respiratory distress, chest wall ecchymoses, facial edema or cyanosis, subconjunctival and retinal hemorrhages, and pinpoint petechiae of the head, neck, and chest. Cerebral hypoxia or anoxia may lead to altered mental status, seizures, or coma. The morbidity and mortality of traumatic asphyxia is largely due to prolonged respiratory embarrassment or anoxic neurological insult.

Rapid extrication and release from compression is the single most important factor in improved survival. The violent compressing forces needed to cause traumatic asphyxia are sufficient to warrant extreme caution in these individuals, as there is a high likelihood of potentially lethal associated injuries. Mortality from asphyxia results primarily from pulmonary constriction, whereas morbidity is primarily caused by neurological damage. Treatment should thus focus on aggressive support of the respiratory and neurological systems. Control of the airway and ventilatory support are paramount.

6.7.5   Traumatic Amputation

Traumatic amputation or mangling due to primary blast injury has become one of the two signature injuries of asymmetric warfare in the Middle East, the other being blast-related traumatic brain injury. Until recently, American civilian rescue personnel have generally been taught to avoid using tourniquets, except as a last resort, due to the near certainty of distal tissue ischemia associated with their use. However, American military experience with tourniquets in response to blast-related traumatic amputation or mangling due to land mines and improvised explosive devices (IEDs) has led to reconsideration of this device. Unfortunately, published data on tourniquet use in the civilian environment is scant. Even so, in cases of traumatic amputation or severe mangling of an upper or lower extremity in domestic civilian practice, tourniquet use is indicated, based on extrapolation from military medical experience with commercially manufactured tourniquets, such as the Combat Application Tourniquet® (C-A-T®). Commercially manufactured tourniquets are strongly preferred to provider-improvised tourniquets due to the time required to deploy the latter as well as their uncertain efficacy.[55,56] A detailed protocol for application of the Combat Application Tourniquet® (C-A-T®) may be found in the *Advanced Disaster Life Support Course Manual 3.0*, Chapter 7, "Mass Casualty Management," or by accessing the manufacturer's Web site.[57,58]

6.7.6 Crush Injury

Crush injuries are common when explosions or traumatic disasters cause structural collapse, as individuals may become pinned beneath debris. Compression of a large mass of skeletal muscle for as short a time as 20 minutes impedes tissue perfusion and leads to tissue ischemia and rhabdomyolysis. Direct injury to the sarcolemmal membrane causes sodium, calcium, and water to enter muscle cells, while potassium, phosphorous, lactate, myoglobin, thromboplastin, and creatine kinase are released from them. Sufficient quantities of the latter substances can be toxic in the systemic circulation. Persistent crushing force, ironically, serves temporarily as a protective mechanism, preventing these potential toxins from reaching the central circulation until the force is removed.

Crush syndrome is an ischemia reperfusion injury and refers to the systemic complications of traumatic rhabdomyolysis. When an entrapped individual is extricated and blood flow into the damaged tissue is restored, toxins are released, leading to the various metabolic derangements characteristic of this potentially deadly syndrome. The syndrome consists of: 1) destruction of muscle mass; 2) compromise of local perfusion; and 3) prolonged compression.[59,60] Severe hyperkalemia may also occur due to massive muscle breakdown (75% of body potassium is stored in skeletal muscle), potentially leading to cardiac dysrhythmia and cardiac arrest. Hypocalcemia is another early complication that can be triggered by the release of large amounts of phosphate from lysed muscle cells. Massive sodium and water shifts cause third space loss of fluid into damaged muscle tissue. This relative hypovolemic state, together with the negative inotropic effects of hyperkalemia and hypocalcemia, can lead to profound shock.

Acute renal failure and disseminated intravascular coagulation (DIC) are late complications of crush injury, and both are associated with high rates of morbidity and mortality. Any delay in resuscitation following a crush injury will increase the likelihood of renal failure. Acute renal failure in this setting is due to a combination of several factors, including volume depletion, metabolic acidosis, renal vasoconstriction, released nephrotoxins, and the precipitation of myoglobin in the distal renal tubules. Release of tissue thromboplastin from damaged muscle may lead to coagulopathy or DIC, further complicating the clinical picture. Myoglobinemia in sufficient quantities creates a pinkish tinge to the plasma and a brownish, tea-like color to the urine, which gradually turns green when exposed to sunlight. An electrocardiogram may show changes due to hyperkalemia, including peaked T waves or wide-complex ventricular tachydysrhythmias.

Prevention of crush syndrome by early and aggressive management of crush injury is the key to effective treatment. The principles of management of crush injury include urgent volume expansion, recognition and treatment of major metabolic derangements, prevention of acute renal failure due to rhabdomyolysis, and management of established acute renal failure. Fluid management in this setting is controversial, with some experts advocating for immediate intravenous cannulation and saline infusion as soon as a limb is exposed, and, if possible, prior to full extrication.[61] Certain guidelines even advocate delaying full extrication until volume resuscitation has begun.[59]

Monitoring of blood pressure, central venous pressure, and urine output should be employed as soon as possible in order to guide fluid resuscitation, resources permitting. Normal saline is the crystalloid of choice. Lactated Ringer's solution should not be used, as it has added potassium and may trigger the development or worsening of hyperkalemia. The infusion rate should be approximately 1 to 1.5 L per hour, with an ultimate goal of 200 to 300 mL/hr of urine output until myoglobinuria has ceased. This aggressive infusion rate dilutes the various constituents such as myoglobin and uric acid that might otherwise precipitate in the distal renal tubules and lead to acute renal failure.

Massive amounts of fluid may be required, but in a mass casualty, it may be prudent to administer a more limited amount of fluid to avoid complications resulting from a lack of close medical supervision. Some authorities have suggested alkalinization of the urine via the infusion of bicarbonate in order to correct acidosis, prevent renal precipitation of myoglobin, and reduce the risk of hyperkalemia. This approach, however, is controversial, because it may worsen hypocalcemia or cause calcium phosphate deposition in various tissues and has not shown added benefit in prospective trials. Similarly, the use of mannitol to stimulate osmotic diuresis remains controversial, as it is mostly supported by experimental animal studies and retrospective clinical studies.

Treatment of hyperkalemia (the most proximate cause of mortality in crush syndrome) should be initiated if there is any evidence of hyperkalemic cardiotoxicity (peaked T waves or QRS prolongation greater than 0.12 seconds). Intravenous glucose and insulin (1 ampule $D_{50}W$ and 10 units regular insulin intravenously) or an inhaled β_2-agonist (such as albuterol) may help to temporarily shift the extracellular potassium into the intracellular space. The potassium exchange resin sodium polystyrene sulfonate (Kayexalate®), 30 to 60 g PO/PR, may be used to promote intestinal elimination of potassium, but its actions are delayed. Intravenous administration of calcium to treat hyperkalemia may be ineffective in the presence of the hyperphosphatemia caused by muscle necrosis, as the calcium may rapidly combine with the extracellular phosphate to cause metastatic calcification. Thus, its use should be reserved for severe hyperkalemia or symptomatic hypocalcemia (tetany, seizure). For individuals with persistent hyperkalemia, acidosis, or acute renal failure, emergent hemodialysis is necessary. Peritoneal dialysis and continuous arteriovenous hemofiltration have been used successfully in disaster situations when dialysis machines or electricity were in limited supply.

6.7.7   Compartment Syndrome

The development of compartment syndrome is a complication of crush injury. Tissue edema inside of the confining fibrous sheath of a muscle compartment can cause an increase in pressure within the compartment, resulting in decreased blood flow and additional injury to the nerves and muscles within the compartment. The injury may not be immediately apparent, and the compressed region may initially appear normal. One of the earliest signs of compartment syndrome is severe pain, especially with passive flexion of the extremity. Erythema at the wound margins and blistering of the adjacent skin may also occur. As the compartment syndrome evolves, the individual may become hypotensive or show symptoms of shock. Marked tenderness, bruising, and swelling can be seen, and the patient may experience numbness and flaccid paralysis which can mimic spinal cord injury, although sphincter tone should be preserved. Distal pulses may or may not be present. Field fasciotomies are controversial, and the risk of bleeding and infection must be weighed against the potential benefit.[62,63] However, they should be performed as soon as possible by a qualified first receiver upon arrival at a definitive care facility.

6.7.8   Gastrointestinal Blast Injury

Gas-containing abdominal organs are injured in a similar manner and at similar over-pressures as the lung. However, primary blast injuries to the abdomen or "blast belly" may be overshadowed by the more immediately life-threatening manifestations of "blast lung." Gastrointestinal injuries are even more common than pulmonary injuries in immersion or enclosed space blasts.[33,64,65] A gastrointestinal blast injury tends to affect the colon and spare the small bowel, owing to the greater amount of gas in the former. Damage may range from edema to hemorrhage to frank rupture. Colonic rupture, although possible acutely, is generally occult and delayed, occurring after stretching and ischemia lead to bowel wall weakening. Shear forces caused by the blast may occasionally tear the mesentery, but nonbowel or solid organ injuries after explosions are more likely due to conventional blunt or penetrating mechanisms. Signs and symptoms are nonspecific and include abdominal pain, nausea, vomiting, diarrhea, tenesmus, decreased bowel sounds, rebound tenderness, guarding, and rectal bleeding.

6.7.9   Auditory Blast Injury

A blast injury to the auditory system occurs at much lower overpressures than pulmonary or gastrointestinal injuries. As a frame of reference, extremely loud acoustic waves, such as those generated at a rock concert, are generally <0.04 psi. An increase in pressures as little as 5 psi may cause tympanic membrane rupture.[66] Blast-related damage to the inner ear can cause an acute sensorineural hearing loss that can be quite incapacitating in the moments following an explosion, often leading those affected to ignore oral instructions or even secondary explosions due to acute hearing loss. Other common symptoms of auditory PBI include vertigo, tinnitus, and otalgia. Although rupture of the tympanic membrane was once thought to be an effective marker for underlying pulmonary or gastrointestinal blast injury, a recent Israeli study reported that 18 patients with underlying pulmonary blast injury did not have tympanic membrane rupture.[66] However, if such a rupture is present, these casualties should undergo chest radiography and an observation period to rule out underlying pulmonary or gastrointestinal injury. Initial treatment involves avoiding probing or irrigation of the canal. If the ear canal is full of debris, then a course of antibiotic drops is recommended.[6] Most perforations involving less than a third of the tympanic membrane surface will heal spontaneously. Individuals with larger perforations or ossicular chain disruption should be referred to an otorhinolaryngologist for further management.

6.7.10   Ocular Blast Injury

Eyes of blast casualties are most vulnerable to secondary and tertiary blast injuries with up to 28% of these casualties experiencing serious injuries.[6] Symptoms include eye pain or irritation, foreign body sensation, altered vision, periorbital swelling, or contusions. Some of these injuries include lid lacerations, hyphemas, retinitis, orbital fractures, and ruptured globe. Up to 10% of eye injuries may involve perforations, some of which may occur with minimal initial discomfort; therefore, these individuals may not present for care for days, weeks, or even months after the event. Referral to an ophthalmologist is mandatory.

6.7.11   Flash Burns

Flash burns may result from the short-lived but intense heat of the blast, which may reach 3000°C. In the absence of secondary fires, such burns usually only affect the individuals closest to the blast, tend to be superficial, and are confined to exposed areas of the body such as the face and hands. Deeper or more extensive burns may occur if the clothes ignite. Burns have been reported as high as 31% in some explosions.[67]

Burns from explosions or traumatic disasters should be managed as other burn wounds. Fluid resuscitation should be initiated as soon as possible to maintain a urine output of 30 to 50 mL/hr as per the Parkland formula (4 mL × weight in kg × % body surface area with second and third degree burns, half of which should be administered within the first eight hours following the time of injury).[68] Considerations in children less than 30 kg should include maintenance fluid in addition to the Parkland formula. However, because blast burns often coexist with blast lung, for which fluid restriction may be necessary, care should also be taken to avoid overzealous fluid resuscitation. Wounds should be covered with clean, dry dressings to prevent heat loss and contamination. Tetanus prophylaxis should be provided, but antibiotic prophylaxis should be avoided unless there is evidence of gross contamination.

6.7.12   Blunt Ballistic Injury

Blunt ballistic injuries are commonly seen after riots and are caused by rubber bullets, beanbag shotgun shells, or by standard bullets impacting a protective vest. Rubber bullets are used by police agencies around the world for crowd dispersal and "nonlethal use of force." Beanbag shotgun shells are nylon bags filled with pellets, which are fired from a standard shotgun. Both of these projectiles have the potential to cause serious injury despite their classification as "nonlethal." Bullet-resistant vests are usually capable of stopping penetration by the low-velocity missiles typical of most handguns, but the kinetic energy of the missile can be transmitted through the layers of protective clothing or armor, producing significant injury without penetration. Although missile penetration is usually prevented, the heart, liver, spleen, lung, and spinal cord remain vulnerable to blunt ballistic injury that may occur beneath benign-appearing skin lesions. Casualties may present with erythema, ecchymoses, and tenderness to palpation over the affected area. Subcutaneous emphysema, crepitus, or bony stepoffs may be present.

Individuals with nonpenetrating ballistic injuries should be closely observed, particularly those with injuries over the abdomen. Plain film radiography will identify any retained foreign bodies or fractures, and serial abdominal examinations or CT scans can help to detect internal injuries that can have a delayed presentation.

6.7.13   Penetrating Ballistic Injury

Large numbers of penetrating injuries have been seen following civil unrest (such as the 1992 Los Angeles riots), urban warfare (such as in Israel and Mogadishu), school or workplace shootings (Columbine, Colorado, and Beslan, Russia), and explosive events (Alfred P. Murrah Federal Building, Oklahoma City). Injuries are produced when a missile dissipates energy to body tissues as it passes through them. The nature of the wound depends on the specific biologic properties of the tissue involved and the physical characteristics of the projectile. The key characteristics of the projectile are its mass, shape, velocity, and propensity to deform or tumble. The degree of wounding correlates with the amount of kinetic energy transferred from the penetrating object to the target tissue. The release of energy causes tissue stretch and cavitation, and the damage done depends heavily on tissue density and elasticity.

Projectiles are customarily described as either "low velocity" or "high velocity," with the arbitrary cutoff equal to the speed of sound in air (approximately 343.2 m/sec, or 1,126 ft/sec, in dry air, at standard temperature and pressure). High-velocity weapons of war tend to produce exponentially greater tissue destruction and cavitation than the low-velocity weapons typically used by civilians. A low-velocity projectile, however, may cause great penetrating trauma if it strikes a bone, deforms, then tumbles and drags so that the tissue absorbs all its energy. Likewise, a high-velocity bullet may pass cleanly through a tissue bed without slowing significantly and produce a relatively mild wound. Some ammunition is specifically designed to fragment or "mushroom" upon entering tissue and will cause increased destruction. Therefore, the complex interaction of projectile and tissue ultimately determines the amount of harmful energy actually delivered and the resultant clinical injury.

In contrast to traumatic amputation or mangling due to severe blast injury, tourniquet application should be avoided in penetrating ballistic injury unless warranted by otherwise uncontrolled hemorrhage from an extremity, in which case it should be expeditiously applied. Treatment decisions at the hospital are based on an estimation of the type and location of the wound, the amount of tissue disruption, and the patient's hemodynamic status. An estimate of the missile's path can be made from the locations of the entrance and exit wounds or the position at which the projectile came to rest within the body. Data from the physical examination and radiographic studies provide the information necessary to make these decisions, allowing prediction of structures that may be damaged. Any penetrating abdominal or thoracic wound in a hemodynamically unstable patient requires emergent surgical intervention.

Penetrating ballistic wounds are generally extensively contaminated, especially when due to an SBI. Adequate debridement is mandatory, and deep wounds should not be closed acutely, as delayed primary closure at 5 days is more appropriate. Because of the high velocity of metal fragments that emanate from exploding bombs, the superficial appearance of entry wounds can appear deceptively small. All penetrating wounds to the chest or abdomen should be adequately explored. Tetanus prophylaxis and broad-spectrum antibiotics should be given.

6.7.14   Penetrating Stab or Impaling Injury

Stab or impaling wounds result from the force caused by a sharp object that disrupts tissue. The clinical injury depends upon the size, shape, depth of penetration, and force with which the weapon strikes the body, and which part of the body is struck. Penetrating chest wounds require careful observation for the development of tension pneumothorax, open pneumothorax, massive hemothorax, and cardiac tamponade. Abdominal wounds require careful observation for the development of hemodynamic instability or peritoneal irritation. Impaled objects should not be removed in the field, but should be stabilized manually or with bulky dressings. Penetrating soft tissue wounds require little field management other than controlling hemorrhage and covering the wound to avoid further contamination. However, they, too, usually require tetanus prophylaxis and broad-spectrum antibiotics.

6.8   PUBLIC HEALTH CONSIDERATIONS

Individuals with preexisting mental health and substance abuse disorders are at high risk for sudden exacerbation of these disorders in an explosion or traumatic disaster and should be identified for surveillance of symptoms. Among preexisting medical diseases, cardiac patients taking β_1 blocking agents and patients taking warfarin or heparin for treatment of hypercoagulability disorders are at higher than usual risk of injury, the former due to a potentially dampened response to shock, and the latter due to a far higher than usual probability of intracranial hemorrhage associated with traumatic brain injury (TBI). Individuals with preexisting injuries or disabilities are also at higher than normal risk of injuries following explosions and traumatic disasters owing to their relative immobility in the setting of blast trauma.

6.9   MENTAL HEALTH CONSIDERATIONS

One mental health challenge unique to blast trauma is the considerable overlap in symptomatology that exists between PTSD and mild TBI due to concussive forces. Veterans of the wars in Iraq and Afghanistan who have sustained mild blast-related TBIs exhibit symptoms of PTSD in very high numbers, similar to veterans of World War I, among whom the terms "commotio cerebri" and "shell shock" were used to describe the syndrome.[69] A debate has raged among military health experts since that time regarding the precise etiology of battle-related PTSD, with most experts favoring a psychological rather than a physiological explanation. The experience in Iraq and Afghanistan has rekindled this debate, with more experts now judging mild blast related TBI to be an important cause of PTSD-like symptoms following explosions and traumatic disasters.[69] Much additional research will be needed to resolve the issue.

6.10 PEDIATRIC CONSIDERATIONS

Children are frequent casualties in disasters, due to direct physical injury as well as mental and social injury and the disruption of the family social infrastructure following the death or serious injury to parents, guardians, and siblings. Although their experiences are not consistently reported separately from those of adults, reports of pediatric casualties are increasingly being found in the medical literature. For example, recall the three children who died in the Avianca plane crash on the North Shore of Long Island, New York, on January 25, 1990; the 19 children who died in the day care center at the Alfred P. Murrah Federal Building in Oklahoma City, Oklahoma, on April 19, 1995; and the innumerable young lives lost during bus bombings in Israel.[70-75] Data from the Israeli Trauma Registry have documented in a series of investigations that older children are more often affected by blast terror–related injuries, the average age of such children being 12.3 years compared with 6.9 years for unintentional injuries in childhood.[72-75] Head injuries also appear to be more common following blast terror–related injuries, which are two to three times more severe, and consume two to three times more hospital resources in terms of pediatric intensive care days, overall length of stay, and need for long-term care than unintentional injuries.

The approach to pediatric casualties of blast terror is no different from that in adults, and the spectrum of injuries observed following blast terror is similar, with the previously noted caveat that head injuries are somewhat more common than in adults. However, critically injured children require the services available in pediatric specialty hospitals for optimal outcome, especially a fully staffed and equipped pediatric intensive care unit.[76,77] Because not all hospitals have the ability to provide such services, specialized hospital disaster resources as well as an internationally recognized training program called fundamental pediatric critical care support, have been developed to permit nonpediatric hospitals and providers to prepare themselves for the care of children in disasters.[78-82]

6.11 SUMMARY

Explosions can occur unintentionally or as a result of a conflict or terrorism. Across the globe, the threat of terrorism involving the use of explosive agents in urban or otherwise crowded environments has become a reality. Increasing population density and urbanization, coupled with the ubiquity of large buildings, mass transit, and mass gatherings, create the potential for a serious disaster involving multiple casualties.

Bombings are blatant and emphatic and, by their very nature, gain immediate public attention. Explosive events are inherently unpredictable. Despite widespread concerns regarding biologic and chemical attacks, conventional explosives are the most commonly used terrorist weapons because they are the easiest to create, obtain, and use. The medical consequences of the detonation of a conventional explosive include death and acute injury, as well as destruction of critical infrastructure such as buildings, roads, and utilities. Health care needs include immediate emergency trauma care, follow-up medical and surgical care, forensic disposition of bodies and body parts, and mental health care.

Explosions cause multiple mechanisms of injury, nearly simultaneously, to a given casualty. An understanding of the types of explosions, as well as the circumstances in which an explosion occurs, can be important in predicting and managing injuries and illnesses following an event. The impact of an explosion or other traumatic disaster depends largely on the composition and amount of explosive materials involved, the surrounding environment, delivery method (if a bomb), distance between the individual and the blast, and any intervening protective barriers or environmental hazards. Blast-related injuries can present unique triage, diagnostic, and management challenges to physicians and other health professionals. First responders run the risk of being caught by subsequent explosions specifically timed to target them, called *secondary devices*. After an explosion or traumatic disaster, health professionals and hospitals must be prepared to treat scores or hundreds of casualties. Their response, however, may be complicated by the loss of utilities (eg, electricity, water), difficulty in transporting casualties, lack of trained personnel, and damage to the hospital infrastructure. Similar effects can be encountered in natural disasters such as tornadoes, earthquakes, and industrial or gas main explosions.

Clinical decision making following an explosion or other traumatic disaster reinforces the all-hazards approach to immediate lifesaving interventions, as well as highlights the importance of organ system–specific injury and illness management. Populations with access or functional needs may be at greater risk if affected by these events. Rapid identification and timely delivery of appropriate interventions are the mainstays for all populations at significant risk following an explosion or other traumatic disaster.

6.12 DISCUSSION POINTS

Explosions and Traumatic Disasters: Putting the PRE-DISASTER Paradigm™ into Practice	
P Planning and Practice	Every disaster plan should include explosive and large-scale traumatic events. Considerations for likely industrial mishaps, transportation incidents, military bases or posts, mass gatherings, and other terrorism targets are important. The likelihood of utilizing alternate care facilities and sizable casualty volumes are important considerations for surge management.
R Resilience	The continuity of governance, law and order maintenance, and functional health care infrastructure are vital to community and individual resilience. Centric to this is access for the ill, injured, and community at large to timely medical, surgical, and mental health services following explosions and traumatic disasters, or any disaster or public health emergency.
E Education and Training	Explosions and traumatic disasters are common worldwide, including in the United States. A basic understanding of the mechanisms of injury and the resulting

blast-related injuries themselves is important for all responders and receivers. A solid fundamental knowledge of current basic and advanced trauma care principles and practices is important.

Explosions and Traumatic Disasters: Putting the DISASTER Paradigm™ into Practice

D	Detection	Although obvious, the initial explosions and traumatic disasters may only disclose part of the actual event. Astute clinicians, public health measures, and technology are all important in gaining situational awareness and threat or etiology assessment.
I	Incident Management	Coordination, role definition, and communication with incident management are important for all health and medical personnel.
S	Safety and Security	Workforce protection is the highest priority and requires responders to be aware of their surroundings and remember that the scene of an explosion or traumatic disaster is dynamic. Situational awareness must be maintained.
A	Assess Hazards	Review Table 6-3 for a list of questions each responder should consider when at the scene of explosions and traumatic disasters. The possibility of secondary devices and/or contaminant materials ("dirty bombs") must always be considered.
S	Support	What outside assistance is needed (eg, police, fire, emergency medical services, government, other)? Can adequate surge capability and capacity be established to meet local public safety and health needs and priorities?
T	Triage and Treatment	Are protocols, procedures, and resources in place for the rapid triage and immediate treatment of casualties? What public health interventions are needed?
E	Evacuation	Planning and operational considerations for an emergency evacuation is a prime consideration. Casualty evacuation must address proper triage and casualty selection, medical provider vehicle type utilization, protocol-guided medical care delivery en route, and communication between vehicles and the destination health facility.
R	Recovery	Following an explosion or traumatic disaster, recovery begins immediately. Access for the ill, injured, and community at large to timely medical, surgical, and mental health services following an explosion or traumatic disaster, or any disaster or public health emergency, is the first step to recovery.

REFERENCES

1. US Department of State. Country Reports on Terrorism. Washington, DC: US Department of State, 2010. Available at http://www.state.gov/s/ct/rls/crt. Accessed April 4, 2011.

2. Arnold JL, Tsai M-C, Halpern P, Smithline H, Stok E, Ersoy G. Mass casualty, terrorist bombings: epidemiological outcomes, resource utilization, and time course of emergency needs (Part I). *Prehosp Disaster Med.* 2003;18:220-234.

3. Halpern P, Tsai M-C, Arnold JL, Stok E, Ersoy G. Mass casualty, terrorist bombings: implications for emergency department and hospital emergency response (Part II). *Prehosp Disaster Med.* 2003;18:235-241.

4. Arnold JL, Halpern P, Tsai M-C, Smithline H. Mass casualty terrorist bombings: a comparison of outcomes by bombing type. *Ann Emerg Med.* 2004;43:263-273.

5. Mallonee S, Shariat S, Stennies G, Waxweiler R, Hogan D, Jordan F. Physical injuries and fatalities resulting from the Oklahoma City bombing. *JAMA.* 1996;276:382-387.

6. DePalma RG, Burris DG, Champion HR, Hodgson MJ. Blast injuries. *N Engl J Med.* 2005; 352:1335-1342.

7. Feeney J, Parekh N, Blumenthal K, Wallack MK. September 11, 2001: a test of preparedness and spirit. *Bull Am Coll Surg.* 2002;87(5):12-17.

8. Lisagor P. 9/11: Jersey City Medical Center—lessons learned. *Bull Am Coll Surg.* 2002; 87(7):8-12.

9. Cushman JG, Pachter HL, Beaton HL. Two New York City hospitals' surgical response to the September 11, 2001 terrorist attack in New York City. *J Trauma.* 2003;54:147-155.

10. Kirschenbaum L, Keene A, O'Neill P, Westfal R, Astiz ME. The experience at St. Vincent's Hospital, Manhattan, on September 11, 2001: preparedness, response, and lessons learned. *Crit Care Med.* 2005;33:S48-S52.

11. Yurt RW, Bessey PQ, Bauer GJ, et al. A regional burn center's response to a disaster: September 11, 2001, and the days beyond. *J Burn Care Rehab.* 2005;26:117-124.

12. Feeney JM, Goldberg R, Blumenthal JA, Wallack MK. September 11, 2001 revisited: a review of the data. *Arch Surg.* 2005;140:1068-1073.

13. Wang D, Sava J, Sample G, Jordan M. The Pentagon and 9/11. *Crit Care Med.* 2005;33:S42-S47.

14. Jordan MH, Hallowed KA, Turner DG, Wang DS, Jeng JC. The Pentagon attack of September 11, 2001: a burn center's experience. *J Burn Care Rehab.* 2005;26:109-116.

15. Galea S, Ahern J, Resnick H, et al. Psychological sequelae of the September 11 terrorist attacks in New York City. *N Engl J Med.* 2002;346:982-987.

16. Cohen Silver R, Holman EA, McIntosh DN, Poulin M, Gil-Rivas V. Nationwide longitudinal study of psychological responses to September 11. *JAMA.* 2002;288:1235-1244.

17. Boscarino JA, Galea S, Adams RE, Ahern J, Resnick H, Vlahov D. Mental health service and medication use in New York City after the September 11, 2001 terrorist attack. *Psychiatr Serv.* 2004;55:274-283.

18. Bureau of Alcohol, Tobacco, Firearms, and Explosives. US Bomb Data Center. Washington, DC: United States Department of Justice, 2011. Available at http://www.atf.gov/explosives/groups/usbdc. Accessed April 4, 2011.

19. auf der Heide E. *Disaster Response: Principles of Preparation and Coordination.* Chapter 1, "The Problem." Available at http://aresalaska.org/docs/Disaster_Response_Principals.pdf. Accessed April 4, 2011.

20. Dallas CD, Coule PL, James JJ, et al., eds. Chapter 3: Traumatic and explosive events. In: *Basic Disaster Life Support Provider Manual.* Version 2.5. American Medical Association; 2004

21. Stuhmiller JH, Phillips YY, Richmond DR. The physics and mechanisms of primary blast injury. In: Bellamy AFR, Zajtchuk R, eds. *Conventional Warfare: Ballistic, Blast, and Burn Injuries.* Washington, DC: Office of the Surgeon General of the United States Army; 1991:241.

22. Cullis IG. Blast waves and how they interact with structures. *J R Army Med Corps.* 2001;147:16-26.

23. Boffard KD, MacFarlane C. Urban bomb blast injuries: patterns of injury and treatment. *Surg Ann.* 1993;25(Part 1):29-47.

24. Phillips YY, Mundie TG, Yelverton JT, Richmond DR. Cloth ballistic vest alters response to blast. *J Trauma.* 1988;28(1 Suppl):S149-S152.

25. Bean JR. Enhanced blast weapons and forward medical treatment. *US Army Med Department J.* 2004;April/May/June:48-51.

26. Frykberg ER, Tepas JJ, Alexander RH. The 1983 Beirut airport terrorist bombing: injury patterns and implications for disaster management. *Am Surg.* 1989;55:134-141.

27. Maningas PA, Robinson M, Mallonee S. The EMS response to the Oklahoma City bombing. *Prehosp Disaster Med.* 1997;12:9-14.

28. Feliciano DV, Anderson GV, Rozycki GS, et al. Management of casualties from the bombing at the Centennial Olympics. *Am J Surg.* 1998;176:538-543.

29. Gutierrez de Ceballos JP, Turegano-Fuentes F, Perez-Diaz D, Sanz-Sanchez M, Martin-Llorente C, Guerrero-Sanz JE. Casualties treated at the closest hospital in the Madrid, March 11, terrorist bombings. *Crit Care Med.* 2005;33(1 Suppl);S107-S112.

30. Gutierrez de Ceballos JP, Turegano-Fuentes F, Perez-Diaz D, Sanz-Sanchez M, Martin-Llorente C, Guerrero-Sanz JE. 11 March 2004: the terrorist bomb explosions in Madrid, Spain—an analysis of the logistics, injuries sustained and clinical management of casualties treated at the closest hospital. *Crit Care.* 2005;9:104-111.

31. Redhead J, Ward P, Batrick N. Perspective: the London attacks—response prehospital and hospital care–a chronicle. *N Engl J Med.* 2005;353:546-547.

32. Aylwin CJ, Konig TC, Brennan NW, et al. Reduction in critical mortality in urban mass casualty incidents: analysis of triage, surge, and resource use after the London bombings on July 7, 2005. *Lancet.* 2006;368:2219-2225 (editorial, 2188-2189).

33. Staten CL. *A Comparison of the Afghan Mujahideen (1979–89) and the Iraqi Insurgency (2003): A Review of the Tactics, Weapons, Training, and Composition.* Chicago: Emergency Response & Research Institute. http://www.authorstream.com/Presentation/Brainy007-53155-afghan-Comparison-Mujahideen-1979–89-Iraqi-Insurgency-2003-Review-Tactics-Weapons-Train-as-Entertainment-ppt-powerpoint. Accessed November 17, 2011.

34. Gans L, Kennedy T. Management of unique entities in disaster medicine. *Emerg Med Clin North Am.* 1996;14:301-326.

35. Mellor SG, Cooper GJ. Analysis of 828 servicemen killed or injured by explosion in Northern Ireland 1970–84: the hostile action casualty system. *Br J Surg.* 1989;76:1006-1010.

36. Mines M. Ocular injuries sustained by survivors of the Oklahoma City bombing. *Ophthalmology.* 2000;107:837-843.

37. Kuwagata Y, Oda J, Tanaka H, et al. Analysis of 2,702 traumatized patients in the 1995 Hanshin-Awaji earthquake. *J Trauma.* 1997;43:427-432.

38. Sorkin P, Nimrod A, Biderman P. The quinary (5th) injury pattern of blast. *J Trauma.* 2004;56:232 (abstract).

39. Kluger Y, Peleg K, Daniel-Aharonson L, Mayo A, The Israeli Trauma Group. The special injury pattern in terrorist bombings. *J Am Coll Surg.* 2004;199:875-879.

40. Centers for Disease Control and Prevention (CDC). *Explosions and Blast Injuries: A Primer for Clinicians.* Atlanta: CDC. Available at http://www.bt.cdc.gov/masstrauma/explosions.asp. Accessed April 4, 2011.

41. Klein JS, Weigelt JA. Disaster management: lessons learned. *Surg Clin North Am.* 1991;71:257-266.

42. Frykberg ER, Armstrong J, Weireter LJ, eds, for the Disaster Subcommitee, Committee on Trauma, American College of Surgeons. Disaster Management and Emergency Preparedness Course. Chicago, IL: American College of Surgeons, 2010.

43. Salomone JP, Pons PT, McSwain NE, eds. *PHTLS-Prehospital Trauma Life Support*, 6th ed. St. Louis: Mosby Elsevier, 2007.

44. American College of Surgeons Committee on Trauma. *Advanced Trauma Life Support® for Doctors (ATLS®) Student Course Manual*, 8th ed. Chicago, IL: American College of Surgeons, 2008.

45. American Burn Association. *ABLS-Advanced Burn Life Support Course Provider Manual.* Chicago: American Burn Association, 2005.

46. Society of Trauma Nurses. *ATCN®–Advanced Trauma Care for Nurses®*, 2008 ed. Lexington, KY: Society of Trauma Nurses, 2008.

47. Emergency Nurses Association. *TNCC-Trauma Nursing Core Course Provider Manual*, 6th ed. Des Plaines, IL: Emergency Nurses Association, 2007.

48. Quenemoen LE, Davis YM, Malilay J, Sinks T, Noji EK, Klitzman S. The World Trade Center bombing: injury prevention strategies for high-rise building fires. *Disasters.* 1996;20:125-132.

49. Wightman JM, Gladish SL. Explosions and blast injuries. *Ann Emerg Med.* 2001;37:664-678.

50. Phillips Y, Zajtchuk J. The management of primary blast injury. In: Bellamy AFR, Zajtchuk R. eds. *Conventional Warfare: Ballistic, Blast and Burn Injuries.* Washington, DC: Office of the Surgeon General of the U.S. Army, 1991;295-336.

51. Ripple G, Phillips Y. Military explosions. In: Cooper GJ, Dudley HAF, Gann DS, Little RA, Maynard RL, eds. *Scientific Foundations of Trauma.* Oxford, England: Butterworth-Heinemann; 1997; 247-257.

52. Mellor SG. The pathogenesis of blast injury and its management. *Br J Hosp Med.* 1988;39:536-539.

53. Maynard R, Coppel D, Lowry K. Blast injury of the lung. In: Cooper GJ, Dudley HAF, Gann DS, Little RA, Maynard RL, eds. *Scientific Foundations of Trauma.* Oxford, England: Butterworth-Heinemann; 1997.

54. Meredith W, Rutledge R, Hansen AR, et al. Field triage of trauma patients based upon the ability to follow commands: a study in 29,573 injured patients. *J Trauma.* 1995;38:129-135.

55. Beekley AC, Sebesta JA, Blackbourne LH, et al. Members of the 31st Combat Support Hospital Research Group. Prehospital tourniquet use in Operation Iraqi Freedom: effect on hemorrhage control and outcome. *J Trauma.* 2008;64:S28-S37.

56. Kragh JF, Walters TJ, Baer DJG, et al. Practical use of emergency tourniquets to stop bleeding in major limb trauma. *J Trauma.* 2008;64:S38-S50.

57. Slone FL, Armstrong JH. Mass casualty management. In Armstrong JH, Schwartz RB, eds. *Advanced Disaster Life Support Course Manual 3.0.* Chicago: American Medical Assocation, 2012.

58. Composite Resources. C-A-T® Combat-Application-Tourniquet®. Available at http://www .combattourniquet.com. Accessed October 23, 2011.

59. Gonzalez D. Crush syndrome. *Crit Care Med.* 2005;33(1Suppl):S34-S41.

60. Sever MS, Vanholder R, Lameire N. Management of crush-related injuries after disasters. *N Engl J Med.* 2006;354:1052-1063.

61. Federal Emergency Management Agency (FEMA). *FEMA US&R Response System Task Force Medical Team Training Manual.* Washington, DC: FEMA; April 1997. Available at http://www .fema.gov/emergency/usr/medmanual.shtm. Accessed April 4, 2011.

62. Oda J, Tanaka H, Yoshioka T, et al. Analysis of 372 patients with crush syndrome caused by the Hansshin-Awaji earthquake. *J Trauma.* 1997;42:470-476.

63. Kazancioglu R, Cagatay A, Calangu S, et al. The characteristics of infections in crush syndrome. *Clin Microbiol Infect.* 2002;8:202-206.

64. Huller T, Bazini Y. Blast injuries of the chest and abdomen. *Arch Surg.* 1970;100:24-30.

65. Harmon JW, Haluszka M. Care of blast-injured casualties with gastrointestinal injuries. *Military Med.* 1983;148:586-588.

66. Leibovici D, Gofrit ON, Shapira SC. Eardrum perforation in explosion survivors: is it a marker of pulmonary blast injury? *Ann Emerg Med.* 1999;34:168-172.

67. Stein M, Hirshberg A. Medical consequences of terrorism: the conventional weapon threat. *Surg Clin North Am.* 1999;79:1537-1552.

68. Cancio LC, Chavez S, Alvarado-Ortega M, et al. Predicting increased fluid requirements during the resuscitation of thermally injured patients. *J Trauma.* 2004;56:404-414.

69. Elder GA, Cristian A. Blast-related mild traumatic brain injury: mechanisms of injury and impact on clinical care. *Mount Sinai Med J.* 2009;76:111-118.

70. van Amerongen RH, Fine JS, Tunik MG, Young GM, Foltin GL. The Avianca plane crash: emergency medical system response to pediatric survivors of the disaster. *Pediatrics.* 1993;92:105-110.

71. Quintana DA, Jordan FB, Tuggle DW, Mantor C, Tunell WP. The spectrum of pediatric injuries after a bomb blast. *J Pediatr Surg.* 1997;32:307-311.

72. Waisman Y, Aharonson-Daniel L, Mor M, Amir L, Peleg K. The impact of terrorism on children: a two-year experience. *Prehosp Disaster Med* 2003;18:242-248.

73. Aharonson-Daniel L, Waisman Y, Dannon YL, Peleg K. Epidemiology of terror-related versus non-terror-related traumatic injury in children. *Pediatrics* 2003;112:e280-e284.

74. Amir LD, Daniel-Aharonson L, Peleg K, Waisman Y, The Israel Trauma Group. The severity of injury in children resulting from acts against civilian populations. *Ann Surg.* 2005;241:666-672.

75. Jaffe DH, Peleg K, The Israel Trauma Group. Terror explosive injuries: a comparison of children, adolescents, and adults. *Ann Surg.* 2010;251:138-143.

76. American College of Surgeons Committee on Trauma. *Resources for Optimal Care of the Injured Patient 2006.* Chicago: American College of Surgeons, 2006.

77. Hannan E, Farrell L, Cooper A. Severity of injury and mortality associated with pediatric blunt injuries: hospitals with pediatric intensive care units vs. other hospitals. *Pediatr Crit Care Med.* 2004;5:5-9.

78. American Academy of Pediatrics (Foltin GL, Schonfeld DJ, Shannon MW, eds). *Pediatric Terrorism and Disaster Preparedness: A Resource for Pediatricians.* AHRQ Publication No. 06-0056-EF. Rockville, MD: Agency for Healthcare Research and Quality; 2006. Available at http://www.ahrq.org/research/pedprep/resource.htm. Accessed April 4, 2011.

79. Centers for Bioterrorism Preparedness Program Pediatric Task Force, New York City Department of Health and Mental Hygiene Pediatric Disaster Advisory Group, New York City Department of Health and Mental Hygiene Healthcare Emergency Preparedness Program: *Children in Disasters: Hospital Guidelines for Pediatric Preparedness,* 3rd ed. New York, NY: New York City Department of Health and Mental Hygiene, 2008. Available at http://www.nyc.gov/html/doh/downloads/pdf/bhpp/hepp-peds-childrenindisasters-010709.pdf. Accessed April 4, 2011.

80. Anonymous. *Pediatric Tabletop Exercise Toolkit for Hospitals,* 2nd edition. New York, NY: New York City Department of Health and Mental Hygiene, 2008. Available at http://www.nyc.gov/html/doh/downloads/word/bhpp/hepp-peds-tabletoptoolkit-010709.doc. Accessed April 4, 2011.

81. Foltin G, Tunik M, Treiber M, Cooper A, eds. *Pediatric Disaster Preparedness: A Resource for Planning, Management, and Provision of Out-of-Hospital Emergency Care.* Washington, DC: EMSC National Resource Center; 2008. Available at http://www.cpem.org. Accessed April 4, 2011.

82. Mejia R, Fields A, Greenwald BM, Stein F, eds. *Pediatric Fundamental Critical Care Support-PFCCS.* Mount Prospect, IL: Society of Critical Care Medicine, 2008.

CHAPTER | SEVEN

Nuclear and Radiologic Disasters

CHAPTER CHAIR

Cham Dallas, PhD

CONTRIBUTING AUTHORS

William Maliha, MD

Glen I. Reeves, MD, MPH

John C. White, CNMT

Jim Lyznicki, MS, MPH

William Bell, PhD

7.1 PURPOSE

This chapter describes principles and practices for the management of individuals and populations affected by nuclear and radiologic disasters. It focuses on the specific clinical response for treating injuries and illnesses resulting from these events, including the unprecedented challenge of dealing with mass casualties from a nuclear detonation. The chapter reinforces the general concepts of situational awareness, hazard assessment, incident management, workforce protection, casualty management, and public health response, which were introduced in Chapters 1 through 5 of this manual. This chapter describes the application of these general concepts in the context of nuclear and radiologic disaster preparedness, mitigation, response, and recovery.

7.2 LEARNING OBJECTIVES

After completing this chapter, readers should be able to:

➤ Discuss the difference between nuclear and radiologic disasters with respect to magnitude and health outcomes.

➤ Define basic radiation terms, types, and units of measure that are important to health personnel.

➤ Describe the rationale for time, distance, and shielding in radiation protection.

➤ Identify early clinical signs and symptoms suggestive of significant radiation exposure.

➤ Discuss general considerations for the clinical management of radiation casualties, including trauma care, hospital management, diagnostic testing, and therapeutic interventions.

➤ Summarize the clinical features and treatment of acute radiation sickness and cutaneous radiation syndrome.

➤ Discuss decorporation techniques and countermeasures for the management of internal contamination with radioactive materials.

➤ Discuss the purpose of emergency public health response actions during a nuclear or radiologic disaster, including risk communication, care of populations with access or functional needs, and population exposure monitoring.

Learning objectives for this chapter are competency-based, as delineated in Appendix B.

7.3 BACKGROUND

As the threat of use of weapons of mass destruction on civilian populations continues to increase, clinical and public health providers and their supporting infrastructures are facing considerable preparedness challenges from the resulting mass casualties. Radiologic and nuclear events represent a unique challenge in this regard. The increased risk posed by the proliferation of nuclear weapons is particularly worrisome, as it is widely recognized that the health care system and the whole societal infrastructure will be completely overwhelmed by the massive scale of destructive outcomes.[1,2] This recognized lack of preparedness to date is of great concern.

According to the federal interagency document Planning Guidance for Response to a Nuclear Detonation, "Local and state community preparedness to respond to a nuclear detonation could result in life-saving on the order of tens of thousands of lives."[2] While nuclear preparedness is indeed very difficult, costly, and currently deficient, this makes the incremental effort for improvement that much more productive in light of the very significant numbers of individuals who could be helped and lives saved with this investment.

Nuclear and radiologic events are often confused with each other, but the two are vastly different in the magnitude and severity of health outcomes. Basically, nuclear events involve very large numbers of deaths and severe injuries, while radiologic events can be expected to have a much smaller or even no impact on morbidity and mortality in an affected population. Either event could be expected to cause significant societal and financial disruption, even change the political landscape. The following definitions and descriptions illuminate these differences:

➤ *Radiologic events* are defined as those that involve the release of radioactive materials into human-populated areas (without a nuclear explosion), where panic and environmental contamination, but not necessarily human injury, are significant hazards.[3] This could involve an addition of radioactive materials to food or water, dispersion of radionuclides into the air, hiding a lethal radiation source (a radiation emission device [RED]), or use of a "dirty bomb," in which radioactive agents are distributed in an area by the explosion of an ordinary (nonnuclear) explosive device (radiation dispersal device [RDD]). Radiation sickness may result in radiologic events if there is a high degree of exposure, but in most radiologic scenarios this will be limited. Other less deadly but more likely events could involve a transportation incident, releasing radionuclides and presenting hazards to limited populations and emergency responders, or inadvertent loss of an industrial source.

➤ *Nuclear events*, in stark contrast, involve a nuclear detonation and an accompanying massive explosion, devastating fireball, mass fires, shock wave, pulse of gamma radiation, and the production of radioactive fallout.[4] Affected individuals sustain extensive thermal burns, trauma, blindness, and short- and long-term radiation sickness. There would be tens of thousands of deaths and significantly more injuries, even for relatively small nuclear weapons. Larger devices could increase those numbers by 10- to 100-fold, which would cripple the capacities and capabilities of most systems.[5,6]

A nuclear detonation in an urban setting will present a disaster of unprecedented magnitude. To mitigate some of the societal effects that the incident will cause, emergency planners must prepare an action plan in advance of any possible event. Planning must involve a collaborative approach among local, state, and federal authorities, as well as a host of private agencies and organizations that provide support and counseling services under normal circumstances. Adequate education and training programs must be an integral part of this process. As there is little doubt that a nuclear disaster will exceed the emergency medical response system capacity, particularly in the first hours of the event, it is obvious that an expansion of properly trained personnel to meet this glaring deficiency needs to be considered. Waiting to develop this capacity until the actual occurrence of an event is a prescription for disaster.

7.4 RADIATION BASICS

Ionizing radiation is electromagnetic energy or energetic particles emitted from an atomic source. Various materials are used commercially as sources of ionizing radiation in applications as diverse as medical diagnostics, medical therapy, sterilizing food and medical instruments, inspecting welds, and drilling for oil. The nature of the potential health effects of nuclear radiation depends on the character of the radiation source. There are three principal types of radioactive decay products:

> *Alpha* (α) *particles* have a very short range and are easy to shield against (even by a single sheet of paper). Alpha particles cannot penetrate the outer layers of skin and are not an external hazard. Radioactive materials that emit them are an internal hazard if ingested or inhaled.

> *Beta* (β) *particles* have a longer range and are harder to shield against. Aluminum foil or glass will stop most beta particles. They can penetrate the outer layers of skin and are both an external and an internal hazard. Beta radiation travels only a short distance in tissue, depending on its energy, and can be a significant source of dose to the skin.

> *Gamma* (γ) *radiation* has a very long range and is very difficult to shield against. Unlike alpha or beta particles, gamma rays are electromagnetic energy waves similar to X rays. Concrete, lead, or steel is needed to shield against sources of gamma rays. Gamma radiation can penetrate through the whole body. It is an external and an internal hazard. High-energy gamma radiation can penetrate deeply into tissue. Most radioactive materials with current commercial applications emit high-energy gamma rays.

Another radiation hazard arises when neutrons impact materials such as metal, soil, rock, and buildings that are in proximity to ground zero during a nuclear detonation. The absorption of neutrons in these materials can make them radioactive, emitting beta and gamma radiation. Combined with radiation fallout, neutron-induced radiation could render the immediate area around ground zero radioactive for several weeks or months.

7.4.1   Radiation Measurement Terms and Units

In the radiation literature, radiation dose is measured in terms, defined by the International System of Units, as both the gray (Gy; the unit of measurement for the absorbed dose) and the sievert (Sv; the unit of measurement for the effective dose), which is the absorbed dose multiplied by factors accounting for the biologic effect of different types of radiation and the radiation sensitivities of different tissues. For high-energy gamma radiation and whole-body exposures, 1 Gy equals 1 Sv. In the United States, the terms for radiation dose, rad (radiation absorbed dose) and rem (roentgen equivalent man) are still used by some groups for Gy and Sv, respectively. The conversion from these terms is straightforward: 1 Sv = 100 rem; 1 Gy = 100 rad.

All radioactive materials have a characteristic *half-life*, defined as the time it takes for the substance undergoing decay to decrease by half. Radioisotopes may have a very short half-life (eg, 67 hours for molybdenum 99) to a very long half-life (eg, 24 400 years for plutonium 239). Iodine 131 (half-life of 8 days) can be an important source of morbidity because of its prevalence in nuclear reactor discharges and its tendency to settle on the ground. Once it enters the body, iodine 131 rapidly accumulates in the thyroid gland, where it can be a source of substantial doses of beta radiation. The amount of radioactivity in a source is measured by the number of nuclear decays per second and is expressed with a unit called the *curie* (Ci), which equals 37 billion decays per second.

7.4.2 Radiation Exposure and Contamination

Human radiation exposure is generally characterized as total- or partial-body exposure (as a result of proximity to a radiation source), external contamination, and internal contamination.

Total- or partial-body exposure occurs when an external source irradiates the body either superficially to the skin or deeply into internal organs, with the depth depending on the type and energy of the radiation involved. Persons who have had total- or partial-body exposure but no contamination are not radioactive and therefore cannot expose their caregivers to radiation. This occurs when radiation penetrates the body from an external source, such as with a chest X ray. The radiation may either be absorbed by the body or pass through the body. Radiation exposure can potentially result in short-term and long-term effects in every organ system in the body.

Contamination occurs when radioactive material, which may be in the form of a gas, liquid, or solid, gets onto the skin or into the lungs, gut, or open wounds. Buildings, motor vehicles, and other inanimate objects also can become coated with radioactive particles. A person contaminated with radioactive materials will be irradiated until the source of radiation is removed. *External contamination* occurs when the radioactive material settles on skin or clothing. *Internal contamination* occurs when radioactive material is ingested or inhaled or enters the body through open wounds.

During a radiation disaster, people should seek to limit exposure by increasing their *distance* from the affected area; increasing the distance decreases the intensity of immediate health effects from the blast, heat, and emitted radiations. The next concern should be to *shield* oneself from the blast and heat and from the emitted radiations by seeking shelter. Depending on the type of radioactivity, effective shielding could be as thin as a piece of paper (for alpha radiation) or as thick as a lead-lined wall (for gamma radiation). The more shielding between an individual and the radiation source, the less the radiation intensity. Individuals also will want to minimize the *time* exposed to the radiation emitted from the blast.

7.4.3 Biologic Consequences of Radiation Exposure

At a molecular level, the primary consequence of radiation exposure is DNA damage. This damage will be fully repaired or innocuous or will result in dysfunction, carcinogenesis, or cell death. The extent of injury and risk of long-term health effects are proportional to the dose received and the rate of delivery. Cellular repair mechanisms can handle injuries caused by a given dose received slowly. The same dose, received more rapidly, can overwhelm cell repair mechanisms, leading to cell death and possible cancer. High exposures, received acutely, can kill cells in the body. If the cells are not critical for survival, the clinical effects may be negligible. However, acute doses that kill large numbers of cells or kill cells essential for organ function will cause clinical symptoms. Rapidly dividing cells, such as those of the gastrointestinal mucosa and the bone marrow, are most sensitive.

The type of radiation and the dose rates that are involved in an RDD would typically be very different from those seen in the detonation of a nuclear bomb, which is why the biologic consequences of these events may differ substantially.

7.5 CHARACTERISTIC INJURIES AFTER NUCLEAR AND RADIOLOGIC DISASTERS

On detonation of a nuclear device or RDD in an urban area, a series of events would occur that would result in a spectrum of injuries requiring medical response. These include traumatic injuries, thermal injuries, and radiation toxicity.

7.5.1 Trauma Injuries

As occurs with conventional explosion blasts, a nuclear blast would cause pressure change (albeit far exceeding that of a conventional blast in both peak intensity and duration) that would decrease in intensity the greater the distance from the blast. It would also cover a much larger area.[7] A shock wave accompanies the pressure change resulting in the destruction of buildings (generally decreasing in intensity the greater the distance from ground zero), causing damage to eardrums and other structures in humans and resulting in the intense movement of enormous quantities of air containing radioactive materials and massive amounts of debris.[8] The destruction of buildings and the movement of materials within the shock wave can be expected to generate thousands of trauma casualties in a densely populated urban area.[1,9] The recognition and management of trauma injuries is discussed in much greater detail in Chapter 6, "Explosions and Traumatic Disasters."

7.5.2 Thermal Burns

A daunting spectrum of thermal burn injuries will be incurred from a nuclear blast as a result of the heat and electromagnetic radiation released by the explosion. Thermal burn injuries (flash burns), which would occur immediately after the detonation (resulting in both fatalities and survivors), should be distinguished from flame burns and also cutaneous radiation burns, which will not appear until hours and days after the event.[10] A nuclear fireball is at least 10 000 times hotter than that produced by a conventional explosion, with a resulting dramatic increase in fires and thermal burns in the affected population.[11] The large release of radiant heat, as well as the generation of many fires in the blast area, will cause a large number of burn casualties, which will create one of the most perplexing logistical medical issues in a nuclear weapon response.[1]

The most difficult aspect of nuclear disaster casualties to address appropriately in terms of health outcome is the overwhelming number of burn casualties that will result.[12] It has been estimated that the burn casualties from just one medium-sized nuclear weapon event could fill every burn bed in the eastern United States. The speed with which burn casualties need to be treated to avoid high levels of pain and increase the chance of survival is almost certain to preclude the successful transport of large numbers (ie, hundreds of thousands) of these casualties to the permanent facilities capable of treating them. About one in eight burn casualties will die as a direct result of the event, slightly less than half will die of infection, and most of the remaining will be lost because of organ failure. The high degree of mortality from infection dictates the use of antimicrobials. The elimination of infection reservoirs on the patient is critical, as is ensuring the infection is not transferred to other sites or other patients. In the Chernobyl experience, beta radiation burns were the primary cause of death in patients dying within the first 2 or 3 weeks and increased the severity of acute radiation syndrome in others (these were mostly firefighters who worked in proximity to the reactor fire).

In the nuclear blasts in Japan in World War II, about 90% or more of thermal burns were from flash burns (direct line of sight exposure to the bomb), rather than flame burns from the fires that were kindled. Thermal burns appear immediately after exposure, unlike radiation burns. These are categorized according to depth of the burn (superficial or first degree, involving the top layer of skin, like a sunburn; partial thickness or second degree involving the first two layers of skin; and full thickness or third degree), and by percentage of total body surface area involved.

Indeed, the predicted phenomenon of mass fires in large urban areas will result in a large proportion of fatalities among the affected area in addition to burn casualties.[13] With the detonation of a large nuclear weapon in a major urban area, several hundred thousand serious burn casualties could need intensive medical treatment. The intense flash of visible light at detonation can itself ignite fires as well as cause external flash burns in humans.[14,15] The most common result of this initial flash is flash blindness, which is a temporary loss of sight. A far more serious (but less common) injury is retinal burn, which can result in permanent blindness. The distances at which burn and flash injuries will occur can be calculated on the basis of the size of the nuclear detonation.[16,17]

7.5.3 Radiation Toxicity

Both immediate and delayed radiation exposure occur after nuclear detonations. Gamma irradiation is released by the detonation, as well as from fission products resulting from the blast.[18] Neutrons emitted in the blast are more hazardous than a similar dose from gamma rays and can also cause other materials (including living tissue) to become radioactive.[19] This can increase the risk to first responders in the area around ground zero. Both gamma and neutron radiation can pass through average walls to cause radiation damage in people. Exposures to delayed radioactivity can occur over very wide areas secondary to the airborne dispersion of fission products, which condense and return to the ground as what is known commonly as "fallout." Airborne detonations produce considerably less fallout than surface bursts.

The dispersion of fallout is dictated primarily by the prevailing winds in the first days after the detonation, with winds at higher altitudes often traveling in very different directions than those on the surface. In the first 24 hours (early fallout), most hazardous exposures are due to activation products from external radiation sources and the larger fallout particles.[20] The smaller particle size of the subsequent late fallout stays aloft longer, but the levels of radioactivity are lower. Less penetrating beta particles and low-penetration (but high-energy) alpha particles are more of a hazard when introduced into the body, as they cause internal contamination.[21] Some higher-energy beta radiation can also be an external hazard.

Internal contamination by radiation-emitting materials will result in considerable human health hazards. For example, radioactive iodine entering the food chain can induce thyroid cancer; immediate treatment (within the first hour after exposure if possible) with potassium iodide (KI) tablets can be highly effective in preventing thyroid cancer.[22,23] Radioactive iodine can be inhaled by rescue workers, who also should take KI.

7.5.4   Electromagnetic Pulse

Detonation of a nuclear weapon above the atmosphere can generate a significant radiofrequency flash of 30 000 to 100 000 kV/m intensity with a rise time of less than 10 nanoseconds. This flash, called *electromagnetic pulse*, can disable or destroy medical equipment, communications equipment, computer-controlled vehicles, and power control systems. Persons with pacemakers, other implanted electrical devices, and those dependent on monitoring or assistance devices can suffer immediate injury.

7.6   SITUATIONAL AWARENESS AND DETECTION

After an explosion, first responders may not be aware they are entering an area in which radioactive material has been dispersed. A high index of suspicion, backed by appropriate radiation survey equipment, will enable them to detect the presence of radiation and deal with themselves, casualties, and uninjured bystanders appropriately. Unlike radiologic events that may be challenging to detect, a nuclear detonation will be readily detected. Most responders will know almost immediately what has occurred. A nuclear detonation will have a staggering impact on societal systems and infrastructures. In the high-dose radiation fallout plume area, many thousands of people will die and become seriously ill.

7.6.1   Scene Assessment

When an event involving ionizing radiation occurs, the first priority is to assess the threat the scene presents to response personnel so they can adequately protect themselves and assess the risks to casualties. Reliable assessment requires using suitable radiation detection equipment. Visible cues such as package or vehicle markings can hint at the possibility of radioactive contamination, but characterization of the radiation environment and threat to personnel requires equipment that can detect the levels of ionizing radiation and identify the specific isotopes present. Many varieties of detection equipment are deployed to first responders, and equipment familiar to the responder should be used. The presence of airborne dust, usually visible, will be an indication for immediately donning personal protective equipment (PPE) before scene assessment. Two major elements of scene assessment are required:

➤ Detection of the radiation field present

➤ Identification of the radioactive isotopes present

Equipment to detect the radiation field is well deployed and usually readily available to responders. An alarm or higher-than-background reading from any radiation detector should alert response personnel to the possibility that radiation is present. Less prevalent is equipment that will identify the isotope present. It is important that when a radiation field is detected, an early call be made to hazardous materials responders or another resource to bring an isotope identifier to the scene to assess the isotope present. This facilitates early identification and appropriate specific treatment. When a reading is taken and confirmed, it is essential to report not only the reading on the instrument but the distance from the source, if this can be determined.

7.6.2   Radiation Detection Technology

The types of detection to be used are grouped generally into these categories: field detection devices (meters), isotope identifiers, and airborne particulate detectors. Some field equipment may not be calibrated. It is important to confirm the dose rate, or radiation field present, with a calibrated meter. Regulations require that calibration information be posted on the device if it is a calibrated instrument. The date the calibration expires should be reported along with the radiation field information and the distance from the source. Reporting the calibration date will enhance the veracity of the report on the scene. Usually, more than one data point is needed to provide approach paths to the scene for response planning and management. Knowing whether the detector is a Geiger counter (which detects beta radiation and gamma radiation) or a scintillation detector (which detects gamma radiation only) is useful for scene management and can affect response personnel management. If an alpha detector is available, it should be brought to the scene as soon as possible. Geiger counters and scintillation detectors generally poorly detect alpha particles. Airborne alpha radiation can be extremely dangerous to response personnel and the affected population because of the potential of high specific activity and significant internal doses from ingestion of alpha-emitting isotopes.

As the response progresses, an airborne particulate detector should be located and brought to the scene to determine the levels of airborne contamination. Because airborne radioisotopes can generally increase the detected background and contaminate detectors, determination of the airborne environment can be very useful. In addition, if a significant airborne environment is present, a general wash-down of the scene by fire equipment may be required to effect a lower general level of contamination.

7.7   HAZARD ASSESSMENT

In any emergency response environment, it is essential to understand that there are multiple hazards present. Any explosion will generate heat and a blast wave, which can create chemical and physical hazards. Firefighters are well trained to assess hazards and risks from structure fires and buildings on the verge of collapse. It is important to recognize that radioactive contamination will travel with any person, or with the wind, or with water drainage. The potential for widespread environmental contamination must be addressed. Emergency operations planning for radiation disasters generally incorporates similar risk assessment considerations as for other hazardous materials incidents (chemical hazards).

In a nuclear detonation, first responders need to be aware of two types of hazards: (1) *activation products* (materials made radioactive by the neutron flux from the weapon) and (2) *fallout (fission) products.* Activation products are present near ground zero and are created almost immediately after detonation. *Fallout* is formed from fission products (ie, what uranium or plutonium atoms "split" or fission into), as well as from activation products created in the nonfuel materials in the device that are vaporized, then cool, condense, agglomerate, and also coat nonradioactive particles in the cloud. They fall from the cloud, hence the name *fallout*. Larger particles fall nearer ground zero; smaller particles get carried by prevailing winds dozens of miles from the point of detonation. Fallout is therefore delayed, from seconds to minutes near the site and for up to several hours downwind. Wind patterns may be complex, and the cloud, which can rise to several thousand feet, may actually be blown in different directions at different altitudes. Although larger fallout particles can often be seen as dust and dirt, radiation itself is invisible and not detectable without survey instruments. These instruments must be used after detonation. Responders should not rely solely on plots of likely fallout patterns. The models will show symmetric, cigar-shaped plumes; in reality, micrometeorology will show "hot spots," irregular contours, and other features. Hence, their predicted radiation levels must be verified.

In a nuclear detonation, casualties will have been exposed to prompt radiation from the device. As prompt radiation occurs only within the first few seconds of device disassembly, this will not be a risk for first responders. However, fallout of fission products begins after the first minute and both casualties and first responders will be affected. In addition, there will be activation products from neutron interaction with materials in the environment and in the tissues of exposed casualties. Activation products are formed within the first few hundred meters from the point of detonation of a nuclear device, though fission products can fall out dozens of miles from the site.

For an RDD, there are, of course, no activation products. As a rule, the lethal radius from the blast far exceeds that from the radiation; so uninjured persons will generally have relatively little radiation exposure. Radiation from contamination, both of the environment and deposited on an individual's clothing and body, can affect first responders. However, it is environmental contamination, not that on the casualties, that provides the greatest risk to first responders. The highest radiation dose received by medical personnel at facilities from the contaminated materials on or inside the injured firefighters at Chernobyl was only 0.01 Sv (1 rem).

Hazards present in a radiologic or nuclear incident may not be limited to radiation or contamination. Incorporated radioactive material can be distributed throughout the body or physiologically

Radiation Exposure Risk

The risk from radiation is identical regardless of radiation type and cause; all that needs to be known to define risk is the dose rate and accumulated dose from all sources.

bioconcentrated into a specific organ system. An example of the latter is the presence of radioactive iodine, which is selectively taken up by the thyroid gland after being ingested or inhaled. Radiologic hazards also can cause eventual stochastic effects, such as cancer.

7.8 INCIDENT MANAGEMENT CHALLENGES

A radiation disaster would likely be followed by a massive, integrated federal, state, and local response. Numerous federal agencies would be involved, including the Federal Emergency Management Agency (FEMA), the Department of Homeland Security (DHS), the Environmental Protection Agency (EPA), the Nuclear Regulatory Commission (NRC), the Department of Energy (DOE), the Department of Health and Human Services (HHS), and the Department of Defense (DOD). State and local departments of health, working closely with the private sector and other public sector entities, would coordinate the appropriate local health system response in initiation of the emergency broadcast system, implementation of disaster or evacuation plans, recommendations for evacuation vs. sheltering in place, instructions to begin the administration of countermeasures (eg, KI), and the creation of local shelters for displaced families. It is essential that first responders know how the deployment of these many assets would cascade from one agency to another or dovetail among agencies to produce a coordinated effort. Federal, state, and local authorities should ensure representation from the medical, mental health, and public health sectors at the emergency operations center (EOC) that is established in response to the incident.

The most notable difference in incident management regarding radioactivity and the management of the disaster scene will be the need to resist nonjustified, and even hysterical, calls for evacuation due to a fear of radioactivity. The visceral fear of radioactivity runs the breadth of the population and unfortunately may include health and political leaders. Incident management personnel will almost certainly be called on to enact dangerous and counterproductive management actions based on fear and inaccurate data coming in.

The early decision that will save thousands of lives is the decision to evacuate vs shelter in place.[3] A good definition of *shelter in place* is to stay where you are, *if* you are inside a stable building that is not at risk of collapse, flooding, or fire. People who are outside or in a building threatened by collapse or fire should get inside the nearest stable building. The dangerous fallout zone can extend 10 to 20 miles or more from ground zero, depending on yield. Large particles of fallout occur nearest ground zero, so there is a critical need to rapidly triage, stabilize, and transport casualties in this zone to avoid their and the responders' accumulation of a lethal dose. This requires controlled evacuation so that all present spend the least amount of time in transit from a dangerously contaminated area to a safe one.

7.8.1 Radiation Field Determination

It is critical to determine the level of a radiation field before sending relief workers into an area. Calculations to determine the radiation field at a given point are simple and easily executed, and responders should be advised of the calculations at the earliest opportunity. It is important for all emergency workers in a radiologic environment to be aware of the radiation field and levels of contamination in their work areas. Entry into the area must be planned before being carried out. Managing the time in the radiation environment is the salient factor controlling an individual's exposure. Radiation exposure is linearly cumulative, ie, twice the time in the scene yields twice the exposure. Less intuitive is the principle of distance. It is important to understand the fundamental principle of the inverse square law: the radiation dose rate decreases as the square of the distance from the source. Doubling the distance from the source reduces the dose rate to one-fourth the level.

In many cases, only emergent or triage-level workers should enter a critical area, and those should have a full range of protection available. Instruments can be used to determine the radiation field, and personnel must be given direction to limit the time present in the work environment. Contamination may be analyzed in the field to determine the level of radioisotopes present, as well as the presence of other contaminants. Respiratory protection should be used as a default to prevent inhalation of any contaminant. Barrier clothing should be used, but the limits of the barrier clothing should be clearly understood and communicated to the workers. A detection instrument that reads an appropriate range of a radiation field should be available to provide duration guidance for the workers. As example, a radiation field of 0.05 mSv/h (5 mrem/h) would be considered a low-threat environment, but a field of 1 mSv/h (100 mrem/h) or higher would require time management to limit exposures. Instruction on the fundamental techniques of managing a radiation risk should be provided as just-in-time training at a minimum. A radiation professional should be available by communication or be present to provide consultation for specific individuals and oversight of response activities.

7.8.2   Logistical Support Services

The movement of supplies in the aftermath of nuclear disaster will be severely hampered by the conditions left by the detonation and fallout, and the subsequent movement of large numbers of people to the very areas where supplies need to be delivered. Resource utilization will be severely impacted and the requirement for reallocation of resources very demanding. Resources must be protected from radioactive contamination as they are in transit and especially after they are brought into the affected areas. Because of the public's widespread and intense fear of radiation, in many instances otherwise uninjured persons who think they have been exposed to radiation will insist on treatment directly from medical providers.

Nuclear events will put strenuous demands on federal emergency support function (ESF) requirements, yet the conduct of these functions is fundamentally the same as in other mass casualty events, relating to the responsibility of government entities assigned to carry out critical duties in a crisis. It is likely, however, that the complete overwhelming of certain ESF resources will result in significant reassignment of duties among available assets in a nuclear event, even though at the end of the assessment, many of the functions will remain insufficient for the event.

7.8.3 Personnel Shortages

Radiologic and nuclear events will require the assignment of various personnel in unfamiliar roles, as these events are so rare as to not require everyday workforce assignment. As an example, the radiologic decontamination component of a hospital's written Emergency Operations Plan will require assignment of security personnel, some prehospital providers, and selected clinical workers, as well as deployment and decontamination assistance of the Regional Decontamination Team. Coordination would be needed between hospital and community agency incident management strategies, which would have to be evaluated for needed improvements in workforce development to achieve these unique goals.

In the larger high-consequence events, not limited to nuclear disasters, it is likely that there will simply not be enough health care workers, even with Herculean efforts with widespread ancillary health care personnel. Particularly problematic is the issue of the security support that this enlarged health care community will require. Finally, the latent period that will certainly extend for many hours or days before substantial regional and federal resources arrive dictates dependence on local personnel, whether health- and/or security-trained or not.

As most high-consequence events are likely to both occur in urban areas and overwhelm (and derange) the available medical response there, the ability to rapidly and safely transfer medical personnel from surrounding areas is indispensable.[24] In most high-consequence events, and especially in a nuclear detonation, medical personnel ingress and patient egress from the affected areas in urban environments are likely to be severely constrained along land routes by panic evacuation, presence of hazardous materials, building and road rubble distortions, and security and/or quarantine restrictions. The need to get medical personnel from outside areas into the affected urban areas would likely be severely constrained, especially in the first hours and days after an event when the medical care is needed the most. These difficulties may be overcome with the utilization of air transport and medical evacuation capabilities, if adequate landing and response areas can be established in a timely manner where they are needed. In these areas, specific locations where airstrips can be rapidly constructed could be identified in advance of a crisis.

7.8.4 Information Sharing

Federal emergency response authorities are coordinated under the DHS, which has a series of notification requirements. Distinct federal agencies have additional responsibilities. The large number of agencies to be notified in a radiation-related crisis may seem daunting, but it is imperative that emergency and other health care responders understand the various federal responsibilities and lines of authority that must be followed. Unfortunately, many people in a disaster will not understand these, and they may attempt to circumvent them and advise others to do so. In most cases, the Federal Bureau of Investigation (FBI), FEMA, and the incident commander will inform people of the proper notification requirements in a particular crisis, but it is incumbent on response personnel to know who to notify in order to maximize response and ensure compliance with the law.

Whenever nuclear reactor materials are involved in a crisis, the NRC must be contacted. An incident of this type involves the release (or potential release) of radioactive agents directly from a functioning reactor, or the dispersion of materials that originated from a nuclear reactor (ie, stolen reactor waste or fuel rods). One of the more frequently ignored federal notification requirements is one governing irregularities in the transportation of nuclear materials. All transportation of nuclear and other radioactive materials is strictly regulated by the Department of Transportation (DOT), and any radiation hazard that results from the release of an agent during or after transport must be reported to the DOT. Considerable concern has been voiced over the large-scale transportation of radioactive waste materials for permanent burial, as such loads could be intercepted by terrorists desiring to use them in radiologic terrorist attacks.

7.8.5   Media Cooperation

One of the greatest potential problems in a nuclear event media response is the appearance of improperly informed "experts" in the immediate aftermath of the event. Among emergency preparedness myths, radiation and nuclear-related misinformation ranks very high in the incidence of wrong ideas among otherwise highly educated people.

One of the most likely media disasters related to nuclear events is the depiction of radiation plumes over a much wider area than is necessary to protect the public from radiation toxicity. An area where 1 to 100 mSv (0.1-10.0 rem) of radioactivity might appear on the surface for a short time is a very modest radiation plume area and is highly unlikely to cause radiation injury. Yet it is likely to be broadcast by the media in the area surrounding a nuclear event, precipitating mass hysteria. In fact, this action would likely result in many injuries and fatalities as people would unnecessarily flee this area. Those fleeing the low-risk area would be far safer staying right where they were, and by fleeing they create delays and additional danger for those who are in truly contaminated areas.

To prevent this scenario, the actual radiation plume distribution shown by the media should be very carefully selected so that people really are protected and the best actions advised for their safety. This is just one example in which poorly informed and likely even hysterical "experts" will find their way on screen or radio at a critical point.

Another example is the nearly universal, but not scientifically supported, fear of birth defects from airborne dispersion of radionuclides. The very high level of fear of radiation in the public (and among medical personnel who should know better) is likely to be greatly augmented by such improperly informed nonexperts.

7.9   WORKFORCE PROTECTION

Most planning scenarios for radiologic emergency response involve establishing an incident command post at a substantial distance from the radiation source. To accomplish this, it is important to determine the radiation environment and consequent exposures to first responders, so those personnel can be given proper management based on their dose received in the incident and have it recorded as part of their medical record in case of future radiation incidents. Determining the radiation field present should be viewed as an "emergent action" to ensure that emergency responders, including medical personnel, are aware of the steps needed to manage the radiation risk. Because nuclear detonations and dirty bombs create airborne radioisotopes, the use of respiratory protection should be the default instruction to all responders when a radiation environment is detected, until such time as airborne radioisotopes are ruled out.

Panic is an extreme danger. Work-related injuries can result, stranding the injured person in a contaminated environment or in the radiation field. Calming the workforce in a radiation environment can be assisted by stressing that radiation is a manageable risk. Respiratory protection and clearing the radiation environment with due dispatch will reduce radiation exposure. More information on workforce protection, including PPE and decontamination, is available in Chapter 4, "Workforce Readiness and Disaster Deployment," as well as in the Advanced Disaster Life Support™ course (v3.0) and supporting course manual.

7.9.1   Scene Safety and Security

The tendency for workers to enter a hazardous environment regardless of personal risk must be addressed. Any person who enters the hazard zone should be provided, at a minimum:

➤ Universal precautions (gloves, gown, booties)

➤ Respiratory protection (N95 respirator or higher)

➤ Time limit in the hazard zone

➤ Decontamination on exit

A decontamination zone should be set up as soon as possible, at the outer perimeter of the response area.[25] When workers leave the contaminated scene, it is important to reduce contamination to levels that will allow doffing of PPE. The standard exclusion zone response structure (ie, hot zone, warm zone, and cold zone) should be implemented. There must be adequate resources, including detection equipment, to ensure contamination is not carried outside the controlled area so as to provide a safe refuge for exiting workers. It is imperative that the cold zone be kept free from contamination; incident command should not hesitate to modify boundaries or move resources if warranted.

In a nuclear detonation or an RDD event, the possibility of airborne contamination is significant. For that reason, any person entering the warm zone or hot zone should have respiratory protection. A mask meeting National Institute for Occupational Safety and Health (NIOSH) N95 requirements or higher is advised, but in the absence of that level of quality, any respiratory protection can be used.

Levels of radiation must be posted, so workers and anyone else near the scene are warned of a hazard. This is standard practice in radiation environments (industrial, medical, and others). Typical posting levels are 0.02 mSv/h (2 mrem/h) for a warning that radiation is present. Emergency response organizations may have higher levels, and it should be remembered that exposure limits for personnel in an emergency response are different from routine workplace limits.[25] Security personnel can be provided with signage and given instructions as to where to place the signs. Wind direction and drainage slope will carry contamination, so it is important to avoid sending sign-placers into a contamination area without PPE.

First responders must be aware of the radiation hazards in their areas of operation. Two perimeters, or control zones, are recommended to facilitate casualty care[26]:

➤ An outer perimeter of 0.1 mSv/h (10 mrem/h), where casualties should be decontaminated, if medical conditions permit, and then transported as indicated. First responders and other personnel coming inside the outer perimeter must have monitoring devices (film badges, preferably "pagers").

➤ An inner perimeter of 0.1 Sv/h (10 rem/h). Responders should not go beyond this perimeter except to perform time-sensitive, mission-critical activities such as lifesaving. No one should go beyond this point without the explicit permission of the incident commander, and then only for short intervals to save lives. Time spent inside this area must be strictly monitored. The decision dose is 0.5 Sv (50 rem). The incident commander must assess benefit, in terms of lives potentially saved vs increased risk to first responders.

It should be noted that activation products and early fallout near the scene will decay, and the radiation levels will drop, so the perimeters will be slowly but steadily shrinking *except* where the fallout plume passes. Here the radiation dose rate levels will increase, in some cases to very high and even fatal dose levels. First responders should therefore never assume that the radiation dose rate is steady; it will always be changing.

Radiation Protection Measures

Danger for human exposure occurs from the ingestion or inhalation of radioactive particles as well as external exposure from radionuclides. In accordance with the time-honored radiation protection maxim of time, distance, and shielding, the best immediate action is to decrease the duration of the exposure, increase the distance from exposure, and put appropriate shielding between individuals and the source of the exposure.

7.9.2   Personal Protective Equipment (PPE)

In a radiation incident, typical barrier PPE may not be effective, because many isotopes produce gamma radiation capable of penetrating most clothing and protective equipment. In general, firefighters are protected from beta radiation by the heavy nature of "bunker gear" or "turnout gear" (boots, trousers and coat, gloves, hood, mask). This will be sufficient to prevent, or drastically reduce, risk of isotope inhalation. No gear will protect against external gamma radiation. If the gear becomes contaminated, it should be removed and collected as the firefighter (or other personnel) leaves the outer perimeter. Alpha radiation does not penetrate intact skin or clothing and is not an external hazard.

The most significant component of any PPE is respiratory protection. An N95 mask or better is optimal. Keeping radioactive materials out of the body is paramount. A problem with any type of respiratory protection in emergency response and management is that it hampers communication. If N95 protection is not available, any respiratory protection should be used until the airborne contamination is ruled out. The skin is protected with standard infection-control procedures, such as latex or nitrile gloves, surgical gowns and scrubs, and booties. Responders should be instructed to remove respiratory protection last when dealing with contaminated patients to reduce the likelihood of inhaled isotopes. Minor intrusions through the barrier, such as needlesticks, clothing tears, and fastener failure, should not be regarded as a significant source of radiation.

Because level C, B, or A gear can restrict movement and diminish the sense of touch, as well as cause heat stress, it may not be useful to wear such PPE when responding to a purely radiation environment. Use of level C or higher barrier clothing for a purely radiologic event also may hamper delivery of medical care. Despite these limitations, it is necessary to keep radioactive material off the skin for efficient decontamination, so some form of barrier clothing is needed. Examples are level D PPE, such as surgical gowns, scrubs, Tyvek suits, or other inexpensive and easy-to-remove clothing. Another challenge is how to hydrate a responder. Water intake requires removing respiratory protection and ensuring that the drinking vessel's edges and contents are not contaminated. Radiation specialists can assist in determining the specific type of PPE required for the situation.

It is important to know whether there are contaminants in the environment other than radioisotopes. Other contaminants may require the use of level C, B, or A PPE, which could further hamper medical treatment of casualties, shorten the time the responder can remain in the response environment, and complicate triage and treatment. One of the early determinations by the safety officer should be the level of PPE needed by persons entering the hot zone, persons staffing the decontamination area, and even security personnel dealing with the numbers of the public approaching treatment facilities. The contamination zone could be regarded as containing airborne "radioactive dirt," which should not be ingested but otherwise may be removed by thorough mechanical means and then tested by means of routine radiation detection equipment.

7.9.3   Radiation Exposure Monitoring

According to guidance from the US Environmental Protection Agency (EPA), situations may occur in which a dose in excess of 0.25 Sv (25 rem) for emergency exposure would be unavoidable to carry out a lifesaving operation or avoid extensive exposure of large populations (see Table 7-1).[27,28] This limit may be exceeded only under the explicit direction of the incident commander, and only when the risks to responders would clearly result in benefits in terms of lives saved. Close monitoring of radiation levels received by responders between the perimeters and inside the inner perimeter is mandatory.

In general, the amount of contamination that could enter the body is extremely small but should be evaluated on a case-by-case basis. In all cases, a detection device should determine the radiation field from the exposed individual. A portal monitor or handheld meter can determine the radiation field level. If the individual has been shown to have a minimal field reading, PPE will prevent internal exposure to medical personnel.

TABLE 7-1 Radiation Exposure Limits for Responders[27,28]

Response Function	Exposure Limit
All personnel	50 mSv (5 rem)
Protecting major property	100 mSv (10 rem)
Lifesaving/protecting large populations	250 mSv (25 rem)
Lifesaving/protecting large populations	>250 mSv (>25 rem); only on a volunteer basis to persons fully aware of the risks involved

If lifesaving emergency responder doses approach or exceed 0.5 Sv (50 rem), emergency responders must be made aware of both the acute and the chronic (cancer) risks of such exposure.

Regulations require that a person in an area with radiation above 0.02 mSv (2 mrem) have monitoring with radiation detection equipment, called *dosimetry*. In a practical application, one individual in a group is required to have some sort of device that records a reading for those in the area. In an emergency, there may not be sufficient dosimetry equipment for either the individual or a group. The critical item then becomes an actual measurement of the radiation field, because the radiation exposure of the workers must be accounted for. A field measurement taken by a radiation specialist can be used for those responding to the event. Documentation is critical. When the measurements are taken, the readings should be communicated to incident command as soon as possible.

It should be noted that radiation exposure limits vary. The National Council on Radiation Protection and Measurements (NCRP) recommends 0.5 Sv (50 rem) as a decision dose for the incident commander to decide whether to remove first responders from further radiation exposure.[25,26] US military guidance allows up to 1.25 Sv (125 rem) in certain special situations.[29] International agencies such as the International Committee on Radiation Protection and the International Atomic Energy Agency (IAEA) also have independently made recommendations. It is not that the biologic effects of ionizing radiation are understood differently among these well-informed scientific bodies or that there are significantly different estimates of risk to responders and casualties; rather, other considerations (political, economic, uncertainties in actual dose received vs estimated likely dose accumulation) enter into decisions for setting such limits.

7.9.4   Casualty Decontamination

A significant problem with delivery of clinical care in a radiologic event is reluctance by medical personnel to handle or be near contaminated persons. The medical provider should understand that contaminated persons are unlikely to present a radiation hazard to the personnel. It is not necessary or advised to delay emergent treatment to decontaminate the casualty.[10,30-34] No medical provider has ever received a radiation exposure from a contaminated casualty sufficient to cause any symptoms.[25,31,32]

Decontamination of the casualty is a matter of mechanical removal of radioactive contamination. Casualties who are ambulatory and contaminated should be provided with any type of privacy clothing, a disposal bag such as a plastic trash bag, and any type of respiratory protection. They should be instructed to don the respiratory protection, doff their clothing and place it in the trash bag or disposal bag, proceed through a same-sex shower, and don the privacy clothing. Respiratory protection could be discarded during or after the shower. Washing the individual with copious water and detergent is an effective method, but any mechanical technique that removes foreign material from the skin without damaging the skin is indicated. Cleaning agents, such as sanitizing or antibacterial agents, may assist with the mechanical removal but will have no other effect on the radioactive nature of the material. If little water is present, contamination can be scraped off the person's skin, and any agent that will absorb materials from the skin can be used. Examples are cornmeal, dry detergent, toothpaste, flour, and virtually any absorbent material.

Small amounts of water should be used to rinse the mouth and nose without swallowing. Special attention should be paid to cleaning the hair. Use shampoo only. The use of conditioner should be avoided, as this can fix radioactive materials to the keratin in the hair. If the hair cannot be washed, it may be cut. The key is to get the material off the contaminated individual and into a containment device. If at all possible, decontamination washoff and residue should be captured after the initial response effort; however, in a mass casualty situation, this may not be possible. Lack of complete runoff containment capability should not be used as a reason to preclude adequate washing for decontamination.[26]

Once the individual has been decontaminated, standard casualty care management guidelines are followed. Observation of the individual with respect to radiologic effects should be continued, with established planned treatment protocols.

7.10 CASUALTY MANAGEMENT

Casualties with conditions requiring emergent intervention, such as arterial injury, can receive emergency treatment with little risk to the provider. With appropriate protective measures, medical response personnel are unlikely to suffer major radiation exposure from the contaminated patient. In a radiologic emergency, lifesaving is separated into two considerations:

➤ Providing emergency care in a radiation field or contamination environment

➤ Providing intervention to ameliorate the effects of the radiation field or ingestion of radioisotopes

7.10.1 Mass Casualty Triage

The goal of triage is to evaluate and sort individuals by immediacy of treatment needed to do the greatest good for the most people.[33] The first responder team needs to sort, assess, perform lifesaving interventions, then treat or transport the casualty. Risks to health care providers from contaminated patients, while greater than zero,

Resources for Radiation Casualty Management Assistance

For immediate help in assessing clinical effects from radiation exposures, health professionals can contact:

➤ Radiation specialists (eg, health physicist, radiation safety officer, nuclear medicine physician, radiation oncologist, radiologist)

➤ Radiation Emergency Assistance Center/Training Site at the Oak Ridge Institute for Science and Education (http://orise.orau.gov/reacts/)

➤ Armed Forces Radiobiology Research Institute and its Medical Radiological Advisory Team (http://www.usuhs.mil/afrri/)

➤ HHS/National Library of Medicine "Radiation Emergency Medical Management" Web site (http://www.remm.nlm.gov/)

➤ Radiation Injury Treatment Network (http://www.ritn.net/)

are very low. Decontamination can often be done simultaneously with treatment if the situation permits, but if sequencing of lifesaving care is necessary, decontamination comes last. Assessments made and actions performed must be documented to guide those down the line in administering appropriate care. Casualty information, incident circumstances (including radiation-specific parameters such as time of onset of emesis after exposure), injuries, and initial treatment should be documented and kept with the individual.

No immediate lifesaving skills are pertinent to radiation exposure alone. Lifesaving procedures are based on conventional trauma injuries: hemorrhage control, airway restoration and maintenance, chest decompression, and antidote injection (for anaphylaxis or chemical agent exposures). In a nuclear detonation, most casualties will have combined injury, consisting of radiation exposure along with burn or traumatic injury. Burns involving 20% to 25% or more of the total body surface area can cause shock. Initial treatment involves steps to prevent shock, elevation of burned areas if appropriate, and covering of the burned areas with sterile gauze or clean cloth. For flame burns around the head and neck area, the airway should be protected.

Triage categories for patients with combined injury will vary by resource scarcity. The problem will be compounded by the fact that an exact or even workable dose exposure estimate may not be known for several hours, while most life-threatening trauma requires treatment within the first hour after injury.

7.10.2   Casualty Transport to Receiving Facilities

The injured public and many of those who are contaminated will require evacuation to a suitable medical treatment or decontamination facility. Once stabilized for transport, casualties should be transported on litters covered by a blanket or sheet and covered with a sheet themselves. This will contain the radioactive materials that may be on the casualties, thus reducing material remaining on the litter and within and contaminating the ambulance. The incident commander or staff will have to direct travel from the scene to the appropriate medical treatment facility and possibly specify what route to take. Civilian vehicles (cars, trucks, ambulances) offer little if any radiation protection factor to those inside compared to someone standing outside the vehicle. This should be kept in mind when traveling in or traversing the dangerous fallout zone.

Even in a nuclear detonation, there may be thousands of casualties who have injuries that require care but are not immediately life threatening (eg, sprains, strains, moderate to severe bruising, eardrum damage, cuts, and lacerations). These persons also may be contaminated by fallout. Because of the massive numbers of casualties with severe injuries requiring prompt care, their care will need to be deferred. Principles of emergency medical care in transit are the same as for a nonirradiated casualty. Except at extremely high and unsurvivable radiation doses, in which a casualty may be at risk for cardiovascular collapse, there is no injury caused by radiation that will require special care in transit. Special care is dictated by the nonradiologic injuries.

The incident commander should notify the receiving facility of the number and types of casualties as well as estimated time of arrival, to allow it to prepare. The procedures are entirely the same as for a conventional mass casualty situation, with the exception that the receiving facility be informed if possible whether there is any residual contamination. Contamination is never allowed to delay urgently required treatment; however, the facility needs to be aware so that casualties can be appropriately routed through the facility and the radiation safety officer and staff can be informed. If the casualties are stable, they should go to a separate area and be decontaminated before entering the treatment facility. The Centers for Disease Control and Prevention (CDC) estimates that half of all initial casualties will seek medical care over a 1-hour period; those less injured will clearly have the advantage in terms of rapidity of access to the closest receiving facility. Plans need to be made in advance for where to place these people who require deferred or minor care.

7.11 CLINICAL MANAGEMENT OF RADIATION CASUALTIES: BASIC CONCEPTS AND PRINCIPLES

After a nuclear or radiologic disaster, there is a good possibility that casualties will arrive at health care facilities unaware they have been exposed to radiation or that they may be contaminated. This is exacerbated by the fact that most casualties with light or moderate injuries, and also those uninjured but concerned they have been exposed to radiation (including those who are contaminated), will self-transport. Exposed individuals may present with fatigue and weakness, nausea, anorexia, emesis, diarrhea, headache, and possibly rash or burns. The astute clinician may notice several patients presenting with these symptoms, some of which are not characteristic of conventional explosives injuries. With an RED, in which the source of radiation exposure is intentionally hidden with the design of irradiating as many people as possible for as long as possible, this will most likely be the case. The astute clinician will have to rely on preincident threat assessment reports combined with his or her clinical judgment, again backed by appropriate instrumentation.

The inundation of hospitals and other emergency provider sites by a mixture of injured casualties, with or without contamination, and uninjured people who will be concerned that they will be harmed by radiation if not treated, requires a rapid, accurate, and established protocol for distinguishing between the two groups. In the case of a nuclear disaster in a major urban area, it is conceivable that the latter group would number in the hundreds of thousands or even millions. Radiologic disasters would generate far fewer casualties than a nuclear weapon attack, but the number of persons concerned that they were exposed and potentially injured from exposure to the disseminated radioactive materials could still be quite high.

While the thousands or even millions of casualties resulting from a nuclear detonation would, in itself, overwhelm current medical response capabilities, the response dilemma is further exacerbated in that these resources themselves would be significantly at risk. There are many limitations on the resources needed for mass casualty management, such as access to sufficient hospital beds, including specialized beds for burn patients; respiration and supportive therapy; pharmaceutical intervention; and mass decontamination.

7.11.1   Clinical Clues to Radiation Exposure

The first symptoms of significant radiation exposure are generally nausea, vomiting, fatigue, and lassitude; these are rather "soft" symptoms that present with other illnesses as well as acute radiation sickness (ARS). Diarrhea also occurs, though usually not until doses of 4 Sv (400 rem) or more.[30] As shown in Table 7-2, symptom severity relates directly to the level of exposure, and the interval from the beginning of exposure to the development of symptoms is inversely related to the dose received. These symptoms abate *if* the casualty is removed from the source. If the sources of radiation are on or within the patient (ie, contamination), the symptoms may resolve more slowly.

The clinical effect of radiation exposure will depend on numerous variables, including the following:

➤ Type of exposure (total- or partial-body exposure vs internal or external contamination)

➤ Route of exposure (eg, skin contact or breathing in or ingesting contaminated material)

➤ Type of tissue exposed (tissue that is sensitive to radiation vs tissue that is insensitive)

➤ Type of radiation (alpha, beta, gamma)

➤ Depth of penetration of radiation in the body (low vs high energy)

➤ Total absorbed dose

➤ Period during which the dose is absorbed (dose rate)

The best laboratory test to determine level of exposure is the complete blood cell count (CBC) with differential. Lymphocytes are the most sensitive tissue in the body to radiation exposure, and a serial drop can tell roughly how high a dose was

TABLE 7-2 Initial Signs and Symptoms of Significant Radiation Exposure[2,30,35,36]

Sign/Symptom	Mild 1-2 Sv (100-200 rem)	Moderate 2-4 Sv (200-400 rem)	Severe 4-6 Sv (400-600 rem)	Very Severe >6 Sv (>600 rem)
Emesis	<35%	35%-72%	72%-95%	·100%
Emesis (time to onset)	≥2 h	1-2 h	<1 hour	<30 minutes
Survival (Chernobyl data)	41/41	49/50	15/22	1/21
Absolute lymphocyte count 24 hours after exposure (% normal)	78%-100%	60%-78%	50%-60%	<50%

Dose ranges cited in references are similar but not exact.

received. Neutrophils spike shortly after acute radiation exposure before dropping, so a high neutrophil-lymphocyte ratio 4 hours or so after exposure is also a very good, though less quantitative, tipoff to significant radiation exposure.[31] As a rule, if the lymphocyte count drops to less than 50% of normal baseline within the first 24 hours, the individual has received a significant dose.

Probably the earliest observable sign of high radiation exposure is erythema of the skin, which can occur a few hours after high levels of exposure. Skin changes and hair loss can be caused by exposure to external radiation, or the presence of beta particles on the skin. However, as these signs do not appear for days or weeks after exposure, they will not be helpful in the early detection of a radiation incident (Table 7-3).

Obviously, if large numbers of people with the above signs and symptoms present in the same time frame, this should increase the astute clinician's index of suspicion of an RDD or RED event and direct their diagnostic procedures and examinations on individual patients to detect possible radiation contamination or exposure.

7.11.2 Patient Assessment and Clinical Decision Making

Patient assessment is primarily based on conventional injuries (eg, mechanical trauma and burns), not on radiation dose received, which will be an unknown initially. For example, if a patient has symptoms that could be associated with either trauma or radiation (eg, hypotension, mental status changes), it is to be presumed that the symptoms are a result of traumatic hypovolemia or traumatic brain injury and not a result of a massive radiation dose. Significant radiation exposure lowers the prognosis, aggravates the symptoms from conventional trauma, decreases wound healing, and increases the risk of infection.

No specific signs or symptoms are pathognomonic for radiation exposure, especially in the first several hours after the incident. The caregiver should ascertain, however, whether nausea and emesis are or have been present and how soon after

TABLE 7-3 Skin Effects of Radiation Exposure[33]

The CDC grades cutaneous radiation injury as follows: Grade 1: >2 Sv (200 rem) Grade 2: >15 Sv (1500 rem) Grade 3: >40 Sv (4000 rem) (Note: these dose levels are local, not whole body)	

Threshold Radiation Dose	Skin Effect
3 Sv (300 rem) Grade 1	Epilation, 2 weeks or more after exposure
6 Sv (600 rem) Grade 1	Transient erythema, followed by secondary erythema in 2 or 3 weeks
10-15 Sv (1000-1500 rem) Grade 1	Dry desquamation of the skin due to damage of the germinal layer, usually appearing 3 weeks after exposure
20-50 Sv (2000-5000 rem) Grade 2 or 3	Wet desquamation, a partial-thickness injury, resulting in edema with bullae and a wet, fibrin-coated dermal surface appearing 2 to 3 weeks postexposure
>50 Sv (5000 rem) Grade 3	Overt ulceration and necrosis with permanent damage to the endothelium and necrosis of the small blood vessels. Time of appearance is inversely related to dose.

exposure emesis began. Also, the patient should be assessed for diarrhea in terms of severity and time of onset after exposure, as well as the presence of blood. Skin and corneal irritation shortly after exposure indicate contamination of these organs.

Regarding the radiation dose effect on triage, it is important to remember that high radiation dose levels will affect prognosis and response to treatment, not immediate casualty care. In a major catastrophe, exposed patients may need to be sorted into one of three groups:

➤ Those who cannot survive even with prompt treatment

➤ Those who will recover without treatment or with treatment that can be delayed

➤ Those who require prompt treatment to save life

This will be especially important in situations in which patients rapidly exceed the surge capabilities and capacities for limited resources (eg, intensive care units, burn unit beds, ventilator support). It is important to remember that palliative care and appropriate utilization of resources should be provided to patients who are deemed unable to survive.

The medical history obtained should mention the time of the incident, where the patient was located, and what his or her movements have been since then. It is important to note whether the individual has had nausea or emesis, when these symptoms began after exposure, and how severe they are; these parameters are helpful in estimating dose received. Other symptoms that may occur in the first minutes or few hours after exposure include diarrhea (ascertain whether blood is present), skin and corneal irritation (may indicate fallout particles), parotitis (inflammation of the parotid gland), anorexia, headache, and, in severe cases, fever, hypotension, mental status changes (disorientation, ataxia, loss of consciousness), and temporary loss of consciousness. With high, but often survivable, radiation exposures, early fatalities (first week to second month) are due to hemorrhage and sepsis; later fatalities are due to specific organ system(s) failure.

Early development of erythema, in the first few hours after exposure, is an ominous sign. Hypotension, tachypnea, and loss of consciousness are suggestive of a lethal exposure, assuming there are no other possible causes of these symptoms. Vital signs (temperature, pulse, blood pressure) must be taken. A high radiation dose can cause fever, though other trauma (burn, infection) can cause these signs as well. It is very important to complete an appropriate all-hazards-minded physical examination. Radiation exposure is only one important aspect to be assessed. Other mechanisms of injury or signs of other illnesses or disease processes must be sought.

In establishing the acceptance of casualties into overburdened health facilities after nuclear events, medical treatment for nuclear and radiologic trauma would be similar to other conventional trauma treatment approaches in that life-threatening complications like airway blockage and shock must be addressed before other issues, including radiologic concerns. The major difference in triage of significantly (defined as more than 1.5 Sv [150 rem]) irradiated patients is that individuals requiring surgical intervention should undergo surgery within 36 hours (48 hours at most) after the exposure. Other surgical procedures should not be performed until after 6 weeks. In a mass casualty situation, treatment of ARS is not indicated when exposure dose is very low (<1 Sv [100 rem]) or very high (>10 Sv [1000 rem]).

Major clinical decisions regarding the timing and extensiveness of surgical procedures need to be made early on. Operative procedures, which include chest tube thoracostomies and venous cutdowns, need to be performed within the first 24 to 48 hours. If done after this time, the probabilities of wound dehiscence, infection, and delayed healing or nonhealing increase dramatically. Reconstructive surgery will need to be deferred for several weeks or months until fibroblasts, osteoblasts, white blood cells, and other radiosensitive immune system components have recovered sufficiently to repair surgical injuries. These are tissues that are sensitive to radiation and become depleted or dysfunctional within hours or a few days after high exposure and therefore are unable to repair or restore necessary surgical trauma after this point.

7.11.3 Trauma Care

The traditional basic skills for care of injuries resulting from the traumatic mechanisms or conventional weapons are employed regardless of presence or level of radiation exposure. Individuals with traumatic injuries to the spine should be stabilized before transport. Management of fluid and electrolytes is important, as are other basic trauma support procedures. It should be noted again that even minimally invasive procedures such as cutdowns, light debridement, and wound closure with suturing should be performed within the first 36 hours after radiation exposure, to decrease the risk of sepsis and wound dehiscence. Unfortunately, in a nuclear attack many burn and trauma patients will have access to medical care significantly delayed by the attendant effects of the blast damage and fires in urban areas.

Adherence to routinely advanced trauma and medical skills is the mainstay of care delivery. Interestingly, RDDs can release fragments requiring surgical removal, especially if radioactive isotopes (like cobalt 60) that fragment rather than pulverize are used. Surgical staff will require medical physics support and radiation monitoring. Fragments should be handed off to the radiation safety officer or designate, then placed in a suitable (lead) container. If blood component transfusions are required, they should be irradiated to 25 Sv (2500 rem) beforehand, to prevent graft vs host disease. Otherwise the principles of surgical and intensive care do not vary from those that apply to nonirradiated patients. Mass casualty burn care will require that a very wide variety of health care personnel acquire burn care treatment skills, including many clinicians who have not treated burns in clinical practice for a long time.

7.11.4   Diagnostic Testing

For a nuclear device, radiation exposure will be assumed; the only uncertainty will be the actual dose received. There is a possibility, particularly with a dud (no nuclear yield but dispersal of weapon fuel) or fizzle (incomplete yield), that plutonium or uranium will be inhaled. As the treatment for these radioactive isotopes is different (chelating agents for plutonium, alkalinization of urine with sodium bicarbonate for uranium), it is important to discern via bioassays of urine and stool which if either of these isotopes may have been inhaled. This can become complicated, as there are devices that contain both uranium and plutonium.

For external radiation exposure, the critical parameter is dose received; what isotopes caused this exposure is not important. For internal radiation contamination, it is essential to know what isotope(s) was/were involved so appropriate decorporation therapy can be inititiated.[11]

Once the patient has been received at a medical treatment facility, serial CBCs with differential should be done as soon as possible after exposure. Leukopenia, particularly lymphopenia, in serial CBCs is probably the quickest and easiest way to diagnosis significant radiation exposure, though confirmation by bioassays or cytogenetics may be necessary. Location of the source(s) confirms the diagnosis. CBCs should initially be repeated three or four times daily until trends in the values warrant less frequent testing. Serum amylase measurement should be done. Cytogenetic testing should be performed; however, at the time of this writing only two institutions in the United States, the Armed Forces Radiobiology Research Institute and the Radiation Emergency Assistance Center/Training Site at Oak Ridge Associated Universities, are accredited to do these procedures.

If external contamination is detected, spectroscopic analysis can determine the isotope involved. This would be appropriate for an RDD but not a nuclear explosion, in which dozens of isotopes could be present. For internal contamination, urinary and fecal samples should be taken. Whole-body counting can be done for gamma-emitting isotopes (most likely cesium 137 and cobalt 60, less likely iridium 192, radium 226, and the beta-emitter strontium 90) and can discern which ones are present.

7.11.5   Therapeutic Interventions

Care of patients exposed to high doses of radiation is complex, particularly if other trauma, toxins, or illness is present. The course of therapy for ARS and cutaneous radiation syndrome is long. As with long-term care in general, mental health support and social support, particularly for patients in isolation because of infection precautions, is important. In addition, there is the fear of the unknown associated with ARS, as well as the fact that the risk of future cancers is known even to the lay public, albeit usually exaggerated.

In any toxic exposure, the first step in therapeutic intervention generally includes stopping further exposure to the toxin. This is true in radiation exposure as well. For external whole-body irradiation, this means removing the patient from the area of radiation exposure and removing external contamination. There is no way at present to reverse or remove radiation damage, only to mitigate its consequences. For internal contamination, this involves decorporation of the radionuclide(s). However, there are often other concomitant injuries that may take precedence over evacuation, shielding, decontamination, and decorporation.

Casualties presenting with symptoms suggestive of neurovascular syndrome have been exposed to extremely high doses of radiation (>20 Sv [2000 rem]).[33] These symptoms include vomiting and diarrhea within minutes of the event, confusion and disorientation, hypotension, edema, convulsions, coma, and hyperpyrexia. This syndrome is fatal within 24 to 48 hours, even with state-of-the-art medical treatment and resources. In a mass casualty situation, treatment for these casualties should focus on palliation of symptoms rather than resource-intensive and ultimately futile efforts at prolonging life. However, an important caveat is to ensure that there is not some other treatable condition that is causing this complex of symptoms.

7.11.6   Altered Care Environment

Nuclear events are likely to cause a very significant change in standards of care because of the enormous casualty loads and the unusual nature of these casualty distributions (ie, hundreds of thousands of casualties, radiation illnesses unfamiliar to most medical personnel, large numbers of burn casualties). It is important to emerge from this extraordinary diversion from the desired standards of care as soon as possible after a nuclear event. *Altered care environment* (ACE) refers to the concept of treating large numbers of casualties outside of a traditional setting because of limitations in existing traditional health care facility capacity. The most striking difficulty will be with mass casualty burn care, as the ratio of medical personnel to patients will be so adverse relative to standard care.

Under normal circumstances, the current standard of care for burn casualties is to transfer any individuals with significant burns to specialty burn centers. This is especially true for pediatric patients. The American Burn Association lists 132 burn centers in the United States with a total of about 1900 beds.[37] However, only a small fraction of these beds are available for new patients at any one time. Various models have predicted that a small nuclear weapon detonated in a large urban area may produce upward of 50 000 to 100 000 patients who have suffered significant body burns, many with comorbid trauma injuries.[12,38-40] With this number of potential burn casualties, it becomes obvious that these individuals will have to be treated in facilities other than burn centers.

Major problems in burn treatment for nuclear detonation casualties are transport, time elapsed from injury to treatment, and availability of trained personnel to enable treatment. With only a handful of facilities capable of handling severely burned patients under any circumstances, the prospect of treating thousands of burn casualties requires rapid expansion of burn treatment capabilities in the disaster area and rapid transport to those sites. The key problem is time, as burn casualties will be in severe pain, and infection will begin to set in during this interim period. The arrival of state and federal assistance may be delayed for hours and days after the detonation, and this assistance is critical for large-scale burn treatment. Many analysts, therefore, have concluded that most severely and even moderately burned patients would die before an adequate response can be mounted. This was the case for the severely burned firefighters and other workers coping with the Chernobyl nuclear disaster.

It is essential, therefore, that local authorities devise emergency response plans that mobilize burn treatment, particularly trained health care providers on the immediate periphery of a nuclear detonation disaster area. Transport will be difficult in a devastated urban area, as it is likely that most roads will have considerable amounts of debris hampering or even preventing the required rapid movement of patients.

7.12   MANAGEMENT OF ARS

ARS is now regarded as a multisystem disorder, with radiation damage occurring to all systems at all doses sufficient to induce ARS. Because of the intrinsic differences in radiosensitivity among the tissues, the type of symptoms and signs demonstrated and the time to their expression varies. A man injured in an industrial accident at Nesvizh, Belarus, received 12.5 Sv (1250 rem) of whole-body irradiation, with some areas receiving up to 18 Sv (1800 rem). He experienced severe emesis within minutes after radiation, as well as severe depression of all hematopoietic elements. However, owing to intensive medical and supportive care, he survived the traditional hematopoietic and gastrointestinal ARS subsyndromes and died of pulmonary damage 16 weeks after exposure. On the other hand, radiation-induced emesis at low, survivable doses is due to the effect of serotonin and histamine released by irradiated tissues on the vomiting and chemoreceptor trigger zones, respectively, in the brain. Headache can occur at intermediate doses, while at high doses central nervous system (CNS) effects occur because of hypotension and direct impairment of neurotransmitter functions. While the implications of regarding ARS as a multiorgan dysfunction syndrome or multiorgan failure rather than three subsyndromes are more academic than directly affecting clinical management, it is important to note that radiation damage can occur to all tissues at all levels, and to be alert to the clinical expression and management of these damages.

As shown in Table 7-4, the three subsyndromes of ARS are as follows:

➤ Hematopoietic, generally occurring at 1 to 6 Sv (100–600 rem)

➤ Gastrointestinal, from 6 to 20 Sv (600–2000 rem)

➤ Cardiovascular/CNS, occurring above 20 Sv (2000 rem)

TABLE 7-4 Clinical Manifestations of Acute Radiation Sickness[10,31,32] (Whole-Body or Extensive Partial-Body Exposure)

Dose	Clinical Status	Description
0-1 Sv (0-100 rem)	Generally asymptomatic	White blood cell count normal or minimally depressed below baseline at 3-5 wk after exposure
0.05 Sv		No symptoms
0.15 Sv		No symptoms, but possible chromosomal aberrations in cultured peripheral blood lymphocytes
0.5 Sv		No symptoms (minor decreases in white blood cell and platelet counts in a few people)

>1 Sv (>100 rem)	Hematopoietic syndrome (prodromal phase followed by latent period of 1 d to 2 wk depending on radiation dose)	➤ Prodromal signs and symptoms (generally lasting 24-48 h: anorexia, nausea, vomiting
		➤ Skin erythema, fever, mucositis, and diarrhea also may be present
		➤ Bone marrow suppression (average 2-3 wk after exposure)
		➤ Laboratory analysis in patients with whole-body exposure greater than 2 Sv can show initial granulocytosis, with pancytopenia evident 20-30 d after exposure
		➤ Subsequent systemic effects:
		  ➤ immunodysfunction
		  ➤ increased susceptibility to infectious complications
		  ➤ possible hemorrhage
		  ➤ sepsis
		  ➤ anemia
		  ➤ impaired wound healing

1 Sv		Nausea and vomiting in approximately 10% of patients within 48 h after exposure
2 Sv		Nausea and vomiting in approximately 50% of persons within 24 h, with marked decreases in white blood cell and platelet counts
4 Sv		Nausea and vomiting in 90% of people within 12 h, and diarrhea in 10% within 8 h; 50% mortality within 60 days without medical treatment
6 Sv		100% mortality within 30 d due to bone marrow failure in the absence of medical treatment
>6-8 Sv (>600-800 rem)	Gastrointestinal syndrome (latent period <1 d)	➤ Symptoms may include severe gastrointestinal damage, with nausea, vomiting, and watery diarrhea occurring within minutes or hours of exposure ➤ Hematopoietic syndrome occurs concomitantly ➤ In severe cases, patient may present with shock and possibly renal failure and cardiovascular collapse ➤ Death usually occurs in 2-3 wk after exposure without medical treatment
8-10 Sv (800-1000 rem)		Approximate maximum dose that may be survivable with the best medical therapy available

(Continued)

TABLE 7-4   *(Continued)*

Dose	Clinical Status	Description
>20 Sv (>2000 rem)	Cardiovascular/CNS (no latent period; immediate onset of overt illness)	➤ Medical intervention is supportive ➤ Within minutes of exposure, patients may experience burning sensation ➤ Within the first hour after exposure, patients experience nausea and vomiting followed by prostration, and neurologic signs of ataxia and confusion ➤ Deteriorating state of consciousness follows, with tremors and convulsions, leading to coma, cardiovascular collapse, and death ➤ Significant neurologic symptoms indicate lethal dose ➤ Death is inevitable and usually occurs within 24-72 h

The three phases of ARS are prodromal, latent, and manifest illness. The fourth phase in survivors is recovery, which can be prolonged and is probably never complete at the cellular level. The prodromal period begins shortly after exposure and is characterized by nausea, vomiting, anorexia, fatigue, weakness, possibly low-grade headache or mild fever, and conjunctivitis and transient skin erythema in many cases. At very high and unsurvivable doses, patients may experience a burning sensation immediately after exposure, with very severe and rapid (within minutes) emesis, high fever, hypotension, possible collapse, and neurologic signs such as ataxia, confusion, severe headache, and deteriorating levels of consciousness to coma and death.

7.12.1   Treatment of Emesis and Diarrhea

Treatment of emesis in irradiated casualties is improved by antiemetics, preferably the 5-HT3 antagonists (ondansetron, granisetron). If emesis and/or diarrhea are severe, fluid and electrolyte balance should be monitored carefully. Antidiarrheal agents such as loperamide can be helpful. Once the emesis subsides, oral feeding is recommended over parenteral feeding to restore the immunologic and physiologic integrity of the gut. If diarrhea is present, low-residue diets may be helpful. Because of infection control considerations, the food should be clean or sterile if possible. After Chernobyl, physicians empirically used probiotics such as *Bifidobacteria* and *Lactobacillus* species to suppress pathogenic overgrowth over the gut epithelium and to encourage growth of normal flora involved in this suppression. Although the likelihood of survival was not demonstrably increased, survival time was, and cultures for pathogenic bacteria were negative.

Except after high radiation doses, the patient usually improves after 24 to 48 hours, with emesis and diarrhea much improved or absent and an increased energy level. The duration of the prodromal period is inversely related to exposure received. This latency period's duration and degree of clinical improvement is also inversely related to the radiation dose received.

7.12.2 Infection Control

After a week or two, the patient's condition deteriorates again. The chief causes of death during the first 60 days are generally infection and hemorrhage, and management principles revolve around the control of these two factors. Laminar air flow and reverse isolation precautions (gown, gloves, masks, hand washing before all patient contact) should be instituted for persons receiving 3 Sv (300 rem) or more, or earlier if comorbid conditions predisposing to infection are present. Oral hygiene is very important, though flossing and brushing should be gentle enough to avoid trauma to the gingival mucosa. Mouthwashes should be considered. Skin should be kept clean. Gut decontamination with quinolones (eg, ciprofloxacin) should be begun, for the reasons described above.[41]

It is critically necessary to control infection while the patient is neutropenic. If the absolute neutrophil count is less than 0.5×10^9 cells/L, a fluoroquinolone should be administered, even if the patient is afebrile without an apparent source of infection. A fluoroquinolone with streptococcal coverage, or addition of penicillin or amoxicillin, should be used. Antimicrobial agents should be continued until fever or failure occurs, and then should be changed. Therapy directed at gram-negative bacteria (particularly *Pseudomonas aeruginosa*) should then be instituted (an aminoglycoside should be considered). For resistant gram-positive infections, vancomycin should be added. If burns are present, a broad-spectrum antibiotic should be used, such as imipenem or piperacillin/tazobactam, depending on local hospital flora. Fluconazole is the starting antifungal agent. Acyclovir should be used if the patient is positive for herpes simplex virus, or else started empirically on the basis of patient history. Antimicrobial management is rather complex, so consultation from infectious disease specialists and the guidelines from the Infectious Diseases Society of America should be obtained.

7.12.3 Cytokine Therapy

Recently, hematopoietic colony-stimulating factors (CSF), which are cytokines, have received Food and Drug Administration (FDA) approval for management of medical treatment-induced neutropenia. Though they have not yet been formally approved for management of radiation-induced aplasia, these cytokines are in the Strategic National Stockpile (SNS), and their off-label use should be considered in casualties with significant radiation exposure. The SNS Radiation Working Group has recommended use of these cytokines,[10] as a significant survival advantage has been demonstrated in laboratory animals when they are given within the first 24 hours after irradiation. Neutrophil recovery occurs 3 to 6 days earlier in humans given cytokines after myelotoxic therapies. Ideally, marrow-resuscitation therapy should begin within 24 hours after radiation if the absolute neutrophil count is less than 500×10^9/L, or perhaps at even higher levels for children and the elderly.

Recommendations for cytokine administration are based, for mass casualty scenarios, on doses of 3 to 7 Sv (300-700 rem) in otherwise healthy persons. This essentially means that cytokines will be administered only to those patients with high radiation doses, approaching and even within the fatal dose range for humans. If multiple injuries are present, 2 to 6 Sv (200-600 rem) should be considered as the starting radiation dose for cytokine treatment. If, in extreme situations, laboratory dosimetry information is not available, a rule of thumb such as emesis beginning within the first 4 hours (median dose of approximately 2 Sv [200 rem]) may be used to start therapy. Current CSFs are filgrastim, pegfilgrastim, and sargramostim. Other CSFs such as darbepoetin and epoetin act similarly to erythropoietin to stimulate erythrocyte replacement; however, the laboratory data are not as robust for recommending their usage. Traditional packed erythrocyte and platelet transfusions will be necessary in heavily exposed patients. It is necessary to irradiate these components with 25 Sv (2500 rem) beforehand to suppress the possibility of transfused leukocytes causing a graft vs host reaction.

7.12.4   Stem Cell Transplants

While stem-cell transplantations have been used with success in patients with certain hematologic malignant conditions with success, the success of this treatment for radiation casualties is much less impressive. Of the 13 patients at Chernobyl given stem-cell transplants, 11 died; the two survivors reconstituted their own bone marrow and no persisting transfused tissue was detected.[32,42] Two persons at the Tokai-Mura, Japan, accident (1999) received allogeneic transplantation and demonstrated transient engraftment followed by complete autologous hematopoietic recovery (both died later).[33] A 1997 review of allogeneic transplant experience in 29 patients with bone marrow failure from radiation accidents showed that all patients with burns died and only three lived more than a year. It was unclear whether the transplants even affected survival. It should also be noted that graft vs host disease was thought responsible for two or three of the 11 deaths at Chernobyl. There is no convincing evidence that allogeneic stem-cell transplants would have much of a role in radiation mass casualty events.

7.13   CUTANEOUS RADIATION SYNDROME (CRS)

CRS is a critical feature of highly irradiated casualties, often associated with expectant patients. It should be noted that of the World War II casualties in the Hiroshima and Nagasaki bombings in World War II, two-thirds had combined-effects (radiation and/or thermal and/or mechanical trauma) injuries. The majority of casualties who died in the first month after the Chernobyl incident had skin injuries from radiation.[32,42] The public tends to associate external skin irradiation mainly with hair loss. Hair loss occurs around 2 weeks after exposure. However, the range of skin injuries in CRS ranges from erythema to epilation to desquamation, both dry and moist, and ulceration with eventual fibrosis.

Generally, when there is significant whole-body radiation, there is significant local radiation injury, primarily CRS. Within the first week after exposure, the patient is generally asymptomatic aside from a transient wave of erythema in the first several hours. In the second week, true erythema develops along with damage to the sebaceous and sweat glands, inhibiting their secretions. During the third week the skin is warm, tender, edematous, and sometimes pruritic. (However, these are localized symptoms; a whole-body exposure of this magnitude would be lethal.) Eventually, dry or, at higher doses, moist desquamation develops. As depicted in Table 7-3 page 7-214, the CDC uses the following grading system for cutaneous injury: grade 1, greater than 2 Sv (200 rem); grade 2, greater than 15 Sv (1500 rem); and grade 3, greater than 40 Sv (4000 rem). Recently new modalities of assessing high-level skin doses, such as Doppler or laser flow profiles, ultrasound visualization of the lesions, and positron emission tomography and magnetic resonance imaging, have been used.

The two main approaches to managing CRS are conservative and surgical treatment. For relatively intact skin, appropriate treatment is corticosteroid ointments, topical antibiotics with dressings if blistering is present, and other emollients. In moist desquamation or ulceration, silver sulfadiazine should be used. The key is to control infection and inflammation. Hyperbaric oxygen, pentoxifylline, and vitamin E preparations are also used in the management of radiation necrosis. If severe pain or necrosis or ulceration without signs of regeneration are present, surgical intervention should be performed. The surgeon needs to be aware that the damage to cutaneous microvasculature extends well beyond the clinically apparent lesion, and there is most likely less vascular support for repair or graft sustainment than would be the case for an ordinary burn of similar extent. It is important to make the procedure more extensive than for conventional burns; otherwise one runs the risk of serial amputations.

During the triage process, including the ongoing patient sorting at medical treatment facilities, clinicians must be aware that CRS will lower the prognosis for survival in casualties with ARS and other major injuries. This, plus the consideration of resource shortages, may indicate less aggressive treatment and treatment with palliative intent.

7.14 MANAGEMENT OF INTERNAL RADIOISOTOPE CONTAMINATION

Internal contamination is the third major radiation injury likely to be encountered, particularly with an RDD. In catastrophic events involving external whole-body exposure and internal contamination (such as major reactor accidents and nuclear detonations), the former is far more predominant. At Chernobyl, when lung and thyroid intake/uptake were measured, the total internal dose was less than 5% of the total external exposure, with the exception of two men who had severe burns and had absorbed radioactive materials through their breached skin. The key parameter in determining injury from *external* irradiation is the dose received; the particular isotopes involved do not substantially affect medical management. The key factor in *internal* contamination is the isotope(s) involved; decorporation procedures are highly isotope dependent.

7.14.1 Isotope Determination

Whenever internal contamination is suspected, it is important to rapidly detect and identify the isotope(s) involved. If the isotope is also present outside the body, a sample can be taken and the isotope identified through mass spectroscopy or similar means. A whole-body counter can identify gamma-emitting isotopes inside the body.

Thyroid scanning is useful in determining whether the thyroid has taken up a significant amount of one or more radioactive iodine isotopes (primarily a beta emitter). Sampling of the nose (obtained by using one swab for each nostril, with care taken not to cross-contaminate) can detect isotopes that have been inhaled. If a swab is not available, the patient should be asked to blow his or her nose onto a cloth; this will be not only diagnostic but therapeutic in that it will remove isotopes caught in the nasal airways before they enter the aerodigestive tract. Finally, bioassays of the urine and stool will detect isotopes that are excreted; 24-hour urine and fecal collections are important in monitoring the remaining body burden if appropriate. Highly water-soluble isotopes such as tritium and cesium (probably the RDD "isotope of choice") are excreted through the sweat; this is useful in identification but not quantification.

7.14.2   Decorporation Techniques and Countermeasures

Once the isotope is identified, countermeasures can be employed for decorporation. It helps to understand the following terms, which are often used when discussing countermeasures for internal contamination:

➤ *Intake* refers to the means of entry into the body.

➤ *Uptake* is when the contaminant gets into the extracellular fluid (primarily blood circulatory system) and lymphatic system.

➤ *Deposition* occurs when the contaminant enters the cells of the target organ or organs. (For example, iodine heads for the thyroid; strontium for bone and milk; and cesium, being water soluble, is deposited into muscle and many other organs as well.) *Elimination* occurs in one of two ways: physical decay of the isotope and biological removal, both of which have a half-life. The combined half-life equals the product of the physical and biologic half-life divided by their sum.

➤ *Lavage,* or rinsing out a cavity (nose, nasopharynx, stomach, and even lungs) prevents uptake of isotopes that have entered the body. (Removal of radioactive fragments, such as from an RDD using cobalt 60, would also fall in this category.)

Elimination of uranium can be increased by alkalinizing the urine. (This also prevents deposition in the renal tubules.) Hydrating the patient can increase the excretion rate of water-soluble isotopes; this therapy was employed in treating patients in Goiânia, Brazil (1987), who had incorporated cesium 137. Accelerating the passage of certain ingested materials by enemas, laxatives, or cathartics will also reduce the time available for uptake.

Certain materials can be rendered insoluble, or much less soluble, by putting in chemicals or ion exchange resins that bind the isotope and reduce uptake:

➤ Prussian blue is useful for ingested cesium, thallium, or rubidium.

➤ DTPA (diethylentriamene penta-acetate) binds to plutonium, and the chelated plutonium is then removed from the body. Chelating agents such as DTPA can also sometimes remove or reduce the body burden of radioisotopes already deposited in the target tissues or organs.

➤ Deposition of radioactive iodine into the thyroid is blocked by administering KI, which saturates the thyroid, thus preventing the absorption of radioactive iodine from the circulation into the thyroid gland.

The sooner the isotope is identified, the sooner the countermeasure can be applied and the more likely its success. For example, if KI is taken within 1 or 2 hours after a single acute exposure, more than 90% of the uptake of radioactive iodine is blocked. If taken within 3 hours of acute exposure, 50% of the uptake is blocked. If taken more than 4 hours after acute exposure, only 10% is blocked. Patients should continue taking KI daily for 1 to 2 weeks after exposure ceases. The daily iodine dose depends on age (Table 7-5).[10]

Use of DTPA also should be initiated early. It can be given via nebulization in adults, assuming the only actinide contamination was via inhalation, as in a "dud" (dispersion of plutonium weapon fuel by the explosives but without a critical yield) or "fizzle" (incomplete yield owing to explosives misfiring). If administered within the first 24 hours, DTPA can remove 80% of soluble incorporated actinides. It is much less effective for insoluble (oxide) actinide compounds or if initiation of therapy is delayed. The first dose should be calcium-DTPA, then zinc-DTPA daily. If the casualty has significant pulmonary injury or preexisting disease, the DTPA should be administered intravenously.

NCRP Report 161 provides a complete list of decorporation therapy recommendations for almost every imaginable isotope, certainly for all those likely to be used in an RDD.[34] (Though there is no "official" list, the ones most likely to be used in an RDD are cesium 137, cobalt 60, iridium 192, americium 241, strontium 90, and possibly iodine 125 and 131. This listing is based on the activity of the isotopes, the energy of the photons they emit, and their relative ease of availability in quantities sufficient to cause harm.) The information in Table 7-6 may be used for quick reference.

The intention of pharmaceutical approaches is to lower the relative risk by decreasing the subsequent body burden of the toxins that the patient will carry over a lifetime. These interventions, therefore, do not in all cases necessarily have to be initiated during the medical crisis response period. Once patients are under the care of a medical provider, enhanced elimination could be used when the response workload allows.

TABLE 7-5 Daily KI Dose

Age	Predicted Thyroid Dose	Daily KI dose
>40 y	>5 Sv (500 rem)	130 mg
18-40 y	0.1 Sv (10 rem)	130 mg
Pregnant or lactating women	0.05 Sv (5 rem)	130 mg
4-17 y	0.05 Sv (5 rem)	65 mg
1 mo to 3 y	0.05 Sv (5 rem)	32 mg
Birth to <1 mo	0.05 Sv (5 rem)	16 mg

TABLE 7-6 Radioisotope Decorporation Therapies[33,34,36]

Isotope	Countermeasure	Dose*
Americium 241	DTPA	Ca-DTPA: IV 1 g over 5-30 min; can nebulize with 1 g in 1:1 dilution with saline or water. Day 2 and thereafter, use Zn-DTPA Children under 12 years: 14 mg/kg IV as above, not to exceed 1.0 g
Cesium 137	Prussian blue, hydration	3 g PO TID for 2 wk (adults and adolescents); 1 g PO TID (children 2-12 y old). Force fluids 3-4 L/d if tolerated
Cobalt 60	DTPA; alternate DMSA, EDTA, NAC	DTPA: see above DMSA: 10 mg/kg PO every 8 h for 5 d, then BID for 2 wk EDTA: 1000 mg/m^2 IV over 8-12 h NAC: 300 mg/kg IV over 24 h
Iodine isotopes	KI	As per Table 7-5
Iridium 192	Consider DTPA, EDTA	As per cobalt 60
Phosphorus 32	Nonradioactive phosphorus	1-2 250-mg tabs QID with water
Plutonium	DTPA	As per DTPA above
Radium 226	Aluminum hydroxide and calcium gluconate	Aluminum hydroxide: 200 mg to 1 g IV slowly every 1-3 d Calcium gluconate: 10 g powder in 30 cc vial; add water and drink
Strontium 90	Aluminum hydroxide and calcium gluconate	As per radium 226
Tritium	Hydrate	3-4 L/d if tolerated
Uranium	Bicarbonate	Administer IV slowly until urine pH is 8-9, for 3 d

Abbreviations: BID, twice daily; DMSA, dimercaptosuccinic acid; EDTA, ethylenediaminetetra-acetic acid; IV, intravenously; NAC, n-acetylcysteine; PO, orally; QID, four times daily.

* Treatment guidelines change over time. All countermeasures should be checked for current recommended dosages before administration of the medication. The most updated clinical guidelines and dosages are available through various federal agencies and medical specialty societies.

There are analysts who question the utility of some enhanced elimination strategies, as there are limited human data to validate the findings from animal studies. Clearly, enhanced elimination approaches should be used only when high levels of radionuclide uptake can be substantiated. A general rule of thumb is that when the cumulative exposure dose is less than the annual limit of intake (ALI) set for a worker occupationally exposed to radiation, no attempt at decorporation is warranted. If the cumulative dose is greater than 10 times the ALI, decorporation therapy is indicated. Doses in between these values require a more considered risk-benefit analysis.[43]

7.15 PUBLIC HEALTH IMPLICATIONS OF NUCLEAR AND RADIOLOGIC DISASTERS

Radiologic events present a significant challenge in terms of public health management and information. The general public's fear prompted by any mention of radiation often causes responses out of proportion to the threat. The perceived threat of radiation has been seen to create panic, and the actual threat is often misrepresented by the media. To reduce the perception that the public's health is at risk because of the presence of any radiation, it is critical that health professionals maintain a focus on the manageable nature of radiation risk. Significant benefit to the public as a whole can be gained by a reasoned, clear approach to advice given.

Many casualties will result from the blast, radiation, and burns. Large numbers of fatalities will stress mortuary services. Public health authorities will work with other agencies to coordinate mass fatality management efforts, provide clean water and sanitation, establish mass triage and treatment facilities, and educate the public about radiation and other health aspects of dealing with the disaster. More detailed information on public health interventions and response actions is available in Chapter 2, "Public Health Response to Disasters."

7.15.1 Crisis and Emergency Risk Communication

Experience during the Three Mile Island incident yielded valuable information on what not to do. Nuclear or radiologic "experts" cannot expect the general public, the emergency response community, or elected officials to simply agree to trust them. Explicit explanations must be made in as simple terms as possible, avoiding complex technical arguments, for any recommendations regarding public activity in a radiologic incident. Guidelines for the general public should be couched in terms that provide instruction regarding means to protect the individual or family in a contaminated area and in a noncontaminated area, and should be concise. A simple "shelter-in-place" instruction should be issued with explanation on means to reduce the dose to the affected population.

Effective risk communication is essential to ensure that the public receives appropriate instructions to protect its health and safety. Many factors should be considered when deciding whether to order a protective action based on the projected radiation dose to a population. Evacuation is the most important action after a radiation release has occurred, particularly after a radioactive cloud release in which there is time to escape exposure. The duration of sheltering required will depend on the extent of environmental contamination. To minimize panic, instructions should be issued as soon as possible and with calm confidence that the recommendation will assist the public in protecting itself. A designated spokesperson should provide as much guidance as possible to empower the public with tools to control its environment.

7.15.2   Mental and Behavioral Health Considerations

In most conceivable radiologic and especially nuclear attacks, it is reasonable to expect that the health care system would be overloaded with massive numbers of patients requiring an array of professionals with specialized training. If this already stretched medical community was also severely impacted by the very attack that requires its response, the effects will be even more devastating. In addition to the loss of medical care, among the anticipated outcomes for the general public will be fear of invisible agents and contagion, magical thinking about radiation, anger at perceived inadequacies by government entities, scapegoating, paranoia, social isolation, demoralization, and loss of faith in social institutions.[44] The 2011 Japanese earthquake and tsunami, in which there was severe damage to three nuclear reactors and also to spent fuel rods in cooling ponds, illustrate this concept well. While there was significant release of radioactivity in the Fukushima reactor complex and the immediate surrounding area, the United States did not receive significant radioactive contamination. Despite this, there was massive purchasing of KI by the general public in the United States in the days immediately following the event. Various government agencies joined the fray by submitting new orders to manufacture KI, illustrating that even experts are not immune to the emotional aftermaths of this kind of geographically remote incident. American news media were on the scene for weeks repeatedly pointing out the perceived (and real) inadequacies of the Japanese response. If the event had occurred on US soil, these manifestations of psychological trauma would have been much more profound.

Emergency responders, public health personnel, and medical providers suffer from the same fears and misperceptions as the public does regarding radiation exposure. In a 2002 survey of nurses and physicians in Hawaii, it was found that only 52% of physicians and 45% of nurses would be willing to care for patients in a nonhospital field medical facility after a catastrophic radiologic incident.[43] Similar findings were observed in a survey of 3800 physicians and nurses, in which only 64% stated that they would be able and 57% would be willing to report for their normal hospital duties in the event of a catastrophic radiologic incident. Emergency planners must take into account that up to 50% of emergency and medical response professionals may be either unable or unwilling to report to work during a radiologic disaster. The authors stated that barriers to willingness included fear and concern for family and self and personal health problems. The findings were consistent for all types of medical facilities surveyed.[45]

Mental and behavioral health issues are discussed further in Chapter 3, "Population Health and Mental Health in Disasters."

7.15.3   People with Functional, Access, or Other Special Needs

In a mass casualty situation from a nuclear detonation or (though much less so) an RDD, there will be several factors that will complicate medical care. Some of these are associated with individuals themselves: the aged, those with combined injuries, pregnant women and their babies, those at the extremes of age, and those with preexisting (comorbid) medical conditions. There also are factors associated with the medical treatment facilities, their personnel, equipment, and supplies. These all have a distinct possibility of being damaged or destroyed by a nuclear detonation or rendered unavailable owing to being in the fallout field. Should the facility lie within a heavy fallout region, its patients and staff will have to be evacuated. The same would apply to nursing homes, care centers, assisted living facilities, and also individuals in non-medically related confinement such as prison inmates. It is likely that many people will be unwilling to enter even uncontaminated areas because of fear of radiation. Finally, there are the stresses on mental health and social networks that are created in any disaster situation, particularly one involving releases of ionizing radiation.

One special need will be that of medical staff and all other responders, who will be subject not only to greatly increased workloads, but also to concern for their families, particularly children, aged parents, and those requiring special home care. Another consideration is care of pets. This may seem unimportant to some, but neglecting their needs will result in unintentional cruelty to animals. As noted previously, the unsubstantiated fear of radiation-induced birth defects will likely terrify pregnant women, and they should be counseled that this is not an actual risk.

7.15.4   Age-Related Vulnerabilities

With advancing age, the capacity to repair injuries decreases. The immune system is less able to fight off infections. Inflammation and wound healing capacities decrease. The incidence of coexisting diseases and medication use may affect the ability to recover from radiation exposure increases. The treatment protocols for radiation only and combined injury are the same, but their likelihood of success decreases. The elderly are not more radiation sensitive per se; in fact, the latency period between exposure to radiation and the development of a radiation-induced cancer increases somewhat, and those older than 40 years do not even need to take KI for exposure to radioactive iodine (except at very high levels). It is the ability to repair radiation damage that decreases with age. Pediatric vulnerabilities also need to be considered and are discussed in Chapter 3, "Population Health and Mental Health in Disasters."

7.15.5   Risk to Pregnant Women and Fetuses

One of the most misunderstood issues in radiation-contaminated environments is the relative risk to pregnant women and prenatally exposed infants. For medical providers, a distinction is needed between high-dose X-ray exposures in medical practice and environmental exposure to radioactive fallout from nuclear weapons or other radiologic sources. It is documented that in relation to X-ray exposures in medical care, children exposed prenatally or soon after birth are more sensitive to radiation exposure than older children and young adults. In unfortunate exposures to X rays in utero in the past, fetuses were found to have, depending on the stage in gestation, an increased risk of congenital malformations and microcephaly at birth and mental retardation and cancer in childhood.

One of the most feared long-term effects of radiation exposure is the subsequent development of cancer. While it has been shown that intense radiographic exposure has produced birth defects in humans, a limited number of defects were reported in Hiroshima and Nagasaki atomic bomb survivors. By tracking the survivors of the

Hiroshima and Nagasaki atomic bomb attacks, it has been determined that there is, for radiogenic cancers (some cancers, such as breast and bone marrow, are relatively radiation sensitive, while others, such as prostate, pancreas, and uterus, are relatively resistant to radiation induction),[30] a long latent period followed by a definite increase in the incidence of these cancers. The actual incidence of teratogenic outcomes resulting from radiation exposure has been highly overestimated, according to studies on numerous historical radiation exposures worldwide.

For environmental exposures to radionuclides after the Chernobyl disaster, there was no significant increase in congenital malformations in infants born to women from the highly contaminated areas, compared with matched controls. This is an interesting finding, as more than 100 times as much radioactivity was released into the air at Chernobyl than at Hiroshima and Nagasaki combined. A slight increase in congenital malformations was determined to occur in Japanese atomic bomb survivors, related to the higher-dose range exposures. The uterine and abdominal walls of the mother do provide some shielding against radiation exposure; the dose inside the uterus is roughly two-thirds of the dose at the mother's skin. Even in the high-dose X ray in utero studies, it was found that in the earliest stages of pregnancy, the chances of mental retardation and microcephaly are virtually nil. The fetus either survives the radiation intact, or fails to implant and dies. It is generally considered that the risk is highest for radiation exposure after 8 weeks of gestation. After 25 weeks these risks are minimal; the effect of high doses is to increase the probability of miscarriage and neonatal death. From the lack of statistically significant congenital abnormalities in more than 60 000 children born to significantly exposed mothers at Chernobyl, it appears that the widespread fear of radiation-induced defects from environmental exposures to radionuclides deposited from airborne dispersion is dramatically overblown. Counseling of pregnant mothers from contaminated areas needs to take into account that 30 000 women decided to terminate their pregnancies at Chernobyl for the sole reason of fear of congenital abnormalities.

In light of the very low incidence of birth defects after the atomic bomb detonations in Japan, the fear of significant numbers of birth defects is not justified. In both the immediate aftermath and during the long-term medical response to nuclear weapon and radiologic exposures, therefore, termination of pregnancy secondary to the anticipation of radiation-induced birth defects is not scientifically justified.

There is, however, an elevated risk of childhood leukemia and solid-tissue cancers in childhood that does increase with increasing dose. Fetuses are probably as sensitive to radiation-induced cancer as young children. There is a theoretical possibility, based on animal studies and chromosomal studies in humans, that subsequent generations will be at increased risk for congenital malformations and cancers; however, there are no epidemiologic data at all, in Japan or elsewhere, that have actually demonstrated this. If either or both parents have been irradiated prior to conception, there is no epidemiologic demonstration of increased congenital malformations or cancer in their children.

7.15.6   Population Monitoring

In a radiologic or nuclear incident involving mass casualties, it is necessity to perform long-term monitoring of exposed individuals and populations. There is a risk of stochastic (cancer) and late deterministic (cataracts) disease processes that can occur even at doses insufficient to cause moderate or severe symptoms in the first days or weeks after exposure. A permanent record of exposure and survey instrument recordings should be created for persons for whom dosimetry information is obtained, even at mass screening places where the asymptomatic but possibly exposed are directed to go to. Responsibility for obtaining and maintaining these records resides with the state, tribal, or local public health department.

Substantial effort will be expended on determining dose to the public from a radiation exposure. If dosimetry is available, records should be kept of measured exposures. If no dosimetry is available, broad exposure charts should be developed, and the location of members of the public should be acquired. When individuals identify their location, their exposure should be noted and recommendation for dose effect amelioration should be provided as soon as possible. For this reason, it is important for a radiation professional to be integrated into the public health activity from the beginning of response actions. Precise dosimetry may take years to fully develop, so early records of likely dose to the public determined by location are needed. Documentation of exposed people will provide significant challenges but will be required for long-term health reasons and to address legal issues. The exposure to large doses of radiation will produce an increased long-term risk of cancer for the exposed people. These cases will need to be monitored and treated for many years.

According to the federal interagency *Planning Guidance for Response to a Nuclear Detonation*, state and local agencies should establish a registry system as early as possible after a nuclear event.[2] This would be used to contact people who require short-term medical follow-up as well as long-term monitoring. It is likely that there will be relatively little opportunity for extensive patient information gathering in nuclear events, so initially only basic and critical information will be collected (ie, name, address, telephone number, contact information). It is recommended that collection of address information not slow up the medical care process, as it is likely that many of these addresses may not be relevant in the immediate follow-up period. Of course, if it is feasible to collect further personal data without difficulties in the treatment procedure, then it should be done. The Planning Guidance document suggests:

> . . . federal agencies, specifically CDC and the Agency for Toxic Substances and Disease Registry, will provide assistance in establishing, coordinating, and maintaining this registry. Emergency responders should be registered and monitored through a mechanism provided by their respective employers. State and local authorities must work with ESF #6 (Mass Care, Emergency Assistance, Housing, and Human Services) and the American Red Cross to establish an evacuee tracking database system.[2]

7.16 SUMMARY

A radiation emergency involves the release of potentially dangerous radioactive materials into the environment. Such incidents can occur anywhere radioactive isotopes are used, stored, or transported. Radiation provokes a special fear, but, with appropriate understanding and preparation, effective clinical care can be provided to exposed people. Radiation can be easily detected with equipment carried by many emergency responders. Radioactive materials may contaminate homes, workplaces, and other resources, requiring extensive and costly remediation and the potential disruption of lives and livelihoods for long periods of time. Serious psychological problems can result in those who think they are being, or have been, exposed.

In the event of a terrorist attack or other radiation disaster, clinicians will play vital roles as responders and as sources of accurate information for affected individuals and communities. The immediate clinical effects of large doses of radiation are well known and can be assessed with the use of simple laboratory tests such as blood cell counts.

Externally contaminated individuals may expose or contaminate others with whom they come in close contact and should avoid such contact until they have been appropriately decontaminated. The health threat to response personnel is low, however, and can be minimized by using universal safety precautions (mask, gown, gloves). Persons who have inhaled or ingested radioactive material require medical attention. Currently, there are no reliable antidotes to treat exposed persons once radiation has been inhaled or ingested, but symptoms can be treated effectively. Oral and intravenous agents are available that can help remove certain radioactive materials from the body.

The occurrence and subsequent management of a nuclear detonation or a significant radiologic release disaster is an important consideration for all health and medical personnel. A basic clinically relevant knowledge of the unique terms, principles, mechanisms of injury, as well as the common units of measure associated with ionizing radiation, is a base on which to build understanding that facilitates workforce protection, as well as clinical decision making that fosters good casualty management. Identifying hazard-specific considerations, including mitigation measures, relevant to nuclear and radiologic disasters is essential to preparedness planning and operational readiness. The recognition of characteristic patterns and onset timing of clinical signs and symptoms are useful both to predict and to reduce overall morbidity and mortality. Historically, fear-based thoughts, misconceptions, and simply misinformation concerning the risks associated with managing casualties of nuclear or radiologic disasters have abounded. Non-science-based information regarding cancer risk, pregnancy management, and fetal health among the general public has historically been commonplace as well. It is important that health and medical providers learn the facts based on the scientific literature and make informed decisions for themselves and to educate communities to do likewise.

7.17 DISCUSSION POINTS

Nuclear and Radiologic Disasters: Putting the PRE-DISASTER Paradigm™ Into Practice		
P	Planning and Practice	Radiologic and nuclear disaster planning demands close collaboration and coordination among federal, state, and local officials. Given these special demands, all communities need to develop, implement, and test preparedness plans for these events in ways that engage all appropriate response agencies.
R	Resilience	The psychological effect of a radiologic or nuclear event will be huge. Psychosocial support will be extremely important to restore a sense of calm, reduce public fear, and support the grieving process. *Resilience* is the capacity of individuals and communities to rebound from adversity, become strengthened, and become more resourceful. Gender, age, and previous medical conditions may influence the impact of a radiologic or nuclear disaster on affected families, individuals, and evacuees and should be taken into account by disaster planners and by those providing psychosocial support.
E	Education and Training	To respond appropriately, health personnel must maintain a specified level of proficiency. This includes maintaining appropriate knowledge of the clinical and public health implications of nuclear and radiologic disasters.

Nuclear and Radiologic Disasters: Putting the DISASTER Paradigm™ Into Practice		
D	Detection	Radiologic exposures can result from the deliberate or unintentional release of radionuclides into the air, water, or food supplies, or onto surfaces with which people come in contact. The resulting health hazards can be similar to those experienced after early and delayed fallout. Usually there are few immediate health effects, unless the radiation source is especially intense. If a radiologic source is located in the vicinity of a population, the primary danger is not being able to detect it. Once a hazard has been identified, people can be evacuated relatively quickly (as appropriate) and further exposure avoided. The immediate clinical effects of large doses of radiation are well known and can be assessed with the use of simple laboratory tests such as blood cell counts.

I	Incident Management	Incident management will involve public health, public safety, and other emergency management entities. Health professionals need to work as members of an integrated disaster team under the structure of the incident command system (ICS). They must comply with regulatory and legal principles, as well as accepted moral and ethical principles, during management of the event.
S	Safety and Security	Personal protection is paramount. Health professionals should adhere to proper decontamination protocols and procedures. Key protection factors are as follows: *time*—reduce the amount of time spent near a source of radiation; *distance*—stay as far away from the radiation source as possible; and *shielding*—place some type of barrier between oneself and the source. While severe consequences have been reported on occasion after exposure of first responders and medical personnel to biologically and chemically contaminated casualties, there have been very few reports of medical personnel suffering ill effects from radiologically contaminated casualties. There have been no verified reports of medical personnel suffering acute injury or even symptoms from exposure to radiologically contaminated casualties.
A	Assess Hazards	Health personnel should know scene and clinical assessment strategies to characterize radiation risks. Fortunately, most radiation exposures can be quickly monitored by standard radiation detection devices. In the event of very large numbers of otherwise uninjured persons concerned they have been exposed, many of these individuals can be identified with a limited or in-depth medical interview, which would be followed by a radiation survey only if resources and time permit.
S	Support	Responders and citizens should be aware of local, regional, and national surge capacity and support services that may be available in a nuclear or radiologic disaster.
T	Triage and Treatment	To decrease morbidity and mortality from a radiologic or nuclear disaster, clinicians should have a basic understanding of radiation illness and treatment principles. Radiation effects its toxicity on biologic systems through ionization, which creates tissue damage by the generation of free radicals, disruption of chemical bonds, and direct damage to cellular DNA and enzymes. The health effects of radiation exposure tend to be directly proportional to the amount of radiation absorbed by the body (radiation dose) and are determined by the: ➤ Radiation type (ie, alpha, beta, X ray, or gamma) ➤ Means of exposure, internal or external (absorbed by the skin, inhaled, or ingested) ➤ Length of time exposed

		Because of the extensive number of trauma injuries involved in nuclear disasters, precautions established for advanced trauma life support take precedence over all considerations regarding the presence of radiation. Given the primacy of trauma support issues, verifying the presence and extent of radiation exposure is still an essential initial process in casualties potentially involved in a nuclear or radiologic event. Optimal management of radiation casualties requires the following: ➤ Knowledge of the type and dose of radiation received ➤ Recognition of the manifestations of radiation sickness ➤ Use of standard medical care ➤ Decontamination ➤ Decorporation techniques A daunting spectrum of burn injuries will be incurred from a nuclear blast as a result of the fireball released by the explosion and subsequent dramatic increase in fires and thermal burns in the affected population. The fireball will create a perplexing logistical medical issue, as thousands of serious burn casualties would need to be managed by the local and regional health care system.
E	Evacuation	The early decision that will save thousands of lives is the decision to evacuate vs shelter in place. Evacuation should be done in areas not affected by dangerous levels of fallout. Trusted, accurate, and prompt directions must be given via the media, to prevent people from evacuating into areas of greater radiation risk.
R	Recovery	Recovery begins immediately after the event. Pre-event resilience is key to recovery. The medical and mental health effect of nuclear or radiologic disaster can be significant. Recovery involves a long-term commitment to affected communities and may last for years. Mechanisms for long-term public health monitoring and surveillance must be implemented and maintained.

REFERENCES

1. Dallas CE, Bell WC. Prediction modeling to determine medical response to urban nuclear attack. *Disaster Med Public Health Prep.* 2007;1:80-89.

2. National Security Staff Interagency Policy Coordination Subcommittee for Preparedness and Response to Radiological and Nuclear Threats. Planning Guidance for Response to a Nuclear Detonation. 2nd ed. Washington, DC: Executive Office of the President (National Security Staff and Office of Science and Technology Policy); June 2010. http://www.hps.org/hsc/documents/Planning_Guidance_for_Response_to_a_Nuclear_Detonation-2nd_Edition_FINAL.pdf. Accessed April 12, 2011.

3. World Health Organization (WHO). *Effect of Nuclear War on Health and Health Services*. 2nd ed. Geneva: WHO; 1987.

4. Cockerham LG, Walden TL, Dallas CE, Mickley GA, Landauer MR. Ionizing radiation. In: Wallace Hayes A, ed. *Principles and Methods of Toxicology*. 5th ed. Boca Raton, FL: CRC Press; 2007.

5. Dallas CE. Nuclear detonation. In: Keyes C, Burnstein JL, Swienton R, Schwartz R, eds. *Medical Response to Terrorism*. New York, NY: Lippincott; 2004.

6. Bell WC, Dallas CE. Vulnerability of populations and the urban health care systems to nuclear weapon attack—examples from four American cities. *Int J Health Geographics*. 2007;6:5.

7. Beker WK, Buescher TM, Cioffi WG. Combined radiation and thermal injury after nuclear attack. In: Brown D, Weiss JF, Mac Vittie TJ, eds. *Treatment of Radiation Injuries*. New York, NY: Plenum; 1990.

8. Barnaby S, Rotblat, J. Nuclear war: the aftermath. The effects of nuclear war. *Ambio*. 1982;11:84-94.

9. Office of Technology Assessment, US Congress. *The Effects of Nuclear War*. Washington, DC: Office of Technology Assessment; 1979.

10. Waselenko JK. Medical management of the acute radiation syndrome: recommendations of the Strategic National Stockpile Radiation Working Group. *Ann Intern Med*. 2004;140:1037-1051.

11. Glasstone S, Dolan PJ. Thermal radiation and its effects. In: *The Effects of Nuclear Weapons*. 3rd ed. Washington, DC: US Dept of Defense, US Energy Research and Development Administration; 1977.

12. Yurt RW, Lazar EJ, Leahy NE, et al. Burn disaster response planning: an urban region's approach. *J Burn Care Res*. 2008;29:158-165.

13. Postol TA. Possible fatalities from superfires following nuclear attacks in or near urban areas. In: Soloman F, Marston RQ, eds. *The Medical Implications of Nuclear War*. Washington, DC: National Academy Press; 1986.

14. Brode HL, Small RD. A review of the physics of large fires. In: Soloman F, Marston RQ, eds. *The Medical Implications of Nuclear War*. Washington, DC: National Academy Press; 1986.

15. Eden L. *Whole World on Fire*. Ithaca, NY: Cornell University Press; 2004.

16. Binninger G, Hodge JK, Wright S, Holl S. Development of a Fire Prediction Model for use within HPAC. Unpublished report. San Diego: L3 Titan Corp; 2003.

17. Brode HL. Fire Targeting Methodology Improvements and Automation. Technical Report DNA TR. Washington, DC: Defense Special Weapons Agency; 1996.

18. Fetter SAA, Tsipis K. Catastrophic releases of radioactivity. *Sci Am*. 1981;244:41-47.

19. Mettler FA, Moseley RD. *Medical Effects of Ionizing Radiation*. Orlando, FL: Grune and Stratton Inc; 1985.

20. Gonzalez AJ. Radiation protection in the aftermath of a terrorist attack involving exposure to ionizing radiation. *Health Physics Soc*. 2005;89:418-446.

21. Cerveny TJ, Cockerham LG. Medical management of internal radionuclide contamination. *Med Bull US Army Eur*. 1986;43:24-27.

22. Medvedev Z. *The Legacy of Chernobyl*. New York, NY: Norton; 1992.

23. Dallas CE. Aftermath of the Chernobyl nuclear disaster: pharmaceutical needs in the Republic of Belarus. *Am J Pharm Educ*. 1993;57:182-185.

24. Alexander DA, Wells A. Reactions of police officers to body-handling after major disaster. *Br J Psychiatry*. 1991;159:547.

25. National Council on Radiation Protection and Measurement (NCRP). NCRP Commentary No. 19. Key Elements of Preparing Emergency Responders for Nuclear and Radiological Terrorism. Bethesda, MD: NCRP; 2005.

26. National Council on Radiation Protection and Measurement (NCRP). NCRP Report No. 138. Management of Terrorist Events Involving Radiological Materials. Bethesda, MD: NCRP; 2001.

27. Office of Radiation Programs, US EPA. *Manual of Protective Action Guides and Protective Actions for Nuclear Events*. Washington, DC: EPA; 1991. http://www.epa.gov/radiation/docs/er/400-r-92–001.pdf. Accessed April 12, 2011.

28. US Department of Homeland Security (DHS), Federal Emergency Management Agency (FEMA). Planning guidance for protection and recovery following radiological dispersal device (RDD) and improvised nuclear device (IND) incidents. *Federal Register*. 2008;73:45029-45048. http://www.fema.gov/good_guidance/download/10260. Accessed April 12, 2011.

29. New York City Department of Health and Mental Hygiene, Health Emergency Preparedness Program. *NYC Hospital Guidance for Responding to a Contaminating Radiation Incident*. New York, NY: Dept of Health and Mental Hygiene; 2008.

30. Flynn DM, Goans RE. Nuclear terrorism: triage and medical management of radiation and combined-injury casualties. *Surg Clin North Am*. 2006;86:601-636.

31. Goans RE, ed. *Medical Management of Radiological Casualties*. 3rd ed. Bethesda, MD: Armed Forces Radiobiology Research Institute; 2009.

32. Mettler FA Jr, Upton AC. *Medical Effects of Ionizing Radiation*. 3rd ed. Philadelphia, PA: Saunders Elsevier; 2008.

33. Mettler FA Jr, Guskova AK, Gusev IA. Health effects in those with acute radiation sickness from the Chernobyl accident. *Health Physics*. 2007;93:462-469.

34. National Council on Radiation Protection and Measurement (NCRP). NCRP Report No. 161. Management of Persons Contaminated with Radionuclides: Handbook. Bethesda, MD: NCRP; 2008.

35. Musolino SV, Harper FT. Emergency response guidance for the first 48 hours after the outdoor detonation of an explosive radiological dispersal device. *Health Phys*. 2006;90:377-385.

36. Oak Ridge Institute for Science and Education. The Medical Aspects of Radiation Incidents. 2010. http://orise.orau.gov/files/reacts/medical-aspects-of-radiation-incidents.pdf. Accessed April 12, 2011.

37. New York State Partnership Enhancing Medical Management Capabilities for a Mass Casualty Incident. *Building a Statewide Burn Disaster Response Plan*. US Dept of Health and Human Services (HHS) Catalog of Federal Domestic Assistance (CFDA) No. 93.889

38. NYS EMS Bureau Survey. Ambulance vehicle count by County, September 2005.

39. ABA Board of Trustees and the Committee on Organization and Delivery of Burn Care. Disaster management and the ABA plan. *J Burn Care Res*. 2005:26.

40. New York Medical College School of Health Science and Practice. New York State Department of Health Community-Based Care Center Toolkit. 2009. http://www.health.state.ny.us/environmental/emergency/community_based_care_center/docs/cbcc_toolkit.pdf. Accessed April 12, 2011.

41. Brook I, Ledney GD, Madonna GS, DeBell RM, Walker RI. Therapies for radiation injuries: research perspectives. *Milit Med*. 1992;157:130-136.

42. Mettler FA Jr, Guskova AK, Gusev IA. *Medical Management of Radiation Accidents*. Boca Raton, FL: CRC Press; 2001.

43. Siegrist DW. The threat of biological attack: why concern now? *Emerging Infect Dis*. 1998;5:505-508.

44. American College of Emergency Physicians. SARS-SP Task Force. 2004.

45. Charatan F. US plans drugs stockpile to counter bioterrorism threat. *BMJ*. 2000;320:1225.

CHAPTER | EIGHT

Chemical Disasters

CHAPTER CHAIR

Michael J. Reilly, DrPH, MPH

CONTRIBUTING AUTHORS

Jim Lyznicki, MS, MPH

Greene Shepherd, PharmD

David S. Markenson, MD, MBA

8.1 PURPOSE

This chapter describes principles and practices for the management of chemical disasters. It reinforces the general concepts of situational awareness, incident management, workforce protection, and casualty management, which were explained in Chapters 1 through 5 of this manual. The application of these general concepts in the context of chemical disaster preparedness, mitigation, response, and recovery is described. Specific emphasis is placed on diagnostic and treatment considerations for individuals exposed to blister agents (vesicants), choking or pulmonary agents, cyanide agents, and nerve agents.

8.2 LEARNING OBJECTIVES

After completing this chapter, readers should be able to:

➤ Identify clinical and epidemiologic clues that may suggest the occurrence of a chemical disaster.

➤ Describe actions that can be taken to protect the health, safety, and security of responders and affected populations in a chemical disaster.

➤ Discuss diagnostic and treatment considerations for individuals exposed to blister or vesicant agents, choking or pulmonary agents, cyanide agents, and nerve agents.

Learning objectives for this chapter are competency-based, as delineated in Appendix B.

8.3 BACKGROUND

Release of chemical agents can occur via unintended or deliberate means, such as through a spill from a damaged railroad tank car or an explosion at an industrial facility with resultant contamination of air, food, water, or consumer products. Global concern has increased about potential terrorist attacks involving the use of toxic chemical agents to cause widespread panic and harm. Chemicals could be released as bombs, sprayed from aircraft and boats, or disseminated by other means to intentionally create a hazard to people and the environment.

Health professionals should be aware of principles involved in managing persons exposed to chemical agents. They need quick access to current information on preparing for a chemical emergency, handling contaminated persons, hazard recognition and assessment, health effects, and accessing emergency assistance. With adequate resources and planning, health professionals and the public can better prepare themselves to recognize an emergency situation and react effectively to protect themselves and others from harm.

8.3.1 Chemical Emergencies

Chemical emergencies typically involve an unintentional exposure to toxic industrial chemicals used or stored in various manufacturing and maintenance facilities. All major cities and emergency medical systems have plans and equipment in place to address chemical emergencies. As part of a hazard and vulnerability analysis, emergency planners identify industrial, commercial, research, and educational institutions that possess chemical agents that pose potential risks to public health and safety. With this information, mitigation and vulnerability reduction steps are taken to prepare for the possibility of the release of hazardous materials under various exposure scenarios.

In day-to-day chemical emergencies, when the emergency medical services (EMS) system is activated and prehospital personnel arrive at the scene, standard information regarding the nature of the chemical exposure is usually available, but this may not be the case with smaller packages that are part of a shipment or carried on delivery vehicles. In addition, during off hours or because of the confusion at the scene, sometimes information that is on-site may not be readily available. Employers may have a material safety data sheet available or may be able to obtain the chemical name from a container or health and safety manager in an industrial setting. The exposed person, as well as bystanders who witness the exposure, may have taken initial first steps by removing the chemical from the exposed person or performing cursory decontamination, particularly if the chemical is irritating to the skin. In these cases, EMS is not usually overwhelmed.

Exposed persons can receive a preliminary decontamination on scene (if necessary) without the need for mass decontamination and can be transported to the emergency department through typical EMS mechanisms. Most hospitals have the capacity to handle a single patient who may have been contaminated with a hazardous substance with the use of an internal decontamination team but without activation of the hospital emergency operations plan or external resources. In these cases, both EMS and the hospital have the resources available to manage the needs of the patient and protect themselves from inadvertent secondary exposure or contamination.

8.3.2   Chemical Disasters

A chemical disaster is different from a chemical emergency in several ways. At the fundamental level, a disaster differs from an emergency when the needs of the incident exceed the capacity to respond. This may manifest itself in many different ways. For example, 200 people may have been exposed to a toxic industrial chemical when a tanker truck rolls over on a major interstate highway and there are not enough EMS units to respond to the event. Twenty-two high school students may be brought to a local community hospital after exposure to an unknown odor at their school, which is causing burning in their eyes, nose, and throat along with bronchospasm. An incident involving an organophosphate pesticide may result in several people being admitted to an urban emergency department, and the pharmacy runs out of atropine. In all these scenarios, patient needs exceed the resources of the health system. When this disparity exists, a disaster exists, and it may not be possible to provide a typical standard of care to all patients.

Chemical disasters will typically involve multiple casualties and potentially adverse environmental health effects. This type of "population-level" event requires the involvement of multiple response agencies including police, fire, EMS, hazardous materials (HAZMAT) teams, local health departments, offices of emergency management, environmental protection agencies, and multiple health care facilities. Depending on the nature and scope of the event, the National Guard, the Federal Emergency Management Agency (FEMA), and other federal agencies also may be involved in response and recovery operations.

8.4   SITUATIONAL AWARENESS AND DETECTION

In a mass illness situation, emergency response personnel and clinicians must determine whether casualties have been exposed to chemical, biologic, or radiologic agents, or a combination thereof. Detection is based on characteristic syndromes, signs, and symptom clusters that would normally be observed in individuals after an exposure to these various agents. Detection of radiation and biologic agent exposure is discussed in Chapters 7 and 9, respectively.

The first steps in detection of a disaster involving the release of a hazardous substance involve information gathering. Important elements of information to obtain early in the incident include the following:

➤ Have there been multiple 911 calls in the same geographic area?

➤ If the scene is a workplace, is there a known hazardous material used at the site?

➤ Is the scene location one that has been identified previously in a hazard and vulnerability analysis?

➤ Is the incident site a location of national significance or a potential target for terrorism?

➤ If a transportation incident has occurred, is any substance spilling or leaking from the container?

➤ Are callers giving information to 911 operators that suggests a toxic exposure?

➤ Are people experiencing an acute or abrupt onset of symptoms?

➤ Are there any unusual odors present?

➤ Are there multiple individuals experiencing the same types of signs and symptoms?

These simple questions can assist in gathering key information about the nature and scope of the event even before the first responding units arrive on scene.

When assessing casualties from a potential incident involving a hazardous substance, it is essential to ensure that staff are adequately protected from exposure and secondary contamination. First it should be determined whether there are any liquids or powders on the individual. Is there any noticeable foreign or unusual odor? If the person can talk, responders should ask what he or she was doing when the incident occurred. The answers may suggest an isolated occupational exposure or industrial incident, or perhaps a more widespread situation. Determining how long ago the symptoms occurred (acute vs gradual onset) can give health care workers information regarding the severity of exposure and the possible toxicity of the agent. Generally, high-dose exposures will result in rapid onset of symptoms and incapacitation within a short period of time. If individuals are ambulatory, able to answer questions, and able to speak in full, uninterrupted sentences or with minimal respiratory distress, their relative acuity will usually be low, particularly if they self-referred to the emergency department. Typically, the longer the duration from exposure to symptom onset, the less severe the clinical manifestation of illness.

8.4.1   Chemical Exposure Clues

In a chemical disaster, information about the nature of the exposure may not be readily available. This unknown nature of the emergency can be daunting when there are multiple casualties who present with symptoms of exposure and the need for decontamination, triage, and treatment. In these cases, health responders rely on detection of chemical exposure that may be based on signs and symptoms (and, when possible, history of present illness) and/or on detection technologies. The individual's activities just before the onset of symptoms can provide clues to the nature of the exposure.

Being able to recognize potential chemical agent exposure by signs and symptoms is a critical function to distinguish individuals who present with more routine or day-to-day problems from those who present as a result of an unusual toxic exposure. Chemical agents most often produce signs and symptoms soon after exposure, typically within minutes or hours of the event. After exposure, nonspecific presentations may appear, including altered mental status (confusion), loss of consciousness, seizures, respiratory distress (trouble breathing), and cardiovascular collapse. Early symptoms of chemical exposure can include nausea, vomiting, and diarrhea (which also are symptoms of psychological stress).

With a chemical release, responder safety and casualty survival hinge not only on awareness of clues at the scene, but also on knowledge and recognition of characteristic signs and symptoms of various chemicals and chemical classes. Chemical classes of concern to disaster responders include the following:

➤ Pulmonary, irritant gases (choking agents) (eg, chlorine, phosgene, many industrial chemicals)

➤ Blister or vesicant agents (eg, sulfur mustard)

➤ Asphyxiant agents (eg, cyanide, carbon monoxide, hydrogen sulfide)

➤ Nerve agents (eg, sarin, VX)

➤ Incapacitating or riot control agents (eg, tear gas, mace, pepper spray, 3-quinuclidinyl benzilate [BZ])

Possible Clues of a Chemical Release

➤ An unusual increase in the number of persons seeking care for a rapid onset of symptoms

➤ Rapid onset of illness with little or no warning

➤ Unexplained illness or death among young or previously healthy persons

➤ Presence of an unexplained odor, low-level clouds, or vapors at the scene

➤ Emission of unexplained odors from ill persons

➤ Clusters of illness in persons who have common characteristics, such as drinking water or eating food from the same source

➤ Unexplained death of plants, fish, or animals (domestic or wild)

➤ A syndrome (ie, a constellation of clinical signs and symptoms in patients) suggesting a disease commonly associated with a known chemical exposure

➤ Sudden unexplained weakness, collapse, apnea, or convulsions in previously healthy persons

➤ Dimmed or blurred vision

(Continued)

Possible Clues of a Chemical Release (continued)

➤ Hypersecretion syndromes (eg, tearing, drooling, diarrhea)

➤ Inhalation syndromes (eye, nose, throat, chest irritation; shortness of breath)

➤ Burn-like syndromes (redness, blistering, itching, sloughing)

Source: Centers for Disease Control and Prevention (CDC). Recognition of illness associated with exposure to chemical agents—United States, 2003. *MMWR Morb Mortal Wkly Rep*. 2003;52:938-940. http://www.cdc.gov/mmwr/preview/mmwrhtml/mm5239a3.htm. Accessed May 2, 2011.

Each chemical class causes a typical, specific set of signs and symptoms called a *toxidrome* (a combination of the words *toxic*, or "poison," and *syndrome*). Knowledge of the major clinical syndromes or toxidromes caused by major classes of chemical agents may facilitate detection and treatment. In this process, health care providers will seek to identify the main features of the individual's chief complaint and presenting problem, as well as the onset of signs and/or symptoms of illness. Although more diagnostic testing may be performed, such screening provides good information, particularly when presented with multiple casualties following a disaster. While some chemical agents may have a characteristic odor (eg, chlorine), real-time identification of most chemicals at a disaster scene may be impossible because the specialized detection equipment required may not be available. In addition, identification by smell requires exposure to the agent, and some hazardous materials (eg, phosgene, cyanide) cannot be reliably detected via smell.

8.4.2   Chemical Detection Devices

Detection of specific chemicals involves the use of sophisticated technical monitoring equipment by HAZMAT response teams. These emergency responders will perform sampling and monitoring of a potential site of a toxic substance release and attempt to gather information on the type of chemical (if unknown) and the quantity released. Examples of the types of equipment include multi-gas meters, oxygen sensing equipment, combustible gas indicators, radiation detectors, photoionization detectors, and special types of chemical agent monitors. If this is a particularly volatile chemical, one that dissipates in the air, plume or fence-line monitoring may also be started and projections made using weather equipment and special computer programs.

Various sensors and detectors are available commercially to monitor and identify chemical agents at or near release sites. A simple rapid detection method involves chemical detection paper that reacts with specific chemicals to produce a color change, similar to pH paper. Unfortunately, chemical papers are effective only when in direct contact with liquids or heavy vapors. Other detection systems rely on air sampling, such as Dräger tubes, the Advanced Portable Detector 2000, and other monitors, which can detect very low levels of chemicals. Proper use of these devices requires training and maintenance. As such, they are difficult for most hospitals and public health departments to maintain and operate but are widely used by fire departments and HAZMAT teams. If chemical detection devices are not available, emergency responders and health care workers will need to begin treatment, and decontamination, for possible chemical exposure on the basis of clinical presentation.

8.5 INCIDENT MANAGEMENT AND WORKFORCE PROTECTION

Incident command should be established as soon as possible at the disaster scene. In the case of chemical agent release, the location of the incident command is critical and should be established upwind, uprange, and uphill from the incident location. Some chemical agents that are heavier than air may still affect a command post located upwind if winds are negligible as well as affect a command post located downhill from the incident scene. The command post should be in the cold zone, at a minimum distance of at least 300 ft (preferably more) from the release location or at least double the safe distance with personal protective equipment (PPE). For larger releases or ones where variable-direction winds may be encountered, consideration should be given to keeping greater distances from the release site. Releases inside a confined space present less of a threat and may allow less distance for the establishment of the command post.

> ### Incident Reporting
>
> Any suspicious or confirmed exposure to a toxic chemical agent should be reported immediately to the local health department and the CDC (http://emergency.cdc.gov/emcontact). Any incident related to terrorism or possible terrorist activity also requires telephonic notification to the National Response Center (http://www.nrc.uscg.mil/) and local Federal Bureau of Investigations office (FBI; http://www.fbi.gov). This includes bombings, bomb threats, suspicious letters or packages, and incidents related to the intentional release of chemical, radiologic, and biologic agents.

In a chemical disaster, resources including both personnel and equipment will be depleted rapidly. In addition to medical equipment, supplies, and medications, worker PPE will likely be used up quickly, as will batteries for powered air-purifying respirators, radios, and lighting, and food and water for staff. The logistics function of the community or health care facility emergency operations plan should be activated and consulted to employ the preidentified procedures to locate additional supplies, equipment, and personnel during a chemical event.

More casualties will occur at or near the site of a chemical release than at a sufficient distance away. Additionally, there is generally a greater severity of symptoms in individuals who are contaminated with the hazardous substance than in those who were only exposed but are not contaminated. (People who are contaminated have the chemical physically on their body or clothes. People who are exposed may have inhaled vapors and have symptoms of illness, but may not have physical contamination. In a chemical event, all people with contamination have exposure.)

Protecting responder and health care worker safety is the most important aspect of responding to or caring for casualties of a chemical disaster.[1-3] Some, but not all, chemical agents have a high potential for secondary contamination from victims to responders. In the 1995 sarin attacks in the Tokyo subways, the closest hospital received 500 patients in the first hour after the event. The initial identification of the agent was incorrect, and it took responders 3 hours to determine the actual chemical agent and inform agencies.[1] Additionally, up to 9% of EMS workers and numerous hospital workers were overcome by treating individuals who had not been decontaminated.[1] If responders and health care workers are incapacitated by secondary exposure to a chemical agent, the effect of the disaster will become more severe because of diminished capacity to respond effectively to the event. For this reason, scene and personal safety is paramount. Precautions must be used until thorough decontamination has been performed or the specific chemical agent is identified. Health professionals must first protect themselves (eg, by using protective suits, respiratory protection, and chemical-resistant gloves) because secondary contamination with even small amounts of these substances (particularly nerve agents such as VX) can be lethal.

At the scene of a chemical agent release, affected individuals may be comatose or having seizures; others who are able are likely to try to flee the scene. The minimum time for response and setup after a HAZMAT incident could be 1 hour or longer because of the sequence of events that must occur (notification, response, perimeter setup, and initiation of triage). In most cases, individuals will not wait for emergency personnel to arrive, as often their most realistic option is to self-evacuate from the scene. As a result, health care facilities will require decontamination facilities, PPE, antidotes, and disaster plans to respond to such an incident and must not rely on EMS for these actions. Early notification will allow the hospital to activate specific procedures and staff to prepare for the arrival of multiple casualties. In addition, this notification will allow various systems such as surge capacity to be in place.

More detailed information on worker protection issues, including the use of PPE and decontamination, is provided in Chapter 4, "Workforce Readiness and Disaster Deployment," and in the Advanced Disaster Life Support™ course (v3.0) and supporting course manual.

8.6 GENERAL CASUALTY MANAGEMENT CONSIDERATIONS

Once released, chemical agents can enter the body by ingestion, inhalation, injection, or absorption through the skin. Some chemical agents have a high potential for secondary contamination from exposed persons to responders, which requires that on-scene and other health care personnel who treat these casualties take appropriate safety precautions. Therefore, when multiple casualties present from the same location with the same time of onset of symptoms, a chemical exposure should be suspected. Emergency workers and health personnel must consider the possibility of chemical agent exposure resulting from any mass casualty event. Safety may hinge on awareness of specific clues at the scene and knowledge of the symptoms that various chemicals may cause.

Health effects of chemical agents range from irritation and burning of eyes, skin, and mucous membranes to rapid cardiopulmonary collapse and death. Such effects are usually immediate (a few seconds), but in rare cases, may be delayed (several hours to days). Immediate symptoms of exposure to chemical agents may include blurred vision, eye irritation, difficulty breathing, and nausea. Affected persons may require urgent medical attention. The most important factor in discerning a chemical agent exposure from a biologic agent exposure is acuity of symptom onset. Chemical agents act rapidly, and individuals can feel symptoms shortly after exposure. Hospital personnel need to be prepared for an influx of casualties arriving within a short time period. Clinical effects will vary depending on the following:

➤ Type of agent

➤ Route of exposure

➤ Amount and concentration of agent

➤ Duration of exposure

➤ Preexisting medical conditions in the exposed individual

8.6.1 Triage Considerations

Triage during a chemical disaster will take place in several locations and involves the triage of both contaminated individuals requiring decontamination and those without contamination or who have already been decontaminated. Because nearly two-thirds of casualties are expected to be self-referred after a disaster, hospital emergency operations plans should consider whether to decontaminate all individuals regardless of scene decontamination or only those who present without having been decontaminated at the site of the release.[4]

Predecontamination triage should be performed on all individuals waiting to proceed through decontamination. Triage at this point should be medically oriented and focus on comparing the individual's medical status relative to all others awaiting decontamination. Because the actual decontamination line will likely present a bottleneck at major incidents, decisions will need to be made regarding which individuals of sufficient injury severity could benefit most from postdecontamination treatment, would be able to survive the decontamination process, and should be allowed entry

Exposure Assessment Assistance

For immediate help in assessing clinical effects from chemical exposures, health professionals can contact:

➤ Regional Poison Control Center (http://www.aapcc.org; 800-222-1222)

➤ CDC (http://www.cdc.gov; 770-488-7100)

➤ National Response Center (http://www.nrc.uscg.mil/; 800-424-8802)

➤ Chemical Transportation Emergency Center (http://www.chemtrec.com/)

➤ Agency for Toxic Substances and Disease Registry (http://www.atsdr.cdc.gov/)

➤ Medical toxicologists, clinical pharmacologists, or other drug information specialists

➤ Chemical Hazards Emergency Medical Management, National Library of Medicine (http://chemm.nlm.nih.gov/index.html)

to decontamination first. Triage should be based on the individual's clinical condition at the time of assessment and the likelihood that he or she will survive the decontamination process. Triage tags can be used during this process; however, completing a triage tag while wearing level C or greater PPE will be difficult given the sensory impairment experienced while wearing the suit. For this reason, alternatives to traditional triage tags should be considered, such as colored tape or bracelets, which can identify casualties and be removed during the decontamination process.

Postdecontamination triage will be performed either on-scene or at a health care facility and will be similar to traditional triage performed on noncontaminated patients. This triage is clinically based and will compare each individual to others awaiting treatment. The specific method of triage will vary according to the system used by the local jurisdiction or health agency. Triage is discussed in greater detail in Chapter 5, "Mass Casualty and Fatality Management."

8.6.2   Casualty Assessment

After individuals are triaged and sent through decontamination, a more detailed medical assessment will be performed either in a safe treatment area on-scene or after arrival at a hospital or health care facility. The first step is a quick visual followed by a more detailed casualty assessment. When conducting this detailed physical examination, it is important to consider the presence of following elements, which are of particular interest in a chemical disaster:

➤ *Cardiovascular:* tachycardia, bradycardia, cardiac dysrhythmia, hypotension/hypertension, delayed capillary refill

➤ *Head, eyes, ears, nose, and throat:* miosis, mydriasis, rhinorrhea, increased salivation, redness or irritation of eyes and mucous membranes

➤ *Integumentary:* blistering, erythema, exanthems, cyanosis, pallor, edema

➤ *Gastrointestinal (GI):* increased bowel sounds, diarrhea, emesis, fecal incontinence

➤ *Genitourinary:* urinary incontinence or frequency of urination

➤ *Musculoskeletal:* convulsions, seizures, muscular tremors or fasciculation

➤ *Neurologic:* level of consciousness, Glasgow Coma Scale score, neuromuscular control (ie, skeletal muscle fasciculation, tremors, or seizures), neuroendocrine changes (ie, increased secretion formation), cranial nerve palsies

➤ *Respiratory:* dyspnea, adventitious lung sounds including rales, bronchospasm/wheezing, rhonchi and stridor, acute pulmonary edema; hypoxia and hypoxemia, low oxygen saturation, abnormal capnography readings

In many cases, it may be difficult to identify the specific agent involved. Certain signs, symptoms, and timing may help narrow the choices. Tables 8-1 and 8-2 present some broad guidance on the onset of signs and symptoms for various chemical agents and preliminary identification based on initial signs and symptoms.

TABLE 8-1 Crude Identification of Chemical Agent Class Based on Time Lag Between Exposure and Onset of Symptoms and Signs

Precipitous Onset	Rapid Onset	Delayed Onset
➤ Choking agent (chlorine)	➤ Nerve agent (inhaled)	➤ Nerve agent (absorbed)
➤ Blister agent (lewisite)	➤ Cyanide agent	➤ Blister agent (inhaled)
➤ Incapacitating agent (Agent 15, BZ)	➤ Vomiting (arsine-based agents: adamsite, diphenylchlorarsine, diphenylcyanoarsine)	➤ Choking agent (phosgene)
➤ Riot control agents (mace, tear gas)	➤ Liquid in eye (mustard gas)	

TABLE 8-2 Initial Identification of Chemical Agent Class Based on Early Signs and Symptoms of Exposure

Organ/System Affected	Signs/Symptoms	Chemical Agent(s) to Consider
Central nervous system (CNS)	Convulsions	Nerve; cyanide
	Confusion, odd behavior	Incapacitating
	Stupor	Any agent
Respiratory	Copious oronasal secretions	Nerve
	Chest pain, wheezing	Nerve; choking; blister
	Frothy sputum	Blister; choking
	Hyperpnea, dyspnea	Choking; blister; cyanide
	Apnea	Nerve; cyanide
	Cyanosis	Cyanide; nerve; choking
Circulatory	Bradycardia	Nerve; cyanide
	Tachycardia	Cyanide; nerve; incapacitating
	Shock	Any agent
Skin	Hot, dry, flushed	Incapacitating
	Vesication	Blister
	Pain on contact	Blister (ie, lewisite)
	Muscle tremors	Nerve
	Erythema	Unknown liquid
GI	Involuntary evacuation	Nerve
	Vomiting	Any agent

8.6.3   Treatment Principles for Chemical Casualties

Initial treatment is based on a differential diagnosis made regarding the type of agent, the manifestation and severity of signs and symptoms, and the estimated dose of the chemical received secondary to exposure. A clinician may or may not know the nature of the exposure at the time he or she is asked to care for a victim of a chemical disaster. Certain diagnostic tests may assist in confirming a clinical diagnosis or ruling out possibilities in a differential diagnosis (ie, cholinesterase levels, cyanide levels). Diagnostic testing in the setting of a chemical disaster with multiple people presenting to health care facilities, all with similar signs and symptoms, will be of limited use. Certainly, treating individuals who have been exposed to a known chemical substance will be easier than treating those exposed to an unknown substance. Ultimately, treatment early on in a chemical disaster will be based on the clinical impression and strongest clinical diagnosis and may involve administering treatment without laboratory, radiologic, or other confirmatory diagnostic testing.

Removal of the individual from the toxic environment, thoroughly decontaminating the person, and preventing further exposure to the agent are the first and perhaps the most important lifesaving steps that can be performed at any level or location of care. Principles of care would address immediate threats to life in accordance with triage priority and availability of resources. Other common therapies in chemical disasters include placement of an intravenous (IV) line, administration of bronchodilators and inhaled anticholinergics, and judicious use of oxygenation therapy. Lifesaving treatment may be limited to bleeding control and airway positioning in a contaminated environment. Triage of casualties in respiratory failure for intubation and ventilator support will need to be made on a conservative basis because of the limited number of available ventilators in hospitals and other health care facilities. The only lifesaving interventions possibly performed in the predecontamination setting would be the use and administration of antidotes such as nerve agent antidote kits (eg, Mark I Kits) or cyanide antidote kits, specifically amyl nitrite if available.

The hospital closest to the event is the facility most likely to be overwhelmed because of the geographic effect, a well-observed phenomenon in which casualties go to the closest hospital regardless of on-site direction.[5] Casualties do not distinguish the specialty characterization of hospitals (eg, adult vs pediatrics, cancer vs cardiac), so every health care facility should plan for reception of a demographic cross section of casualties. It is paramount that hospitals be notified early to prepare for mass casualties. Many casualties of a chemical event will arrive at the hospital by private vehicle and thus without having been decontaminated. In fact, the sarin incident in Tokyo demonstrated this reality when approximately four of five casualties presented directly to hospitals without the intervention of HAZMAT or other prehospital personnel.

8.7   CLINICAL MANAGEMENT OF SELECTED CHEMICAL AGENTS

This section discusses four chemical agent categories that are generally regarded by experts as being of greater health concern and also discusses selected toxic industrial chemicals. These agents are categorized by their general mechanism of action: blister agents (vesicants), choking or pulmonary agents, cyanide or asphyxiant agents, and nerve agents. Although these chemicals may be regarded as potential agents of terrorism, they also can represent a serious hazard through unintentional industrial- and transportation-related disasters, such as from a chlorine tank car spill or the release of a toxic plume from a chemical manufacturing plant.[1,3] Thousands of toxic industrial chemicals are in daily use and present myriad potential exposure hazards.

8.7.1   Blister Agents (Vesicants)

Blister agents (also referred to as *vesicants*) are so named because they are characterized by a common blister-like appearance on the skin. Common forms of vesicants include lewisite, mustard agents, and phosgene oxime.[3] These agents are highly persistent and, once aerosolized, settle rapidly out of the air. This makes the skin the primary route of exposure and the pulmonary and GI tracts the secondary routes. Vesicants act at the cellular level and can cause symptoms that include redness and blistering of the skin, shortness of breath, GI symptoms, and burning of the eyes.[3] First used for chemical warfare during World War I, vesicants remain a threat for use as a terrorist weapon or as a chemical warfare agent. In Iraq, vesicants (specifically mustard) were used against Iran during the 1980s war.[6]

Lewisite is an organic arsenical with vesicant properties. Pure lewisite is a liquid that is colorless and oily even in cold weather. It has been described as having the odor of geraniums. Lewisite can be mixed with mustard to form a persistent liquid that has a garlic-like odor. There are no confirmed reports that lewisite has been used in warfare, but some countries may have it stockpiled.

Sulfur mustard (2,2,-dichlordiethyl sulfide) has been used as a chemical weapon since World War I, while nitrogen mustard is a chemotherapy agent and has never been used for chemical warfare. Mustards are oily liquids and have been described as having the odor of mustard, garlic, onion, or horseradish. They penetrate skin, rubber gloves, many textiles, and skin. Exposure to as little as 1.0 to 1.5 teaspoons of mustard liquid is lethal to 50% of adults. However, it is exposure to mustard vapor rather than the liquid that is of greatest medical concern. Mustard is a persistent agent but becomes a major vapor hazard at high ambient temperatures. It is three times more toxic than a similar concentration of cyanide gas.[7] During World War I, 80% of mustard casualties were due to mustard vapor.

8.7.1.1   *Blister Agent (Vesicant) Pathophysiology*

Vesicants rapidly penetrate cells and generate a highly toxic intermediate episulfonium ion. This ion irreversibly alkylates DNA, RNA, and protein. Alkylation disrupts cell function and causes cell death. Depletion of glutathione inactivates sulfhydryl-containing enzymes and causes loss of calcium homeostasis, lipid peroxidation, cellular membrane breakdown, and cell death.[8]

Warm moist tissues are more severely affected because the chemical reaction is temperature-dependent and facilitated by the presence of water. Therefore, exposure of the mucous membranes to vesicant agents results in severe damage. Actively reproducing cells are most vulnerable to alkylation, so epithelial and hematopoietic cells are the most susceptible. Conjunctivitis, chemosis, blepharospasm (eyelid spasms), and corneal perforation result from even low-level vapor exposures to vesicants.

Exposure of the respiratory tract to vesicant vapors results in epithelial sloughing and pseudomembrane formation. The resulting damage to the respiratory epithelium makes the victim unable to clear pathogens and dead tissue. Most affected individuals die of pneumonia, respiratory failure, or sepsis.

8.7.1.2   Diagnosis of Blister Agent (Vesicant) Exposure

There are no laboratory tests to identify acute exposure to vesicants, so detection is based on clinical signs and symptoms. Mustards damage the skin, eyes, respiratory tract, GI mucosa, and hematopoietic system. The clinical effects are dependent on whether there was exposure to liquid or vapor; liquid exposure primarily damages the skin while vapor exposure exerts its toxicity upon the upper respiratory tract.

Initially, chemical burns from mustard appear superficial. Pruritus, burning, and stinging pain over exposed skin are early symptoms. Later, the areas become erythematous and edematous. More extensive contamination causes superficial bullae to appear over 24 hours. Full-thickness burns may occur with severe exposures and resemble scalded skin syndrome or toxic epidermal necrolysis. The blister fluid does not contain active mustard and is thus not toxic. Ocular symptoms may develop in 4 to 8 hours. These include burning pain, the sensation of a foreign body in the eye, photophobia, tearing, and blurry vision. Examination may disclose eyelid edema, conjunctival injection, chemosis, corneal abrasions and ulceration, and decreased visual acuity. Permanent blindness and corneal scarring may occur with severe exposures. Gastrointestinal involvement may result in abdominal pain, nausea, vomiting, diarrhea, and weight loss.[7]

The upper respiratory system is damaged by inhalation of mustard vapor, but the lower respiratory tract and lungs are rarely affected. Initial symptoms include sinusitis or sinus congestion, sore throat, and hoarseness. Lower respiratory tract symptoms such as cough, dyspnea, or respiratory distress may occur if the lower respiratory tract is damaged. Pulmonary edema rarely occurs.

Bone marrow may be suppressed by mustards. Precursors of leukocytes die 3 to 5 days after exposure. Anemia and thrombocytopenia are late findings. Acute exposure to lewisite liquid and vapor causes signs and symptoms similar to those of the mustards.

8.7.1.3   Blister Agent (Vesicant) Treatment Considerations

Treatment after exposure to mustard or lewisite requires immediate decontamination. Exposed people do not attempt early decontamination themselves because signs and symptoms are often delayed. Clothing should be removed immediately and the skin washed with soap and water. Because mustard is relatively insoluble in water, water alone has limited value, and some suggest that the skin should be carefully washed with 0.5% hypochlorite solution or with alkaline soap and water, which inactivates the sulfur mustard; however, hypochlorite may not be appropriate for pediatric patients. Ocular exposure requires copious irrigation with saline or water.

Treatment is mainly supportive (Table 8-3). Because effects are often delayed, exposed individuals may initially be asymptomatic. If there is history of severe exposure, securing an airway should be considered before upper airway obstruction

TABLE 8-3 Clinical Considerations for the Management of Blister Agents (Vesicants)

Blister Agent (Vesicant)	Diagnostic Considerations	Clinical Effects	Treatment Considerations

➤ Sulfur mustard (H)	➤ Symptom onset: delayed 2-48 h
	➤ Primarily liquid hazard
	➤ May be confused with skin exposure to caustic irritants (eg, sodium hydroxide, ammonia)
	➤ Intracellular enzyme, RNA, and DNA alkylating agents
	➤ No specific laboratory tests; detection based on clinical signs and symptoms
		➤ Dependant on whether liquid or vapor exposure: liquid primarily damages skin; vapor affects upper respiratory tract	➤ Immediate decontamination:
			  ➤ Skin: soap and water
			  ➤ Eyes: irrigation (water)
			  ➤ Both skin and eyes: possible impact only if done within minutes of exposure
			➤ Supportive care:
			➤ Thermal burn-type treatment
			➤ Symptomatic management of lesions
			➤ For pediatric considerations, see Section 8.8.

➤ Distilled mustard (HD)	➤ Symptom onset: delayed 2-48 h ➤ Odor: garlic, horseradish, or mustard	➤ Skin: erythema and blisters (may be delayed $\leq$8 h), pruritus ➤ Eye: irritation, conjunctivitis, corneal damage, lacrimation, pain, blepharospasm ➤ Respiratory: mild to marked acute airway damage, pneumonitis within 1-3 d, respiratory failure ➤ GI: nausea, vomiting, diarrhea may be present ➤ Bone marrow stem cell suppression leading to pancytopenia and increased susceptibility to infection ➤ Fever, sputum production ➤ Combination with lewisite (called mustard-lewisite or HL) results in rapid effects of lewisite and delayed effects of mustard agents	➤ No antidote ➤ Skin: silver sulfadiazine ➤ Eye: homatropine ophthalmic ointment ➤ Pulmonary: antibiotics, bronchodilators, corticosteroids ➤ Colony-stimulating factor may be helpful for leukopenia ➤ Systemic analgesic and antipruritics ➤ Early use of positive end-expiratory pressure or continuous positive airway pressure ➤ Maintain fluid and electrolyte balance (do not excessively fluid resuscitate as in thermal burns)

(Continued)

TABLE 8-3 *(Continued)*

Blister Agent (Vesicant)	Diagnostic Considerations	Clinical Effects	Treatment Considerations
➤ Lewisite (L)	➤ Symptom onset: immediate ➤ Odor: fruity or geranium ➤ Organoarsenic compound ➤ More volatile than mustard ➤ Damages eyes, skin, and airways by direct contact	➤ Skin: gray area of dead skin within 5 min, erythema within 30 min, blistering 2-3 h, immediate irritation or burning pain on contact, severe tissue necrosis ➤ Airway: inflammation, respiratory distress	➤ Symptomatic care ➤ Possible antidote: BAL (dimercaprol) for systemic effects in severe cases; the dosing regimen is 3-5 mg/kg intramuscularly (IM) every 4 h for 4 doses ➤ For pediatric considerations, see Section 8.8.
➤ Phosgene oxime (CX)	➤ Symptom onset: immediate ➤ Odor: freshly mown hay ➤ Urticant, nonvesicant agent ➤ Vapor extremely irritating, vapor and liquid cause tissue damage on contact ➤ Immediate burning, irritation, wheal-like lesions ➤ Eye and airway damage ➤ No distinctive laboratory findings	➤ Eyes: pain, blepharospasm, lacrimation, conjunctival, eyelid edema ➤ Airway: pseudomembrane formation, nasal irritation ➤ Intravascular fluid loss, hypovolemia, shock, organ congestion, leukocytosis, miosis; immediate pain on contact	➤ No antidote ➤ Parenteral methylprednisolone may be effective in preventing noncardiogenic pulmonary edema ➤ Experimental: aerosolized dexamethasone and theophylline for pulmonary involvement

occurs. Fluid losses are less than those seen with thermal burns, and it is therefore important to avoid overhydration. Wound care is essential and includes the liberal use of analgesia, debridement, irrigation, and topical antibiotics. Ocular injury requires ophthalmologic consultation. Daily irrigation, topical antibiotic solutions and corticosteroids, and mydriatics may be needed.

There are no antidotes available to treat toxicity from the mustard agents. Antioxidants such as vitamin E, anti-inflammatory drugs, mustard scavengers (glutathione, N-acetylcysteine), and nitric oxide synthase inhibitors (L-nitroarginine methyl ester) have been investigated. Granulocyte colony-stimulating factor is usually recommended for patients with bone marrow suppression.[7]

British antilewisite (BAL) or dimercaprol is a chelating agent that has been used to reduce systemic effects from lewisite exposure. Because of its side effects, BAL should be administered only to those who have signs of shock or pulmonary injury and in consultation with the poison control center. Side effects include pain at the injection site, nausea, vomiting, headache, burning sensation of the lips, mouth, throat, and eyes, lacrimation, rhinorrhea, salivation, muscle aches, chest pain, anxiety, and agitation. Contraindications to BAL therapy include renal disease, pregnancy (except in life-threatening circumstances), and concurrent use of medicinal iron. Alkalization of the urine stabilizes the dimercaprol-metal complex and may protect the kidneys during chelation therapy. Hemodialysis should be considered to remove the BAL if renal insufficiency develops.

8.7.2   Choking or Pulmonary Agents

Pulmonary agents, commonly referred to as *choking agents*, are so named because of the primary effects on lung tissue. Common toxic industrial chemicals that would be classified as pulmonary agents include ammonia, methyl isocyanate, methyl bromide, hydrochloric acid, and chlorine.[9] Pulmonary agents that have been used as chemical warfare agents include phosgene (CG), diphosgene (DP), chlorine (Cl), and chloropicrin (PS). Pulmonary agents are typically inhaled, and their mechanism of action is either on the central or peripheral airways in the lungs.[3] Pulmonary agents such as hydrochloric acid and chlorine will cause burning and irritation to the epithelial lining of the airways resulting in swelling and fluid accumulation in the lungs.[10] Other pulmonary agents will not necessarily cause burning or edema to the upper airways but will cause pulmonary edema, hypoxia, and hypotension.

Pulmonary agents can be broken down into high, moderate, and low water solubility to predict the major sites at which they exert their effects. Highly water-soluble pulmonary agents such as ammonia are used extensively in manufacturing processes and therefore are stored in large quantities and are often transported via rail and tanker trucks. The most common moderately water-soluble pulmonary agent is chlorine. Chlorine is a greenish yellow gas at room temperature that is a pulmonary irritant capable of damaging the upper and lower respiratory tracts. Its first documented use as a chemical weapon was in Ypres, Belgium, in 1915. In addition to its past use in warfare, chlorine gas is one of the most common reported occupational and environmental inhalation exposures. Pulmonary agents with low water solubility are represented best by phosgene and nitrogen dioxide. Originally developed as a chemical warfare agent, phosgene is currently produced at greater than 1 billion tons per year in the United States for use in manufacturing.

Phosgene is considered the most dangerous of the pulmonary agents because it directly damages the lungs with little or no warning. It was used for the first time as a chemical warfare agent in 1917 and accounted for many chemical casualties in World War I. At room temperature, phosgene is a colorless, nonflammable gas with the odor of newly mown hay. When released into open atmosphere, it may appear as a white cloud and the odor may not be detectable because toxic concentrations may be below the olfactory threshold. Because phosgene is denser than air, it accumulates in low areas such as trenches. Rapid olfactory fatigue results, making phosgene's warning properties unreliable. At higher concentrations (>1.5 ppm) phosgene may have an acrid, pungent odor.

8.7.2.1   *Pathophysiology of Choking or Pulmonary Agents*

The effects of pulmonary agents can be predicted by their water solubility, as most of these gases combine with the moisture in the airway tissues and mucous membrane, forming an acid or base resulting in tissue damage.

Highly water-soluble choking or pulmonary agents: Highly water-soluble agents such as anhydrous ammonia, hydrogen chloride gas, sulfur dioxide, and formaldehyde are very quick to combine with the moisture of the mucous membranes of the eyes, nasal passages, and upper airway, forming damaging acids and bases. As a result of their rapid reaction with water, the region of action is the upper airway to the level of the vocal cords. Anhydrous ammonia combines with water to form a potent base that rapidly damages the tissue. Hydrogen chloride gas and sulfur dioxide combine with water to form hydrochloric acid and sulfuric acid, respectively. Contact of these agents with the airway results in direct tissue damage and death. The resulting edema can cause airway obstruction and laryngospasm. This may limit the damage primarily to the upper airway. In large concentrations or prolonged exposures, damage below the vocals cords may occur. Most deaths from inhalation of highly water-soluble pulmonary agents are due to airway obstruction.

Moderately water-soluble choking or pulmonary agents: Moderately water-soluble pulmonary agents are slower than the highly water-soluble agents to combine with the moisture in the airway and damage the tissues. The result is that the gas is inhaled deeper into the airways, causing damage to the moderate-sized airways (bronchioles). Exposed individuals will experience upper airway symptoms similar to those with the highly water-soluble agents, although not as severe. In addition, the irritation of the bronchioles will result in bronchospasm and wheezing. In large concentrations or prolonged exposure, direct damage to the alveoli can occur.

Poorly water-soluble choking or pulmonary agents: The low water solubility of these agents allows them to be inhaled deep into the lungs before combining with moisture to damage the alveoli. Their lack of irritation of the mucous membranes causes them to go undetected, allowing the victim to continue to be exposed unaware. Nitrogen dioxide combines with water to cause nitric acid, and phosgene forms hydrochloric acid in the alveoli.

8.7.2.2   Diagnosis of Exposure to Choking or Pulmonary Agents

There is no specific diagnostic test that can be used in the necessary treatment window for the diagnosis of exposure to choking or pulmonary agents. As such, clinicians will have to make treatment decisions based on the presenting signs and symptoms. General diagnostic criteria and examples of representative choking or pulmonary agents (chlorine and phosgene) are described below.

Chlorine exposure: Individuals exposed to chlorine are often able to describe the typical swimming pool chlorine or "bleach-like" smell. This significantly aids in the detection of chlorine exposures. After exposure to chlorine gas, the person experiences irritation of the conjunctivae, nose, pharynx, larynx, trachea, and bronchi, resulting in inflammation and localized edema. Because it is highly water soluble, chlorine will react with water to form hydrochloric and hypochlorous acid in the airway. Individuals will have upper respiratory symptoms and will experience a significant amount of wheezing from the irritation of the bronchioles. If the individual has received a sufficiently large exposure, the alveoli fill with fluid, causing pulmonary congestion and edema.

Corneal abrasions and burns may be present, but severe ocular injury rarely occurs. Tears buffer the acids formed by the reaction of the chlorine with mucous membranes. Individuals exposed only to gas may not require decontamination. If skin symptoms are present, full decontamination must be performed, as the gas combined with the moisture on the skin may result in skin burns.

Phosgene exposure: At low concentrations, individuals may present with mild cough, chest tightness, and shortness of breath. Moderate concentrations may also produce lacrimation. High exposures may cause noncardiogenic pulmonary edema within 2 to 6 hours after exposure, and death may ensue within 24 to 48 hours.

At the time of exposure, there may be coughing, choking, chest discomfort, nausea or vomiting, headache, and tearing. As phosgene is inhaled, the resulting damage to the alveoli may not be immediately evident. The earliest symptom is the onset of exertional dyspnea. This results from pulmonary edema caused by the tissue damage in the alveoli. The onset of pulmonary edema can be insidious and delayed, with exposed individuals remaining asymptomatic for as long as 72 hours after exposure; most of these individuals with serious exposures will show symptoms within 24 hours of exposure.

The presence or absence of these symptoms does not aid in predicting exposure severity. For example, some individuals with severe choking episodes fail to develop further lung injury. Others, with only minor respiratory tract irritation, have been known to develop fatal pulmonary edema. There also may be a 2- to 24-hour period during which the individuals are symptom free. Substernal chest pain, cough, rapid shallow breathing, frothy sputum, and cyanosis signal the onset of pulmonary edema.

8.7.2.3 Treatment Considerations for Choking or Pulmonary Agents

Individuals exposed to phosgene or chlorine gas do not pose a risk of secondary contamination outside of the hot zone. People exposed to liquid phosgene, however, may contaminate other personnel from off-gassing vapor.

There is no specific antidote for phosgene or chlorine. In cases of suspected ocular injury, the initial pH should be determined. Copious irrigation with normal saline should continue until the pH returns to 7.4. Topical anesthetics may help to limit pain. As shown in Table 8-4, pulmonary symptoms may be delayed up to 4 to 6 hours after exposure, so repeat assessments should be made. Patients with pulmonary edema may require positive end-expiratory pressure either by a mask or by endotracheal intubation. Diuretics and corticosteroids have not been shown to be effective. Individuals with hyperactive airways may require aerosolized bronchodilator therapy. Anticholinergic bronchodilators may provide limited drying of airway secretions. Prophylactic antibiotics are not recommended.

8.7.3 Cyanide Agents

Cyanide and cyanogen chloride essentially mimic carbon monoxide poisoning. The chemicals are transported within the blood and interfere with the body's ability to use oxygen at the cellular level, causing a chemical asphyxiation.[3,10] Cyanide can be absorbed through the skin, although symptom onset would be delayed and it would take 30 to 60 minutes for signs or symptoms to present.[3,10] Cyanide is more commonly ingested or inhaled by affected patients. As a potential terrorism agent, cyanide specifically deserves discussion because of its availability and its potential effects if released into an enclosed space such as a subway tunnel or building.

Cyanide is produced by the combustion of many carbon- and nitrogen-containing compounds, particularly wool, silk, and plastics. Cyanide poisoning often affects individuals who have been trapped in a fire within a confined space, particularly if there were large amounts of synthetic materials and plastics burning. At temperatures below 78° F, hydrogen cyanide (HCN) is a colorless or pale-blue liquid (hydrocyanic acid); at higher temperatures it is a colorless gas that is very volatile and can be

TABLE 8-4 Clinical Considerations for the Management of Choking or Pulmonary Agents

Choking or Pulmonary Agents	Diagnostic Considerations	Clinical Effects	Treatment Considerations

➤ Acrolein
➤ Ammonia (NH₃)
➤ Chlorine (CL)
➤ Chloropicrin (PS)
➤ Diphosgene (DP)
➤ Nitrogen oxides (NO$_x$)
➤ Perfluoroisobutylene (PFIB)
➤ Phosgene (CG)
➤ Sulfur dioxide (SO₂)
	➤ Symptom onset: rapid or delayed; 1-24 h (rarely ≤72 h)
	➤ Odor (CG): freshly mown hay or grass
	➤ Easily absorbed by mucous membranes of eyes, nose, oropharynx; degree of water solubility of the agent influences onset and severity of respiratory injury
	➤ Lung tissue damage may be confused with inhalation exposure to industrial chemicals (eg, HCl, Cl₂, NH₃)
	➤ Chest radiograph: hyperinflation, noncardiogenic pulmonary edema
		➤ Eye and airway irritation, dyspnea, chest tightness, rhinorrhea, hypersalivation, cough, wheezing
		➤ High-dose inhalation may produce laryngospasm, bronchospasm, pulmonary edema, pneumonitis, and acute lung injury with delayed onset (≤48 h) of acute respiratory distress syndrome
			➤ Decontamination:
			  ➢ Fresh air
			  ➢ Skin: water
			➤ No specific antidotes
			➤ Supportive measures; specific treatment depends on the agent
			➤ IV fluids for hypotension; no diuretics
			➤ Ventilation with or without positive airway pressure
			➤ Bronchodilators for bronchospasm
			➤ Methylprednisolone may be effective in preventing noncardiogenic pulmonary edema but has not yet been proven

present in lethal concentrations at room temperature. The vapor is flammable and potentially explosive.

The cyanide ion is ubiquitous in nearly all living organisms that tolerate and even need it in low concentrations. The fruits and seeds (especially pits) of many plants such as cherries, peaches, almonds, and lima beans contain cyanogens capable of releasing free cyanide after enzymatic degradation. Cyanides are widely used in chemical syntheses, electroplating, mineral extraction, dyeing, printing, photography, and agriculture, and the manufacture of paper, textiles, and plastics. In the United States alone, more than 300 000 tons of cyanide are manufactured annually, and its widespread use could provide a readily available source for terrorist activity.

8.7.3.1 Cyanide Pathophysiology

HCN is lighter than air and therefore dissipates when released into open spaces. It is readily absorbed through the lungs, and the onset of symptoms is within seconds to minutes after exposure. Children exposed to the same levels of HCN as adults will receive larger doses relative to body size, as their lung surface area is larger in proportion to their body size. The exposure of skin and mucous membranes to HCN results in rapid absorption, contributing to systemic toxicity. Symptoms of systemic toxicity from skin absorption may be immediate or delayed up to 60 minutes. HCN liquids are also caustic and can result in significant chemical burns similar to the effect of the mustards. The ingestion of cyanide solutions, salts, or cyanogens can be rapidly fatal.

Hydrogen Cyanide (HCN)

Synonyms:

➤ Hydrocyanic acid

➤ Formonitrile

➤ Prussic acid

Sources:

➤ Combustion of urethane, wool, silk, plastics, or any material containing both carbon and nitrogen

➤ Manufactured by oxidation of ammonia-methane mixtures and the catalytic decomposition of formamide

➤ May be formed—cyanide salts + acid

➤ Used in fumigating, electroplating, mining industries

Physical properties:

➤ Description: colorless gas or pale-blue liquid

➤ Boiling point: 78° F (25.6° C)

➤ Gas density: 0.94 (lighter than air)

➤ National Institute for Occupational Safety and Health (NIOSH) "Immediately Dangerous to Life or Health" (IDLH) level: 50 ppm

➤ Water solubility: miscible with water

➤ Flammability: flammable at temperatures >0° F (−18° C)

Cyanide Salts—Potassium Cyanide (KCN) and Sodium Cyanide (NaCN)

Synonyms:

➤ Potassium salt of hydrocyanic acid

➤ Sodium salt of hydrocyanic acid

Sources:

➤ When combined with acid, cyanide salts produce hydrogen cyanide

➤ Fumigant (rodenticide and insecticide)

➤ Gold and silver ore extraction

(Continued)

Cyanide Salts—Potassium Cyanide (KCN) and Sodium Cyanide (NaCN) (continued)

➤ Mining

➤ Electroplating

➤ Steel production

Physical properties:

➤ Description: white solid

➤ Boiling point: 2957° F (KCN); 2725° F (NaCN)

➤ NIOSH IDLH level: 25 mg/m^3

➤ Water solubility: 72% (KCN); 58% (NaCN) at 77°F

➤ Flammability: nonflammable

HCN readily penetrates rubber and barrier fabrics. Butyl rubber gloves provide good short-term skin protection.

People normally have low, nontoxic levels of cyanide in their bodies as they routinely eat foods that contain small amounts of cyanide that form cyanogens. The body eliminates these small amounts of cyanide with a hepatic (liver) enzyme called rhodanese. Rhodanese catalyzes the reaction of cyanide (CN^-) with thiosulfate ($S_2O_3^{-2}$) to produce thiocyanate (SCN^-), which is excreted in the urine. In the case of a toxic exposure, the amount of cyanide present exceeds the body supply of thiosulfate. It is the body supply of thiosulfate, not the rhodanese, that is the main rate-limiting step in detoxifying cyanide.

Before the pathophysiology of cyanide poisoning can be understood, it is necessary to review the manner in which cells use oxygen and glucose to produce energy. Foods are ingested and are converted by the body into glucose, which is transported to the cell for energy production. The result is a series of reactions that occur in mitochondria to produce adenosine triphosphate (ATP). ATP, produced in the mitochondria by a process known as *oxidative phosphorylation*, creates a hydrogen ion gradient between the intermembrane space and the interior of the mitochondria. The hydrogen ion gradient is used by ATP synthetase to produce ATP.

The series of reactions that produce the hydrogen ion gradient is called the *electron transport chain*. The final step in the electron transport chain is cytochrome oxidase, also called *cytochrome a,a3*. Cytochrome oxidase reacts directly with molecular oxygen to produce aerobic metabolism. Cyanide has a high affinity for the ferric ion (Fe^{+3}) contained in the cytochrome oxidase and binds to it, which inhibits the final step in the electron transport chain and substantially decreases the amount of ATP that can be produced (Figure 8-1). In essence, the mitochondria are unable to use oxygen to sustain the life of the cell, and the cell dies. The classic summary of the mechanism of cyanide poisoning is that the cells are unable to use the oxygen in the mitochondria and therefore the venous blood remains oxygenated and bright red in appearance. However, this idea has been disputed, with some studies showing that a majority of patients may present with cyanosis.[11] Cells that are most sensitive to oxygen deprivation, such as the brain and the heart, are the first to show signs and symptoms of cyanide toxicity.

8.7.3.2 Diagnosis of Cyanide Exposure

Unlike the nerve agents, cyanide does not have a well-defined toxidrome, and victims of cyanide poisoning have many nonspecific symptoms. HCN is said to have a faint, bitter almond taste, but 20% to 40% of the general population cannot detect it because of the absence of a gene that governs the ability to smell the gas. Those who can smell cyanide may not describe the odor as that of bitter almonds. Unpublished research presented at the CDC disputes the idea pervasive in the medical community that cyanide has a "bitter almond smell."[11] Researchers found that more than 600 HAZMAT team members, who were exposed to 20 to 30 ppm of HCN to determine whether they had the genetically determined ability to smell cyanide, all described the smell as "musty" or "chlorine-like." No person exposed as part of the project described cyanide as having a bitter almond smell.[11] In addition to the confusion over the smell of cyanide and the genetically determined ability to smell it, rapidly occurring olfactory fatigue can make odor alone a poor detection method. A potential tipoff for the clinician is the characteristic bright-red venous blood that is the result of the inability of the cells to use oxygen, although this finding has been disputed.[11] Detection devices for cyanide are limited, expensive, and lacking in clinical relevance.

Hydrogen cyanide is highly toxic in all routes of exposure but has almost no effect after brief exposure to very low concentrations. Unfortunately, there are no specific distinguishing signs and symptoms after small exposures, and symptoms may resolve when the individual has been removed from a toxic environment to fresh air. In the event of the use of cyanide in a terrorist attack, a large number of casualties from the same location with nonspecific symptoms, reports of fatalities near the epicenter of the attack, and the lack of an organophosphate toxidrome or evidence of irritant gas exposure should lead to the suspicion of chemical agent use and of cyanide as the potential agent. Individuals may experience a variety of symptoms depending on the form of cyanide, the concentration, and the route of exposure. In the event of use of cyanide as a terrorism agent, the most likely scenarios would be the release of hydrogen cyanide gas in a confined or enclosed space, or contamination of the water supply with cyanide salts.

The central nervous and cardiovascular systems are the most susceptible to cyanide poisoning. Extremely low-level exposures may produce few or no symptoms, as the body is able to metabolize the cyanide into nontoxic forms that are eliminated from the body. Moderate-level exposures are nonspecific and may include excitement, dizziness, nausea, vomiting, headache, and weakness. As the exposure continues,

FIGURE 8.1

Cyanide Inhibition of Cytochrome Oxidase on Mitochondria
This figure shows the buildup of oxygen due to cyanide inhibition of cytochrome oxidase.

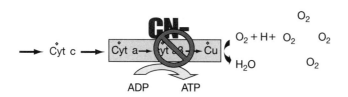

Abbreviations: ADP, adenosine diphosphate; Cyt a, cytochrome A; Cyt c, cytochrome C.

the individual may develop cardiac arrhythmias, hypotension, drowsiness, tetany, seizures, hallucinations, and loss of consciousness. In acute higher-level exposures, loss of consciousness may occur within seconds and death within minutes.

Individuals with severe cyanide poisoning experience intense air hunger, shortness of breath, and chest tightness. Pulmonary findings include increased respiratory rate as well as increased depth of respirations. As the poisoning progresses, respirations may become slow and gasping. Pulmonary edema may occur because of local irritant effects of HCN in the alveoli.

The diagnosis of cyanide poisoning is primarily clinical and is based on the rapid onset of CNS toxicity and cardiorespiratory collapse. Laboratory testing is not useful for guiding clinical therapy in the acute phase. Routine ancillary tests may include complete blood cell count, blood glucose, electrolytes, electrocardiogram, serum lactate levels, arterial blood gases, pulse oximetry, and chest radiograph. After acute treatment, methemoglobin levels may be monitored, but the usual monitoring methods are unreliable in cases of cyanide poisoning and may seriously underestimate the level of inactive hemoglobin. Survivors of a serious exposure should be evaluated for ischemic damage to the brain and heart. Individuals who have serious systemic poisoning may be at risk for CNS sequelae such as Parkinson-like syndromes and thus should be monitored long term.

8.7.3.3   Cyanide Treatment Considerations

Speed is critical in the treatment of cyanide poisoning. Symptomatic individuals should immediately receive supportive care with 100% oxygen and antidote therapy as needed. Treatment should be given simultaneously with the performance of decontamination procedures. In the case of ingestion, emesis should not be induced. If the individual has reflexive gagging, activated charcoal should be administered.

As summarized in Table 8-5, the treatment of cyanide poisoning is twofold: (1) displace the cyanide from cytochrome oxidase and (2) provide a sulfide ion donor to metabolize the cyanide into thiosulfate. The enzyme responsible for the metabolism of cyanide into thiosulfate is rhodanese. The supply of a sulfur donor (and not the rhodanese) is the rate-limiting step in this process. Cyanide that cannot be metabolized into nontoxic forms accumulates and has a high affinity for the ferric ion (Fe^{3+}) of the cytochrome oxidase of the electron transport chain. The removal of the cyanide from the cytochrome oxidase is the aim of treatment. There is a ferrous (Fe^{2+}) ion in each hemoglobin molecule.

Amyl nitrite administered by inhalation should be started as soon as the diagnosis of cyanide poisoning is made. Amyl nitrite is an oxidizer that changes the Fe^{2+} ferrous ion into Fe^{3+}. The product of this change in hemoglobin to the oxidized state is referred to as *methemoglobin* (MET-hemoglobin). Methemoglobin loses its ability to bind oxygen, and water becomes bound at the oxygen-binding sites, but the cyanide is attracted to and binds to the ferric ion in red blood cells. Thus, the cyanide is displaced from the cytochrome oxidase in the mitochondria (Figure 8-2). The administration of sodium nitrite further encourages and maintains the methemoglobin state. Sodium thiosulfate is then administered to provide the sulfur donor group needed for rhodanese to convert the cyanide into thiosulfate, which can be excreted by the kidneys.

TABLE 8-5 Clinical Considerations for the Management of Cyanide Agents

Cyanides	Diagnostic Considerations	Clinical Effects	Treatment Considerations

➤ Cyanogen chloride (CK)
 ➤ Hydrogen cyanide (AC)
	➤ Symptom onset: rapid, seconds to minutes
	 ➤ Odor: smell of "bitter almonds" but also described as musty or chlorine-like
	 ➤ Nonspecific hypoxic and hypoxemic symptoms; no well-defined toxidrome
	 ➤ Binds cellular cytochrome oxidase causing chemical asphyxia, lactic acidosis
	 ➤ CNS effects may be confused with carbon monoxide and hydrogen sulfide poisoning
	 ➤ Laboratory testing: cyanide, thiocyanate, serum lactate levels; venous and arterial partial oxygen pressure
		➤ Respiratory: shortness of breath; chest tightness; tachypnea (early); respiratory arrest
		 ➤ GI: nausea, vomiting
		 ➤ Cardiovascular: hypertension (early and transient); tachycardia (early and transient); ventricular arrhythmias; bradycardia (late); intractable hypotension (late); fatal arrhythmia, shock
		 ➤ CNS: anxiety, dizziness, headache, drowsiness, weakness, apnea, convulsions, seizure, coma
		 ➤ Metabolic acidosis and increased concentration of venous oxygen (patient also may present with cyanosis)
		 ➤ Moderate exposure: nonspecific findings, gasping, flushing, (typically not cyanosis)
		 ➤ High exposure: convulsions, cessation of respiration
			➤ Decontamination:
			   ➤ Fresh air
			   ➤ Skin: soap and water
			 ➤ Immediate treatment of symptomatic patients is critical (airway, breathing, circulatory support)
			 ➤ Antidote: sodium nitrite and sodium thiosulfate; repeat one-half of initial doses of both agents in 30 min if there is inadequate clinical response
			 ➤ Amyl nitrate capsules are available for first aid until intravenous access is achieved
			 ➤ Cyanide Antidote Kits are commercially available
			 ➤ Hydroxocobalamin (vitamin B_{12a}, Cyanokit): 70 mg/kg (maximum of 5 mg)
			 ➤ Activated charcoal for oral exposure
			 ➤ Mechanical ventilation as needed
			 ➤ Circulatory support with crystalloids and vasopressors
			 ➤ Correct metabolic acidosis with IV sodium bicarbonate
			 ➤ Seizures controlled with benzodiazepines
			 ➤ For pediatric considerations, see Section 8.8.

The *Cyanide Antidote Kit*[10] contains three medications: amyl nitrite pearls, sodium nitrite (IV solution), and sodium thiosulfate (IV solution). Amyl nitrite should be administered by crushing the ampule and placing it under the victim's nose for 30 seconds per minute, changing to a new ampule every 3 minutes until IV access is obtained and the sodium nitrite can be administered. The typical adult dose of sodium nitrite is 10 mL of a 3% solution (300 mg) IV over 5 minutes. This should be followed by an IV infusion of sodium thiosulfate, 50 mL of a 25% solution (12.5 g) over 10 to

FIGURE 8-2

Induction of
Methemoglobinemia
(MetHb) to Remove CN
from Mitochondria

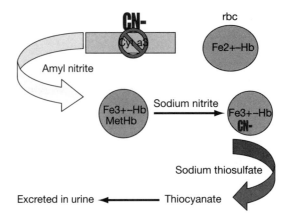

20 minutes. This can be repeated in 30 minutes at half the initial dose if the patient does not respond to treatment. Pediatric doses vary, are weight based, and should be administered in consultation with a pediatric physician.

Hydroxocobalamin (vitamin B_{12a}) has been used for the treatment of cyanide poisoning. Hydroxocobalamin reacts with cyanide to form cyanocobalamin, which is water soluble and nontoxic and can be excreted by the kidneys.

The Cyanokit, approved by the US Food and Drug Administration (FDA) in 2006, consists of two 2.5-g vials of hydroxocobalamin for intravenous injection. The Cyanokit has several advantages over the Cyanide Antidote Kit. Hydroxocobalamin is much less toxic and has been shown to be effective in some cases when the exposed person was in cardiac arrest, with the one limitation of requiring IV administration.

8.7.4   Nerve Agents

Nerve agents are a class of chemical agents that interfere with the ability of acetylcholinesterase (AchE) to break down acetylcholine. The resulting excess acetylcholine causes an overstimulation of skeletal and smooth-muscle contraction, along with glandular secretion. Common agents include household and commercial pesticides such as diazinon and parathion, as well as G- and V-series nerve agents (including sarin, tabun, soman, and VX).

Nerve agents are considered to be the most dangerous of all chemical warfare weapons. Certain pesticides known as carbamates and organophosphates produce similar physiologic effects, but nerve agents are much more potent. The G-agents are one group of this type of agent. The common names for the G-agents are tabun (GA), sarin (GB), and soman (GD). The G stands for German and the A, B, and D represent the specific chemicals. The V-agents are the other class of nerve agents; the most common agent is VX (no common name). The V stands for "venom" and the X originates from chemicals originally synthesized as an insecticide.

The modern use of nerve agents began in World War II when chemist Gerhard Schrader was working on the development of organophosphate insecticides.[12] In 1936 he developed the first nerve agent, tabun (GA), followed by sarin (GB), named for the initials of the scientists participating in its creation.[12] The German Ministry of Defense required that substances with potential military use be reported to the government, so Schrader complied with this regulation, and a large production facility was built at Dyhernfurth. This facility produced tabun and sarin beginning in 1942. Toward the end of World War II, the Soviets captured the Dyhernfurth facility, dismantled it, and moved it to the former Soviet Union, where production continued.

Tabun, sarin, and soman are considered volatile, or nonpersistent, agents. They evaporate readily. VX, however, has a much higher viscosity and an oily consistency, making it more persistent or nonvolatile. All nerve agents can be rapidly absorbed through the skin. Nerve agent vapors are heavier than air and tend to sink into low places such as trenches or basements.[7] Because VX has a higher lipophilicity and a greater persistence than the other agents, it is 100 to 150 times more toxic than sarin when victims sustain dermal exposure. A 10-mg dose applied to the skin is lethal to 50% of unprotected individuals.[7]

8.7.4.1 Nerve Agent Pathophysiology

First, it is necessary to briefly review the mechanism of toxicity to better understand the pathophysiology of nerve agents. Acetylcholine is one of the most important neurotransmitters for skeletal muscle, smooth muscle, and endocrine gland function. After acetylcholine enters a nerve synapse, it attaches to AchE so it can be broken down into acetate and choline. Acetate goes into intermediate metabolism, and choline is taken up presynaptically and recycled to form more acetylcholine. Nerve agents are attracted to AchE, preventing acetylcholine from bonding with the enzyme. This prevents the neurotransmitter from breaking down and causes an excess of acetylcholine throughout the body.

The nerve agents GA, GB, GD, and VX are potent AchE inhibitors. When this enzyme is inhibited, acetylcholine builds up at the nerve synapse. This accumulation results in the characteristic symptoms of nerve agent poisoning. Neurotransmitter excess is manifested in both the sympathetic and parasympathetic nervous systems. Cholinergic excess can result in tachycardia, hypertension, and mydriasis (nicotinic), which may be misleading for the clinician who expects to see the cholinergic (muscarinic) findings of bradycardia, miosis, and "polyrrhea" (secretions from every orifice).

8.7.4.2 Diagnosis of Nerve Agent Exposure

The primary detection of nerve agents is based on the signs and symptoms in exposed individuals. The majority of exposed people will present with miosis in the case of the volatile agents, but victims of VX exposure usually do not manifest miosis. More severely affected individuals will present with vomiting and seizures. When these symptoms are observed, the treating clinician should include nerve agent exposure in the differential diagnosis.

Depending on the agent and the degree of exposure, the effects of nerve agents may be immediate or delayed. Large inhalation exposures to nerve agents are likely to be lethal immediately. Small dermal exposures to these agents may have delayed effects and require a period of observation.

Mnemonics for Symptoms of Nerve Agent Exposure	
SLUDGEM	**DUMBELS**
Salivation	Diarrhea
Lacrimation	Urination
Urination	Miosis
Defecation/diarrhea	Bronchorrhea/bradycardia
Gastrointestinal	Emesis
Emesis	Lacrimation
Miosis	Salivation/sweating

If a nerve agent has been released, there may be unexplained or unusual polyrrhea in various individuals. Additionally, cholinergic signs and symptoms may be present. Symptoms of nerve agent exposure can be recalled by using the mnemonics SLUDGEM or DUMBELS.

Routine toxicology screens do not identify nerve agents in serum or urine. However, there is laboratory testing for the two types of cholinesterase found in the blood, known as *butyrylcholinesterase* (BuChE) and *erythrocyte cholinesterase* (RBC-AchE). These are not identical to the tissue enzyme AchE but provide an accessible source for measuring body cholinesterase activity. Studies that have attempted to relate symptoms of toxicity to AchE levels have found a greater correlation with RBC-AchE than BuChE.[8,13] Additionally, nerve agents tend to inhibit RBC-AchE to a greater degree than BuChE. In the Tokyo sarin terrorist attack, a BuAchE level less than 20% of that predicted was a useful prognostic indicator for patients with a poor outcome.[14]

Cholinesterase levels may vary depending on ethnicity and other genetic factors, nutritional status, and underlying disease states. Symptoms vary in relation to serum cholinesterase levels. Eye and airway signs are caused principally by direct exposure and have little correlation to RBC-AchE levels,[14-17] so that measuring RBC-AchE is not always reliable. While these tests do exist, they are not widely available and will not provide results in the window needed for acute treatment. Treatment decisions should be clinically based, but treatment should never be withheld from a symptomatic patient while awaiting laboratory confirmation. Conversely, decreased cholinesterase activity in the absence of clinical signs of toxicity is not an indication for treatment.[7]

8.7.4.3 Nerve Agent Treatment Considerations

Treatment of nerve agent casualties should be based on the initial signs and symptoms and modified accordingly once the actual agent is identified (Table 8-6). If the exposure was to a volatile agent, such as sarin or soman, individuals will be symptomatic within the first hour after exposure. This usually means that people who are not symptomatic when they are evaluated at the hospital are not likely to be seriously

TABLE 8-6 Clinical Considerations for the Management of Nerve Agents

Nerve Agents	Diagnostic Considerations	Clinical Effects	Treatment Considerations
➤ Cyclohexyl sarin (GF) ➤ Sarin (GB) ➤ Soman (GD) ➤ Tabun (GA) ➤ VX	➤ Symptom onset: vapor (seconds), liquid (minutes to hours); symptom onset: may be delayed up to 18 h, particularly for localized exposures ➤ Odor: none (GB, VX), fruity (GA), camphor-like (GD) ➤ Most toxic of known chemical agents ➤ Irreversible AchE inhibitors (muscarinic, nicotinic, and CNS effects) ➤ May be confused with organophosphate and carbamate pesticide poisoning ➤ Laboratory testing: erythrocyte or serum cholinesterase activity to confirm exposure	➤ Eyes: excessive lacrimation, miosis may be present ➤ Respiratory: rhinorrhea, bronchospasm, respiratory failure ➤ GI: hypersalivation, nausea, vomiting, diarrhea ➤ Skin: localized sweating ➤ Cardiac: sinus bradycardia may be present ➤ Skeletal muscles: fasciculations followed by weakness, flaccid paralysis ➤ CNS: loss of consciousness, convulsions, apnea, seizures	➤ Decontamination: ➤ Liquid: remove clothes; copious washing of skin and hair with soap and water; ocular irrigation ➤ Rapid establishment of patent airway ➤ Antidote: Atropine and 2-PAM Cl; additional doses until bronchial secretions are cleared and ventilation improved ➤ Early administration of 2-PAM Cl is critical to minimize permanent agent inactivation of AchE (ie, aging) ➤ Benzodiazepines to control nerve agent–induced seizures ➤ Airway and ventilatory support as needed ➤ Atropine, 2-PAM Cl, and diazepam are available in autoinjector kits ➤ For pediatric considerations, see Section 8.8.

exposed. For exposure to VX, individuals may not become symptomatic for up to 18 hours and should be observed for a much longer period. If the exposure history is uncertain, it is prudent to institute a longer observation period. The severity of symptoms and the rapidity of their onset will determine the dose of the antidotal therapy.

The acute management of a person with nerve agent exposure involves rapid establishment of a patent airway. The major cause of death is hypoxia resulting from bronchoconstriction and bronchorrhea. In severe cases, it may be necessary to administer atropine before attempting other interventions. Bronchoconstriction creates airway resistance on the order of 50 to 70 cm H_2O, making ventilation difficult before atropine administration. Succinylcholine should be used with caution to assist with intubation, as nerve agents prolong the drug's paralytic effects. Once atropine has been administered and intubation performed, aggressive suctioning of secretions should be performed. Three pharmaceutical agents are considered essential for the management of nerve agent exposure: atropine, pralidoxime, and diazepam (or other benzodiazepines).

Atropine is an agent with both systemic and central effects that combats the effects of acetylcholine excess at muscarinic sites. Atropine dosing should begin with 1 to 2 mg, but much more than the usual amounts may be required afterward (Table 8-7). Lack of response to normal doses of atropine is a hallmark of organophosphate intoxication, and patients with severe muscarinic effects will require larger amounts of the drug. Atropine may be given by various routes including IM, IV, or endotracheal. The efficacy of the endotracheal route has recently been questioned, and it should be used only if no other route is available. The endpoint of atropine administration is the clearing of bronchial secretions and decreased ventilator resistance. This is an essential point to remember because heart rate and pupil diameter are not useful parameters for monitoring the response to treatment with this antidote. Nebulized bronchodilators such as albuterol are not as effective as atropine at treating nerve agent exposure because an anticholinergic effect is needed.[12] More atropine should be administered if assisted ventilation remains difficult or if secretions persist. Additionally, clinicians should not be dissuaded from giving atropine if the individual is tachycardic.

Typical doses for atropine in severely affected nerve agent casualties are 5 to 15 mg given parenterally.[18,19] This dosage is in sharp contrast to the much larger doses required in organophosphate insecticide intoxication, in which several grams of atropine may be required during the first days of treatment.[20,21] In cases of severe organophosphate poisoning, an intravenous drip is begun to meet the continuing requirement for atropinization.[20]

Atropine causes an anticholinergic toxic syndrome when administered in excess of the amount required to reverse muscarinic effects.[22] Mydriasis, tachycardia, hypertension, urinary retention, and dry skin characterize an anticholinergic syndrome. The blocking of perspiration may be a dangerous effect in the setting of high ambient temperatures or continued physical activity. With the inability to dissipate heat, hyperthermia may ensue with resultant rhabdomyolysis and other life-threatening effects of increased corporal temperature. These individuals should be monitored with a rectal probe at frequent intervals and be kept in a cool environment.

Pralidoxime chloride (2-PAM Cl) is a substance that reactivates AchE when it is inhibited by a nerve agent. This oxime is the one most commonly used in the United States, but in other countries other oximes may be used to reactivate the enzyme through the same pathway. When an organophosphate or nerve agent binds to the esteratic site of the enzyme, the bond may either be regenerated by 2-PAM Cl or become permanent in the absence of an antidote. If the bond becomes permanent, the reactivation of AchE is no longer possible. This process, known as *aging*, occurs at different time intervals after exposure to different nerve agents. For example, sarin requires several hours to age, whereas soman ages in only 2 to 6 minutes. VX has the longest aging time of the nerve agents, requiring more than 2 days.

Once 2-PAM Cl has regenerated AchE, the enzyme resumes its critical role in the breakdown of acetylcholine, normalizing neurotransmission. This improves nicotinic symptoms such as fasciculations, muscle twitching, and weakness. The antidote also may improve breathing, although it will not treat muscarinic symptoms such as bronchorrhea and bronchoconstriction. Therefore, 2-PAM Cl is always given in conjunction with atropine and not alone in the treatment of nerve agent exposure.

Usually an exposure to sarin allows adequate time for clinicians to treat the patient if enough antidote is available. The oxime 2-PAM Cl is administered by slow IV infusion over 30 minutes (Table 8-7). The main side effect of rapid infusion is hypertension, which is rapidly responsive to phentolamine.

The oxime 2-PAM Cl has been shown to be ineffective in the treatment of soman poisoning. Because soman has an extremely rapid aging time of 2 to 6 minutes, the bond between soman and the AchE becomes irreversible before the 2-PAM can be administered in most cases. Therefore, 2-PAM Cl is essentially useless in soman poisoning. A group of reactivators known as the *bispyridinium oximes* show some promise in the treatment for soman poisoning. One such agent is HI-6, which is not currently available in the United States. Unfortunately, there is not a perfect oxime reactivator useful for all agents. Nevertheless, the patient should be treated with 2-PAM Cl in all cases where exposure to a nerve agent is suspected. The exact identity of the agent is usually not known early in the course of the incident, and 2-PAM Cl will not harm a soman-intoxicated patient.

Diazepam and other benzodiazepines should be used to treat seizures induced by nerve agents, either IV or with an autoinjector. IV is more practical in the hospital setting. Military sources suggest that in casualties manifesting symptoms of severe toxicity, benzodiazepines should be administered even before the seizures are evident. If three of the MARK I autoinjector kits are used (due to more severe symptoms), diazepam should be administered immediately after the autoinjector kit administration is completed. With the exception of benzodiazepines, conventional treatments for seizures such as phenytoin are considered ineffective in this setting.[22]

Autoinjector usage[23]: As of September 2004, the FDA had approved pediatric autoinjectors of atropine in 0.25-, 0.5-, and 1-mg sizes (Table 8-8).

TABLE 8-7 Nerve Agent Therapy

Patient Age	Mild/Moderate Symptoms[a]	Severe Symptoms[b]	Other Treatment
Infants, children, adolescents	See pediatric considerations (Section 8.8)	See pediatric considerations (Section 8.8)	See pediatric considerations (Section 8.8)
Adult	Atropine: 2-4 mg IM; 2-PAM Cl: 15 mg/kg (1 g) IV slowly	Atropine: 6 mg IM; 2-PAM Cl: 15 mg/kg (1 g) IV slowly	➤ Assisted ventilation as needed. ➤ Repeat atropine (2 mg IM or 1 mg IM for infants) at 5- to 10-min intervals until secretions have diminished and breathing is comfortable or airway resistance has returned to near normal ➤ Phentolamine for 2-PAM Cl–induced hypertension: 5 mg IV ➤ Diazepam for convulsions: 5 mg IV
Elderly, frail	Atropine: 1 mg IM; 2-PAM Cl: 5-10 mg/kg IV slowly	Atropine: 2 mg IM; 2-PAM Cl: 5-10 mg/kg IV slowly	

[a] Tearing, runny nose, mild chest tightness, localized sweating, nausea, vomiting, moderate dyspnea, muscle fasciculations, dyspnea, wheezing
[b] Moderate symptoms plus severe dyspnea, seizure, convulsions, apnea, flaccid paralysis, unconsciousness, cardiovascular collapse

Source: Agency for Toxic Substances and Disease Registry. *Medical Management Guidelines for Nerve Agents.* http://www.atsdr.cdc.gov/MHMI/mmg166.pdf. Accessed May 2, 2011.

TABLE 8-8 Atropine Autoinjector Size Determination[23]

Approximate Age	Approximate Weight	Autoinjector Size
<6 mo	<15 lb	0.25 mg
6 mo to 4 y	15–40 lb	0.5 mg
5–10 y	41–90 lb	1.0 mg
>10 y	>90 lb	2.0 mg (adult size)

Pediatric autoinjectors of pralidoxime are not FDA approved or available. When adult autoinjectors are used, appropriate atropine and pralidoxime dosing for children may be estimated as follows. If pediatric autoinjectors are available and it is operationally practical, the standard 2.0-mg atropine in a Mark-I kit may be replaced with a pediatric atropine autoinjector or the pediatric atropine autoinjector may be combined with a pralidoxime autoinjector. With this approach, Table 8-9 may be used to determine the number of pralidoxime autoinjectors. This approach is not possible with DuoDote, as this is provided as a single unit with both medications.

Each Mark-1 kit contains two autoinjectors (0.8-in needle insertion depth), one each of atropine 2 mg (0.7 mL) and pralidoxime 600 mg (2 mL), to be administered in two separate IM sites. DuoDote provides the same medications, atropine 2.1 mg (0.7 mL) and pralidoxime 600 mg (2 mL), but as a single autoinjector with the need for only one IM injection; while not approved for pediatric use, they should be used as initial treatment in circumstances for children with severe, life-threatening nerve agent toxicity for whom IV treatment is not possible or available or for whom more precise IM (mg/kg) dosing would be logistically impossible (especially prehospital). Suggested dosing guidelines are offered; note potential excess of initial atropine and pralidoxime dosage for age or weight, although within general guidelines for recommended total over the first 60 to 90 minutes of therapy for severe exposures.

TABLE 8-9 Pralidoxime and Atropine Autoinjector Usage[23]

Approximate Age	Approximate Weight	No. of Autoinjectors (Each Type)	Atropine Dosage Range, mg/kg	2-PAM Cl Dosage Range, mg/kg
3–7 y	13–25 kg	1	0.08–0.13	24–46
8–14 y	26–50 kg	2	0.08–0.13	24–46
>14 y	>51 kg	3	≤0.11	≤35

Table 8-9 lists usage of the Mark-1 or DuoDote kits to ages 3 years or greater, based on adherence to recommended dosages for atropine and pralidoxime. If an adult Mark-1 kit or DuoDote is the only available source of atropine and pralidoxime after a bona fide nerve agent exposure, it should be administered to even the youngest child.

8.8 PEDIATRIC TREATMENT CONSIDERATIONS

Chemical agent exposure in the pediatric population presents with several specific problems, which are primarily related to anatomic and physiologic differences[23]:

➤ Children have a higher metabolic rate and breathe at a faster rate, which causes them to inhale a larger dose and to be exposed more rapidly than an equivalent adult.

➤ The child's skin is thinner and more permeable to foreign agents, making the child much more sensitive to a given concentration of chemical.

➤ Many agents are heavier than air, which creates increased concentrations closer to the ground, thus exposing children to greater doses than adults.

➤ The various developmental and cognitive differences in children may limit their ability to recognize the danger and flee from risk. The simple physical differences in height, weight, and strength will alter the child's ability to function in a crowded, hysterical mob situation, all of which may lead to incapacitation and result in a higher exposed dose of agent.

Signs and symptoms: Children's physiology will affect the way they may react to a particular toxin. The constellation of symptoms is the same, although the timing and severity of symptoms and the time of onset may differ. Because of the immaturity of enzyme systems and metabolic rate, they can be much more sensitive to an agent, have more serious and persistent effects, and show a higher mortality. Because children's organ systems may still be developing, they may suffer long-term effects not experienced by adults. They also have an immature blood-brain barrier, so agents may have increased effects in children. Finally, because they have different receptor sensitivities, they may show either earlier or more severe symptoms.

Treatment: The same differences in physiology will affect the selection and dosing of antidote therapy for chemical agents (see Table 8-10). Medication used to treat the effects of chemical agents have all been developed and tested in the adult population, but there is very little data on the response of children to these therapies. As such, dosages may need to be extrapolated from adult dosages or from pediatric dosages for similar agents (organophosphate insecticide poisoning dosing in children used to treat nerve agent exposure). In addition, administration to children will often require weight-based adjustment.

TABLE 8-10 Recommendations for Pediatric Management of Chemical Agents[23]

Agent	Clinical Management[a]

Tabun, sarin, soman, VX	➤ Airway, breathing, circulatory support (ABCs)
	➤ Atropine[b,c,d]: 0.1 mg/kg IV, IM (may use 0.05 mg/kg for mild/moderate symptoms; minimum 0.1 mg, maximum 5 mg); repeat every 2-5 min, as needed, for marked secretions, bronchospasm
	➤ Pralidoxime (2-PAM Cl):[e] 25 mg/kg IV, IM (may use 15 mg/kg for mild/moderate symptoms; maximum 1 g IV, 2 g IM); may repeat within 30 to 60 min, as needed, then again every 1 h for 1 or 2 doses, as needed, for persistent weakness, high atropine requirement
	➤ Diazepam:
	   ➤ 30 d to 5 y of age: 0.05-0.3 mg/kg IV to a maximum of 5 mg/dose
	   ➤ 5 y and older: 0.05-0.3 mg/kg IV to a maximum of 10 mg/dose
	➤ Dosing may be repeated every 15 to 30 min
	➤ Lorazepam: 0.1 mg/kg IV, IM (maximum 4 mg)
	➤ Midazolam: 0.1-0.2 mg/kg (maximum 10 mg) IM, as needed, for seizures or severe exposure
	➤ Phentolamine for 2-PAM Cl–induced hypertension:
	   ➤ 1 mg IV (infants and children)
	   ➤ 5 mg IV (adolescents)

Mustard	Symptomatic care
Lewisite	Possibly British anti-lewisite (BAL), 3 mg/kg IM every 4-6 h for systemic effects of lewisite in severe cases
Chlorine, phosgene	Symptomatic care
Cyanide	➤ ABCs; 100% oxygen ➤ Sodium bicarbonate, as needed, for metabolic acidosis ➤ Sodium nitrite (3%):

Cyanide (continued):

Dosage (mL/kg)	Estimated hemoglobin concentration (g/dL) for lower case Average and Child
0.28	10
0.34	12
0.40	14
Max 10 mL	

➤ Sodium thiosulfate (25%) 1.65 mL/kg (maximum, 50 mL)
➤ Hydroxycobalamin (vitamin B_{12}, Cyanokit), 70 mg/kg (maximum of 5 mg), repeat as needed × 1

[a]Decontamination, especially for individuals with significant nerve agent or vesicant exposure, should be performed by health care providers garbed in adequate PPE. For emergency department staff, this consists of nonencapsulated, chemically resistant body suit, boots, and gloves with a full-face air purifier mask/hood.
[b]Intraosseous route is likely equivalent to intravenous.
[c]Atropine might have some benefit via endotracheal tube or inhalation, as might aerosolized ipratropium.
[d]As of September 2004, the FDA approved pediatric autoinjectors of atropine in 0.25-, 0.5-, and 1-mg sizes (see Section 8.7.4.3)
[e]Pralidoxime is reconstituted to 50 mg/mL (1 g in 20 mL water) for IV administration, and the total dose infused over 30 min, or may be given by continuous infusion (loading dose 25 mg/kg over 30 min, then 10 mg/kg/h). For IM use, it might be diluted to a concentration of 300 mg/mL (1 g added to 3 mL water—by analogy to the US Army Mark-1 autoinjector concentration), to effect a reasonable volume for injection. Pediatric autoinjectors of pralidoxime are not FDA approved or available.

Source: This table was created from recommendations developed at the Consensus Conference, in part based on reviewed reference materials from the American Academy of Pediatrics, CDC, and FDA, and adaptation from published work (Henretig FM, Cieslak TJ, Eitzen EM Jr. *J Pediatr.* 2002;141:311-326), which was updated in 2008 and 2010 and reproduced with permission from D. Markenson, Center for Disaster Medicine, New York Medical College.

8.9 SELECTED LARGE-SCALE CHEMICAL DISASTERS: LEARNING FROM EXPERIENCE

8.9.1 Bhopal, India (1984)

In what is considered by many to be the worst chemical release in history, the Union Carbide plant disaster in Bhopal, India, provides a striking example of the potential for chemical agents to produce large numbers of casualties. On the night of December 23, 1984, 40 tons of methyl isocyanate (MIC) were released into a city of nearly 900 000 inhabitants and spread over 30 square miles.[24] Initial estimates of the dead were 6000, with as many as 400 000 injured.[24] Reports of the morbidity and mortality from the disaster suggested numerous acute and chronic illnesses resulting from the disaster, including ocular trauma and related pathologies, pulmonary edema, miscarriages, fetal abnormalities, chronic obstructive pulmonary disease, pulmonary fibrosis, asthma, emphysema, fevers, psychiatric disorders, and certain types of cancers.[24,25] Long-term follow-up studies are ongoing, with more than 500 000 persons being monitored to date.[24]

While much attention has been paid to nerve agents because of terrorism concerns, many chemical agents such as MIC have great potential to cause mass casualties. Irritant gases are transported by road and rail through communities every day, and although terrorism is indeed a concern, the more likely scenario for a chemical mass casualty event is one of a transportation or industrial incident that releases a chemical agent.

8.9.2 Tokyo Sarin Subway Attack (1995)

The first use of a chemical agent on a civilian population was on June 27, 1994, when the Aum Shinrikyo cult released sarin gas in Matsumoto, Japan, in an attempt to assassinate several key judges. The release resulted in seven deaths and 144 injuries. Following this, the Aum Shinrikyo cult released 30% sarin in a very unsophisticated attack on March 20, 1995. The attack was timed to occur at the rush hour of the heavily commuter-dependent town of Tokyo. Containers of 30% sarin were placed on the floor of the subway cars and punctured by the perpetrators as they exited the subway. This crude method of delivery was successful in producing a large number of casualties. Had pure sarin and a sophisticated delivery device been used, much larger numbers of injured and dead would have been expected. The subway release (while not the first) was more publicized because of the significant numbers of "worried well" who presented to hospitals. Most stories reported 5500 "injuries," but at least 4000 of the 5500 had no effects at all from the attack and were deemed to have not been exposed to the sarin. Six hundred forty-one casualties reported to one hospital alone, St. Luke's International Hospital. Taking into consideration all regional hospitals, and not solely St Luke's International Hospital, there were approximately 900 exposed people who sought care. This included 54 critical patients, 12 deaths, and 135 exposed and injured emergency responders.[26]

There are several important lessons to be learned from the Tokyo sarin incident. The first is that, without a high index of suspicion, the detection of a chemical event can be very difficult. The symptoms of nerve agent exposure where not recognized immediately by responders, and therefore no decontamination was performed and no PPE was used. More than 23% of hospital staff who treated casualties had symptoms that included ocular pain, headache, sore throat, dyspnea, nausea, dizziness, and nose pain, but none was seriously affected. Of the 1364 EMS providers who responded to the scene, 135 were exposed and developed symptoms. If the casualties had merely been undressed outside ("dry decontamination"), this would probably have been sufficient to prevent all health care workers from becoming affected, even if they did not use any PPE. Dry decontamination involves simply undressing the individual to release any trapped vapor or liquid sources that may be on the person's clothing. Other lessons that can be learned from the Tokyo sarin attack is that EMS does not transport the majority of casualties from disasters and that approximately four of five will self-transport to the hospital. The notion that all affected individuals will be decontaminated on the scene is not realistic, as was well demonstrated by this event.

Of the 641 patients seen at St Luke's on the day of the disaster, five were in critical condition. Three patients had cardiopulmonary arrest (CPA), and two were unconscious and had respiratory arrest soon after arrival. Of these five critically ill patients, three were successfully resuscitated and were able to leave the hospital 6 days after admission. One patient with CPA did not respond to cardiopulmonary resuscitation and died with findings of conspicuous miosis that continued even at the time of her death. A second patient with CPA was resuscitated but died 28 days after admission because of irreversible brain damage.

8.9.3   British Petroleum Oil Spill, Gulf of Mexico (2010)

On April 20, 2010, the British Petroleum Deepwater Horizon oil rig exploded, releasing hundreds of thousands of gallons of crude oil into the Gulf of Mexico; 11 rig workers were killed, making it one of the most devastating environmental disasters in US history. The chemicals present in crude oil contain aromatic hydrocarbons, including volatile organic compounds (VOCs) such as benzene, toluene, and xylene. Exposure to these VOCs can cause depression of the CNS, respiratory distress, tachycardia, and headache.[27,28] Additionally, benzene is a known carcinogen, and toluene is a reported teratogen.[29] Crude oil can also release hydrogen sulfide gas, heavy metals, and polycyclic aromatic hydrocarbons, which can contaminate the food supply.[28,29] Burning oil releases particulate matter and can be associated with cardiovascular and respiratory symptoms.[29]

One particular issue in this disaster is the large quantities of chemical dispersants that were used to degrade the oil. No research has been performed on such widespread and prolific use of these chemicals and their potential health effects. These chemicals are mainly composed of detergents, surfactants, and petroleum distillates.[28,29] Some chemical dispersants have been known to cause skin irritation and infections, respiratory problems, nausea, vomiting, and eye irritation. Long-term effects are unknown.[27-29] Case reports of relief workers who sought medical attention for symptoms after cleanup work suggest several common symptoms, including cough, shortness of breath, chest pain, and dizziness, with the most common symptoms being headache, throat irritation, and nausea.[27-29] Although these symptoms can be suggestive of exposure to hydrogen sulfide gas or hydrocarbons, they also can be indicators of other unrelated illness.

Another important issue in this disaster is the risk of exposure to cleanup workers. Many workers who volunteer lack the necessary types of PPE or training on proper PPE use. Additionally, because of the heat and humidity in the region, it is common for workers to remove their protective equipment as a result of heat stress. This puts workers at higher risk for illness secondary to exposure, particularly because they are closer to the chemical hazards and are thus exposed to higher concentrations of the chemicals.

8.10 SUMMARY

Chemical agents can be released via unintended or deliberate means, such as through a spill from a damaged railroad tank car or an explosion at an industrial facility with resultant contamination of air, food, water, or consumer products. Chemicals also could be released as bombs, sprayed from aircraft and boats, or disseminated by other means to intentionally create a hazard to people and the environment. Health effects of chemical agents range from irritation and burning of eyes, skin, and mucous membranes to rapid cardiopulmonary collapse and death. Such effects are usually immediate (a few seconds) or very rarely delayed (several hours to days). Immediate symptoms of exposure to chemical agents may include blurred vision, eye irritation, difficulty breathing, and nausea. Affected persons may require urgent medical attention. The presence of several persons presenting with the same symptoms should alert clinicians and hospital staff to the possibility of a chemical attack. If an attack occurs, most casualties will likely arrive at the hospital within a short time period. This situation differentiates a chemical attack from a biologic attack involving infectious microorganisms, in which time elapses between exposure and the development of symptoms.

Some, but not all, chemical agents have a high potential for secondary contamination from victims to responders. This requires that medical treatment facilities have clearly defined procedures for handling contaminated individuals, many of whom will transport themselves to the facility. Precautions must be used until thorough decontamination has been performed or the specific chemical agent is identified. Response personnel must first protect themselves (eg, by using protective suits, respiratory protection, and chemical-resistant gloves) because secondary contamination with even small amounts of these substances (particularly nerve agents such as VX) can be lethal.

Efficient deployment of HAZMAT teams and other personnel trained in decontamination procedures is critical to control a chemical agent attack. Although all major cities and emergency medical systems have plans and equipment in place to address this situation, health professionals must be aware of principles involved in managing persons exposed to these agents. Health professionals and other responders also need quick access to current information on preparing for a chemical emergency, handling contaminated persons, hazard recognition and assessment, health effects, and accessing emergency assistance. With adequate resources and planning, health professionals and the public can better prepare themselves to recognize an emergency situation and react effectively to protect themselves and others from harm.

8.11 DISCUSSION POINTS

Chemical Disasters: Putting the PRE-DISASTER Paradigm™ into Practice		
P	Planning and Practice	After an actual incident, drill, or exercise, chemical disaster response plans should be reviewed to determine whether the procedures in the written plan were adequate and met the actual needs of the occurrence. Typically, areas for improvement are noted in an after-action report, and revisions to the plan would be made and promulgated by the chief executive.
R	Resilience	When hazards are identified that may produce a potential chemical disaster, any possible mitigation actions that can isolate the hazard from a vulnerable population or critical infrastructure should be considered when feasible. These steps will increase the resiliency of a community or health care facility after any type of disaster.
E	Education and Training	Training should be based on the current, updated version of the jurisdiction's emergency operations plan, and the training evaluated by conducting a discussion or operations-based exercise. Particular emphasis on recognizing the signs and symptoms of chemical exposure, how to take initial personal protective actions, and performing decontamination should be considered for chemical disasters.
Chemical Disasters: Putting the DISASTER Paradigm™ into Practice		
D	Detection	Reliable information regarding the exact nature of the chemical and extent of a person's exposure is unlikely early on in the event. As such, health care providers should be able to identify the type of agent and principles of care on the basis of signs and symptoms of illness, as well as how to determine that a possible chemical event has occurred in the community by using additional resources.
I	Incident Management	Like all disasters, chemical disasters will be managed by using the incident command system (ICS). It is likely, on the basis of the scope of the event, that the jurisdiction's emergency operations center or hospital command center will be activated for a large-scale incident. Adhering to ICS principles and following the chain of command are essential to ensure that all critical functional roles are performed during a chemical disaster.

S	Safety and Security	Preventing personnel and critical facilities from secondary contamination is paramount in responding to a chemical disaster. Rapid site security measures and perimeter control should be put into place as soon as possible, and hospitals should be placed on lockdown. This will ensure better control of how contaminated individuals are handled, and the spreading of contamination and potential for secondary contamination of critical infrastructure will be avoided. Additionally, appropriate PPE should be utilized by first responders and first receivers when performing rescue, triage, or decontamination operations during a chemical disaster.
A	Assess Hazards	Hazard assessment will be based on the availability of information regarding the location, scope, and type of event that has occurred. Identification of the specific hazard and the possibility of contamination spreading from the scene to secondary locations should be considered by responders. Individuals who present to health care facilities who are ambulatory, alert, and talking will have generally been exposed to less of the hazardous substance than those who are unresponsive or have alterations in mental status.
S	Support	Support to manage the incident should be requested through the ICS structure in place either on-scene or at the facility. Individuals in positions to identify and procure resources for incident operations should have procedures in place for rapid execution and deployment of resources as soon as possible. Additionally, individuals in logistics or planning positions who are in charge of resource procurement and allocation should have proper training on their roles and participate in frequent drills and exercises.
T	Triage and Treatment	Triage will be performed twice, both at the scene and at the hospital, particularly when decontamination is being performed. Individuals should be triaged initially to prioritize who goes through decontamination first and then triaged medically after the removal of contamination. The fundamental principle of triage during a chemical disaster is to treat the most people with the best chance of survival using the resources available. In the setting of a mass casualty event treatment will be symptom-based on clinical diagnoses and should not rely on diagnostic testing. Neurologic, pulmonary, and cardiovascular effects will be the most likely to cause mortality in a chemical disaster. Both cyanide and nerve agents have specific antidotes that can be administered to reverse the effects of the agent.
E	Evacuation	Decisions on evacuation or sheltering in place will depend on several factors, including the weather, the time of day, the ability of the facility or building to be prepared for sheltering in place, and the distribution and vulnerabilities of the population affected. The decision for evacuation or sheltering in place will be made within the ICS and include input from HAZMAT teams, public health agencies, and emergency management personnel.
R	Recovery	Recovery from the event will be based on the level of preparedness that existed before the event. If facilities and jurisdictions have comprehensive plans, sound training, and frequent drills, they will generally be more resilient after an event than a facility or jurisdiction that is less prepared. Removal of all traces of contamination, restoration of essential services, and securing critical infrastructure are priorities in recovery from a chemical disaster.

REFERENCES

1. Committee on Research and Development Needs for Improving Civilian Medical Response to Chemical and Biological Terrorism Incidents, Institute of Medicine. *Chemical and Biological Terrorism: Research and Development to Improve Civilian Medical Response*. Washington, DC: National Academy Press; 1999.

2. Occupational Safety and Health Administration. OSHA Best Practices for Hospital-Based First Receivers from Mass Casualty Incidents Involving the Release of Hazardous Substances. Washington, DC: OSHA; 2005. http://www.osha.gov/Publications/osha3249.pdf. Accessed May 2, 2011.

3. US Army Medical Research Institute of Chemical Defense. *Chemical Casualty Care Division: Medical Management of Chemical Casualties Handbook*. Aberdeen Proving Ground, MD: Chemical Casualty Care Office, Medical Research Institute of Chemical Defense; 2000.

4. Rcilly MJ, Markenson D. Hospital referral patterns: how emergency medical care is accessed in a disaster. *Disaster Med Public Health Prep*. 2010;4:226-231.

5. Frykberg E. Principles of mass casualty management following terrorist disasters. *Ann Surg*. 2004;239(3):319-321.

6. Zajtchuk R, Bellamy RF. Medical aspects of chemical and biological warfare. In: Zajtchuk R, ed. *Textbook of Military Medicine*. Washington, DC: Office of the Surgeon General, Department of the Army; 1997.

7. Arnold JL. Chemical Warfare. *E-Medicine J*. 2001;2(10).

8. Ketchum JS, Sidell FR, Crowell EB Jr, Aghajanian GK, Hayes AH Jr. Atropine, scopolamine, and ditran: comparative pharmacology and antagonists in man. *Psychopharmacologia*. 1973;28:121-145.

9. Centers for Disease Control and Prevention (CDC). Choking/Lung/Pulmonary Agents. http://www.bt.cdc.gov/agent/pulmonary/. Accessed May 2, 2011.

10. Agency for Toxic Substances and Disease Registry. Medical Management Guidelines for Hydrogen Cyanide. http://www.atsdr.cdc.gov/MMG/MMG.asp?id=1073&tid=19. Accessed May 2, 2011.

11. Curry S. The truth about cyanide. Paper presented at: Chemical agents of opportunity for terrorism preparedness and response; January 23, 2003; Centers for Disease Control and Prevention, Atlanta, Georgia.

12. Sidell FR. Nerve agents. In: Zajtchuk R, ed. *Textbook of Military Medicine*. Washington, DC: Office of the Surgeon General, Department of the Army; 1997.

13. Grob D, Lilienthal JL, Harvey AM, Jones BF. The administration of di-isopropyl fluorophosphate (DFP) to man, I: effect on plasma and erythrocyte cholinesterase; general systemic effects; use in study of hepatic function and erythropoiesis; and some properties of plasma cholinesterase. *Bull Johns Hopkins Hosp*. 1947;81:217-244.

14. Okumura T, Takasu N, Ishimatsu S, et al. Report on 640 victims of the Tokyo subway sarin attack. *Ann Emerg Med*. 1996;28:129-135.

15. Craig AB, Woodson GS. Observations on the effects of exposure to nerve gas, I: clinical observations and cholinesterase depression. *Am J Med Sci*. 1959;238:13-17.

16. Harvey JC. Clinical Observations on Volunteers Exposed to Concentrations of GB. Medical Laboratories Research Report 114. Edgewood, MD: Army Chemical Center; 1952.

17. Sidell FR. Clinical considerations in nerve agent intoxication. In: Somani SM, ed. *Chemical Warfare Agents*. San Diego, CA: Academic Press; 1992.

18. Sidell FR. Soman and sarin: clinical manifestations and treatment of accidental poisoning by organophosphates. *Clin Toxicol*. 1974;7(1):1-17.

19. Ward JR. Case report: exposure to a nerve gas. In: Whittenberger JL, ed. *Artificial Respiration: Theory and Applications*. New York, NY: Harper & Row; 1962:258-265.

20. Chew LS, Chee KT, Yeeo JM, Jayaratnam FJ. Continuous atropine infusion in the management of organophosphorus insecticide poisoning. *Singapore Med J.* 1971;12:80-85.

21. Vale JA, Meredith TJ, Heath A. High dose atropine in organophosphorus poisoning. *Postgrad Med J.* 1990;66:878.

22. Keyes C. Toxicity of anticholinergic agents. In: Aghababian RV, ed. *Emergency Medicine: the Core Curriculum.* Philadelphia: Lippincott-Raven; 1998.

23. Markenson D, Redlener I. Pediatric Preparedness for Disasters and Terrorism: A National Consensus Conference. Executive Summary and Final Report. New York, NY: National Center for Disaster Preparedness, New York Medical College School of Public Health; 2007. http://www.njcphp.org/legacy/drup/sites/default/files/Pediatric_Preparedness_Conference_Report.pdf. Accessed May 2, 2011.

24. Mishra PK, Samarth RM, Pathak N, Jain SK, Banerjee S, Maudar KK. Bhopal gas tragedy: review of clinical and experimental findings after 25 years. *Int J Occup Med Environ Health.* 2009;22:193-202.

25. Greenberg MI. Methyl isocyanate (MIC). In: Greenberg MI, ed. *Encyclopedia of Terrorist, Natural, and Man-Made Disasters.* Sudbury, MA: Jones and Bartlett; 2006.

26. Beaton R, Stergachis A, Oberle M, et al. The sarin gas attacks on the Tokyo subway? 10 years later/lessons learned. *Traumatology.* 2005;11:103-119.

27. McCauley LA. Environments and health: will the BP oil spill affect our health? *Am J Nurs.* 2010;110:54-56.

28. Slomski A. Experts focus on identifying, mitigating potential health effects of Gulf oil leak. *JAMA.* 2010;304:621-622, 624.

29. Solomon GM, Janssen S. Health effects of the Gulf oil spill. *JAMA.* 2010;304:1118-1119.

CHAPTER NINE

Biologic Disasters

CHAPTER CHAIR

Charles Stewart, MD, MSc(DM), MPH

CONTRIBUTING AUTHORS

Theodore Cieslak, MD

Elin A. Gursky, ScD, MSc

George R. Gentile, RN, BSN, MPH

Apryl Brown, MD, MPH

Jim Lyznicki, MS, MPH

9.1 PURPOSE

This chapter describes principles and practices for the management of biologic disasters. It reinforces the general concepts of situational awareness, incident management, workforce protection, and casualty management, which were explained in Chapters 1 through 5 of this manual. The application of these general concepts to the management of the Centers for Disease Control and Prevention (CDC) category A biologic agents is described. Clinical and public health management of large-scale infectious disease outbreaks, such as an influenza pandemic, is introduced and supports the more in-depth discussion in the Advanced Disaster Life Support™ (ADLS®) course (v 3.0) and supporting course manual.

9.2   LEARNING OBJECTIVES

After completing this chapter, readers should be able to:

➤ Describe six key factors that compose the "chain of infection."

➤ Identify clinical and epidemiologic clues suggestive of a biologic disaster.

➤ Discuss actions that can be taken to protect the health, safety, and security of responders and affected populations in a biologic disaster.

➤ Describe essential infection control strategies to prevent the spread of biologic agents.

➤ Discuss appropriate clinical management guidance for CDC category A biologic agents.

Learning objectives for this chapter are competency-based, as delineated in Appendix B.

9.3   BACKGROUND

Biologic agents are bacterial, viral, fungal, and parasitic organisms and toxins that cause disease in humans, plants, and animals. For humans, these diseases can be spread, directly or indirectly, from one person to another, as well as can be transmitted from animals, insects, plants, or contaminated food and water. Infectious diseases are a continuing threat to all persons, regardless of age, gender, lifestyle, ethnic background, and socioeconomic status. Societal, technologic, and environmental factors have a dramatic effect on infectious diseases worldwide, facilitating the emergence of new diseases and the reemergence of old ones, sometimes in drug-resistant forms or forms with no susceptibilities. Environmental changes can affect the incidence of these diseases by altering the habitats and ecology of disease vectors. In recent years, global concern has increased about bioterrorism, the deliberate use of certain pathogens or biologic products by terrorists to influence the conduct of government or to intimidate or coerce a civilian population.

The specter of bioterrorism is grim. Health professionals need to be prepared to detect, diagnose, characterize, and respond appropriately to use of biologic weapons and to the threat of new and reemerging infections. This requires thoughtful situational awareness, suspicion of new presentations of old diseases, rapid identification of possible biologic warfare or terrorism agents, cogent understanding of new and reemerging diseases as they present within the local area, and careful attention to personal infection control practices.

9.4   BASICS OF INFECTIOUS DISEASE EXPOSURE
AND TRANSMISSION

Exposure refers to the potential to become infected with a biologic agent. Exposure assessment requires understanding of the mode(s) of transmission and the distribution of the infectious agent in human and animal populations and in the environment. This includes the presence of disease vectors and reservoirs, the extent of human encroachment into animal habitats (and vice versa), environmental degradation, and climate change. This also includes the threat posed by emerging infectious diseases moving into new ecological niches and the possibilities of movement of disease agents across borders.

The *chain of infection* involves six key factors that lead to disease (see Figure 9-1). Each of these factors should be characterized when considering prevention and control measures. Environmental factors that may influence disease occurrence also must be evaluated. The goal of any infection control intervention is to break the chain of infection.

Infectious agent: The greater the organism's virulence (ability to grow and multiply), invasiveness (ability to enter tissue), and pathogenicity (ability to cause disease), the greater the possibility that the organism will cause an infection.

Reservoir: A reservoir can be any person, animal, arthropod, plant, or substance (or combination of these) in which an infectious agent normally lives and multiplies, on which it depends primarily for survival, and where it reproduces itself so that it can be transmitted to a susceptible host.

Portal of exit: This is a means for a biologic agent to leave the reservoir. For example, the microorganism may leave a human reservoir through the nose or mouth when the person sneezes or coughs. Microorganisms also can be disseminated from a bowel reservoir via feces.

Mode of transmission: This refers to the mechanisms by which the infectious agent is spread to or among humans. Transmission of microorganisms can occur by one or more of the following means:

➤ *Airborne transmission* may occur if the microorganism can remain suspended in the air for long periods. Airborne transmission takes place through coughing or sneezing, which may disseminate microbial aerosols. Aerosol spray is an effective technique for dissemination of biologic weapons. For many infective agents, the risk is greatest if the agent reaches the target population in the form of particles within the narrow aerodynamic size range where particles are small enough to penetrate the alveoli in the depths of the lungs but are not so small that most of them fail to be deposited and instead are exhaled. Droplets as large as 20 µm can infect the upper respiratory tract; however, these relatively large particles generally are filtered by natural anatomic and physiologic processes,

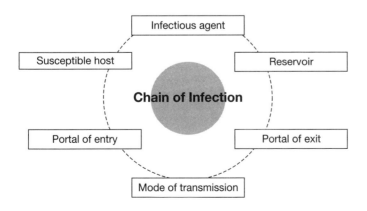

FIGURE 9-1
The Chain of Infection

and only much smaller particles (ranging from 0.5 to 5 µm) reach the alveoli efficiently. These smaller particles are not efficiently retained during respiration and may be relatively unstable under ambient environmental conditions.

This does not mean that larger particles do not enter the alveoli or that larger particles within any other mucous membrane cannot cause disease, but rather that the smaller particles achieve the maximum number of human casualties.[1]

A subset of aerosol contamination is airborne contamination from the patient. The airborne particles may be generated by cough or sneeze. This was clearly a major problem in spreading of smallpox, pneumonic plague, and tuberculosis.[2] In other disasters, it may cause spread of respiratory diseases among survivors of the disaster.

➤ *Droplet contact* results from coughing or sneezing on another person; it is similar to airborne transmission, but the droplets are significantly larger and settle out more rapidly.

➤ *Direct physical contact* is essentially touching or being touched by an infected person. Direct contact with an infected person can spread microbial diseases and has accounted for transmission of multiple diseases. Intact skin provides an excellent barrier for most, but not all, biologic agents. This may be a relatively ineffective method of transmission, but given a highly infective disease with a long latent period, such as smallpox, it may be workable. Mucous membranes and damaged skin such as cuts or abrasions may enhance infectivity.

➤ *Indirect physical contact*, usually by touching contaminated objects or surfaces, is relatively ineffective as a transmission mode. However, anthrax contamination in the mail in 2001 demonstrated that, for at least this disease, indirect contact was a viable means of causing infection.

➤ *Fecal-oral transmission* usually results from contact with contaminated food or water sources.

➤ *Vector-mediated transmission* can occur via infected insects (eg, mosquitoes, fleas), arthropods, other invertebrate hosts, and animals (eg, bats) that bite humans or others, transmitting disease-causing microorganisms. This technique was used successfully for the dissemination of bubonic plague bacteria in China by Japanese Unit 731 during the buildup to and during World War II. This technique also could be employed with a highly contagious disease such as smallpox by using an infected human as a vector. Some experts believe that this method of dissemination is complex, difficult to control, and relatively unreliable. Nonetheless, it has been used successfully.

The distinction between transmission types is an important consideration for intervention. Direct transmission can be interrupted by appropriate individual hygienic practices and precautions and by proper management of infected persons and their contacts. The interruption of indirect transmission requires other approaches, such as adequate ventilation, boiling or chlorination of water, disinfection of surfaces, laundering of clothing or bedding, and vector control.

Portal of entry: Infectious agents may enter the host through the skin, mucous membranes, lungs, gastrointestinal tract, or genitourinary tract; agents may enter fetuses through the placenta. Portals also result from tubes placed in body cavities (eg, urinary catheters) or from punctures produced by invasive procedures such as intravenous fluid replacement. Some biologic agents can cause infection only by entering a specific portal of the body, whereas others cause different infections when entering different portals. *Bacillus anthracis* spores, for example, can be inhaled, causing inhalational anthrax; enter through a cut on the skin, causing cutaneous disease; or be consumed in undercooked infected meats, causing gastrointestinal disease.

Susceptible host: Development of the disease in a host reflects characteristics of the specific agents and is influenced by the following factors:

➤ Host defense characteristics (eg, skin, genetic factors, inflammatory response, immunologic response)

➤ Underlying medical conditions causing immunodeficiency

➤ Malnutrition

➤ Pregnancy

➤ Age

➤ Increased exposure risk (occupational, travel)

➤ Behavioral factors (hand washing, respiratory hygiene, sexual behavior, drug use)

9.5 TYPES OF BIOLOGIC DISASTERS

Disasters caused by biologic agents may have certain characteristics that impose additional challenges compared to other kinds of emergency responses. The event may unfold silently, escaping early detection, and may rely heavily on an integrated health and medical response. The scale of a biologic event may be difficult to predict; there may be one or two casualties or hundreds of thousands. Unlike other disasters that may be limited to a single location, a biologic disaster may spread as disease is transmitted from one person to another. Law enforcement and public health officials will need to work closely together, sharing information and resources.

Modern demographic and ecological conditions that favor the spread of infectious diseases include more frequent and faster movement across international boundaries by tourists, workers, immigrants, and refugees; rapid population growth; increasing poverty and urban migration; alterations in the habitats of animals and arthropods that transmit disease; increasing numbers of persons with impaired host defenses; and changes in the way that food is processed and distributed. In the globalized world, diseases can spread broadly via international travel and trade. Air travel has increased substantially, and more people are visiting remote locations where they can be exposed to infectious agents that are uncommon in their native countries. Added to these developments is the ability of microorganisms to mutate and adapt rapidly, which has facilitated the reemergence of various communicable diseases (eg, tuberculosis), the emergence of new diseases, and the evolution of antimicrobial resistance (which means that previous curative treatments for a wide range of parasitic, bacterial, and viral infections have become less effective).

Notable Epidemics and Pandemics

➤ 541 to 542: the Plague of Justinian (thought to be bubonic plague)[3]

➤ The fourteenth century: the Black Death (bubonic plague)[3]

➤ 1855 to1950s: bubonic plague, Third Pandemic[3]

➤ 1918 to 1920: influenza, Spanish flu. More people were hospitalized in World War I from this epidemic than from wounds. Estimates of the dead range from 20 to 100 million worldwide[4]

➤ 1957 to 1958: influenza, Asian flu[5,6]

➤ 1968 to 1969: influenza, Hong Kong flu[5,6]

➤ 2009 to 2010: influenza, 2009 H1N1 flu pandemic[7]

9.5.1 Epidemics and Pandemics

The terms *epidemic* and *pandemic* refer to the extent to which an infectious disease spreads in a population. An epidemic is defined by an illness or other health-related issue that occurs in higher numbers than would be expected normally within a country or region. A pandemic is a worldwide epidemic of a disease. Three conditions must be met for a pandemic to occur:

➤ A new disease emerges to which a population has little or no immunity.

➤ The disease is infectious for humans.

➤ The disease spreads easily among humans.

Planning requires that health authorities assess possible control measures; drug and vaccine inventories; emergency mechanisms to increase drug and vaccine supplies; legal and liability issues for mass prophylaxis; and research, development, and production capacities for new drugs and vaccines.

Although influenza (flu) is a common illness each year, many underestimate the potential public health effect of this disease. Each year, influenza causes respiratory illnesses in thousands of individuals, with severe problems usually occurring in children and the elderly, as well as those with chronic disease such as heart and lung disease, diabetes, and illnesses that weaken the immune system.

In today's world, a communicable disease in one country is a mandated concern for all. This reality forms the basis of the International Health Regulations (IHR; http://www.who.int/ihr/en/), which give the World Health Organization operational authority to ensure the proper surveillance and control of epidemics and pandemics that threaten the global community.

9.5.2 Bioterrorism

Bioterrorism (BT) and biologic warfare involve the intentional use of a biologic agent or biologic product to cause harm to humans and other living organisms. The distinction between these two is blurry and may be only a matter of scale. BT and biowarfare agents can be inexpensive and relatively easy to produce; delivery devices may be disguised as agricultural sprayers or pest control devices. It is very difficult, if not impossible, for an intelligence service to detect the research, production, or transportation of these agents. It is equally difficult to defend against these agents once they have been released. By preparing for any infectious disease outbreak, health authorities will be better prepared for both intentional BT and naturally occurring epidemics.

An act of BT is fundamentally different from other forms of disasters. A resulting epidemic with a contagious disease capable of spreading from person to person is one of the most dreaded potential outcomes. Because BT, by definition, is a criminal act that causes illness, both law enforcement and public health authorities have responsibilities for responding to the event. Law enforcement authorities must rapidly conduct a criminal investigation to identify and apprehend the perpetrator. Efforts to obtain and preserve forensic evidence may be paramount. This is a federal crime that involves cooperation with federal law enforcement authorities.

To date, the largest and most effective terrorism attacks using biologic weapons have used contamination of food. Uncooked foods such as salads are generally more susceptible. This technique was used by the 1984 Rajneeshee bioterror attack that caused 750 people in the Dalles, Oregon, area to contract salmonella.[8-10] This technique also was used to spread anthrax and glanders to livestock by the German sympathizer Dr Anton Dilger in Washington, DC, in the months before World War I. In both of these terrorist attacks, the very easy-to-develop liquid form of the agent was used to disseminate the disease. An alternative to contamination of the food supply is agricultural attack with an agent that destroys crops or livestock.

Because the United States has superb water purification systems in every city and county, contamination of the water supply would probably be the least effective method for deploying a biologic weapon in the United States. Dilution, filtration, and chlorination processes associated with water distribution significantly decrease the likelihood of a successful distribution of an agent in the water supply. Contamination of an individual water supply such as within a specific building is a more feasible scenario. Distribution through the water supply is possible only with access to a postpurification water distribution system with an agent that requires very few organisms for infectivity and would not be destroyed with residual chlorine from purification.[11] Destruction or bypass of these purification and filtration systems is a possible terrorism scenario, however. Distribution of contaminated water or drink containers at a mass gathering also would be a plausible scenario.

9.6 CHARACTERISTICS OF BIOLOGIC AGENTS

In theory, any organism or its byproducts (eg, toxins) that causes human disease could be used as a weapon against others. However, certain organisms are better suited for this purpose than others. This may be due to the ease with which adequate quantities of the organism can be grown, the ability to spread to large numbers of people, the ability to spread from person to person once released, or the severity of the disease caused by the organism. The CDC categorizes pathogens that present a BT risk into three groups, which are described in Table 9-1.

TABLE 9-1 Potential BT Threats

CDC Category	Characteristics	Examples
Category A: high-priority agents	➤ Can be easily disseminated or transmitted from person to person ➤ Cause high mortality with a potential for a major impact on public health ➤ May cause public panic and social disruption ➤ Require special action for public health preparedness	➤ Anthrax (*Bacillus anthracis*) ➤ Botulism (*Clostridium botulinum* toxin) ➤ Plague (*Yersinia pestis*) ➤ Smallpox (*Variola major*) ➤ Tularemia (*Francisella tularensis*) ➤ Viral hemorrhagic fevers (VHFs): filoviruses (eg, Ebola, Marburg) and arenaviruses (eg, Lassa, Machupo)
Category B: second-priority agents	➤ Are moderately easy to disseminate ➤ Cause moderate morbidity and low mortality ➤ Require specific enhancements of the CDC's diagnostic capacity and disease surveillance	➤ Brucellosis (*Brucella* species) ➤ Epsilon toxin of *Clostridium perfringens* ➤ Food safety threats (eg, *Salmonella* species, *Escherichia coli* O157:H7, *Shigella*) ➤ Glanders (*Burkholderia mallei*) ➤ Melioidosis (*Burkholderia pseudomallei*) ➤ Psittacosis (*Chlamydia psittaci*) ➤ Q fever (*Coxiella burnetii*) ➤ Ricin toxin from *Ricinus communis* (castor beans) ➤ Staphylococcal enterotoxin B ➤ Typhus fever (*Rickettsia prowazekii*) ➤ Viral encephalitis (alphaviruses, eg, Venezuelan equine encephalitis, eastern equine encephalitis, western equine encephalitis) ➤ Water safety threats (eg, *Vibrio cholerae*, *Cryptosporidium parvum*)
Category C: third-priority agents (including emerging pathogens that could be genetically engineered for mass dissemination)	➤ May be easily available ➤ May be easily produced or disseminated ➤ Have the potential for high morbidity and mortality and therefore may have a major impact on public health	➤ Emerging infectious diseases such as Nipah virus and hantavirus ➤ Severe acute respiratory syndrome (SARS)

Adapted from Khan AS, Morse S, Lillibridge S. Public health preparedness for biological terrorism in the USA. *Lancet.* 2000;356:1179-1182; and Bioterrorism Agents/ Diseases (CDC), http://www.bt.cdc.gov/agent/agentlist-category.asp. Accessed April 28, 2011.

9.7 SITUATIONAL AWARENESS AND DETECTION

A clinician who notes that something unusual is happening and seeks assistance for an explanation is likely to be first to detect a covert release of a biologic agent or (re) emerging infectious disease outbreak. The most important aspect is for all health care providers to have a high index of suspicion for biologic events and to avail themselves of public health reporting. Often it is information not from a single provider but from multiple reports seen through the eyes of the public health entity that puts the pieces together to determine the presence of a biologic disaster.

Effective response to a disease outbreak depends on rapid identification of the causative agent and specific diagnosis. When the identity of the biologic agent is known, response is, in some ways, straightforward. Natural outbreaks increase over a period of weeks or months, while a BT incident may produce a large number of casualties in hours to days. A larger problem arises when the identity of an agent is uncertain. In fact, in some cases, an intentional release may be threatened or suspected, but it may remain unclear whether such a release has actually occurred. Recent experiences with West Nile virus,[12] SARS,[13] pneumonic tularemia,[14,15] and monkeypox[16] highlight this problem. In each of these instances, the possibility of BT was properly raised, although each outbreak ultimately proved to be naturally occurring.

Because a biologic agent must reproduce and multiply within a susceptible host organism, these agents have characteristic *incubation periods*. The incubation periods, typically several days in length, allow for the wide dispersion of exposed cases in time and space. Because these are infectious agents, the first response to the threat is generally not recognized by traditional first responders, but rather by clinicians—primary care providers, hospital emergency department staff, and public health officials. Simultaneous outbreaks of a disease in noncontiguous areas should prompt health authorities to consider an intentional release or a new epidemic, as should simultaneous or sequential outbreaks of different diseases in the same locale. It is important to recognize that a biologic agent may have been released in multiple locations.

> ## Epidemiologic Clues of a Bioterrorist Attack
>
> In addition to an increased number of patients, other clues that may signal a biologic disaster include:
>
> ➤ An increase in unexplained deaths
>
> ➤ Unusual age distribution of the patients (eg, severe illness among persons 20 to 50 years old)
>
> ➤ Unusual seasonality (eg, severe widespread respiratory illness during the summer months)
>
> ➤ An unusual manifestation of disease (eg, inhalational anthrax), or the occurrence of an animal die-off

The public health department has the unique ability to monitor multiple hospitals and clinics simultaneously. Community public health officials routinely investigate and analyze disease patterns. In addition to public health personnel, other community health care providers and first responders can provide important epidemiologic clues to the potential disease outbreaks:

➤ Astute first responders, emergency medical technicians, or dispatchers may provide the first clue by noting multiple calls for similar reasons to a specific geographic location or noting calls from patients with similar complaints.

➤ Clinical laboratories can provide advanced notification by monitoring the volume of tests ordered or by reporting any occurrences in which a patient is diagnosed with disease caused by a potential BT agent, novel infectious agent, or agent with epidemic or pandemic potential. Laboratories may be more likely to identify unusually high occurrences of a particular syndrome, because they receive specimens from multiple medical providers.

➤ Emergency (911) call centers can provide information on the volume of calls and types of EMS responses. Any increase in the volume of calls above seasonally expected levels with no obvious explanation could signify the occurrence of a public health event. The nature of the 911 calls can be analyzed for patterns. Mapping the geographic distribution of calls may point to the possible source of agent release.

➤ Medical examiner review of death certificates and investigation of unexplained deaths can provide information on reported deaths, including those caused by a potential biologic agent exposure or any suspicious deaths in previously healthy individuals. Any rapid rise of mortality above seasonally expected levels with no obvious explanation might be an indication of an unnatural public health event.

➤ In 2001, the United States instituted the BioWatch program to monitor and detect the intentional release of biologic agents in the air. The program is currently deployed in more than 30 high-risk metropolitan areas and has been utilized for special events such as the Super Bowl and national political conventions. BioWatch currently monitors for known and well-characterized threats that have the largest potential to do harm to society, including smallpox, anthrax, tularemia (rabbit fever), and plague. The technology, locations, and placement of BioWatch sensors are not made public.

9.8 CLINICAL DECISION MAKING

The existence of a biologic event may be difficult to recognize at first. Typically, persons will begin to visit ambulatory clinics and emergency departments after the onset of symptoms. Many epidemic and bioterrorism diseases, in their prodromal forms, appear as simple, undifferentiated febrile illnesses; sometimes associated with malaise and other nonspecific symptoms, they are difficult to distinguish from other common ailments, such as acute respiratory or influenza-like illnesses. Definitive laboratory diagnostic tests are typically not available or not obtained.

Some infectious diseases have specific characteristic clinical findings and a limited differential diagnosis (Table 9-2). For example, inhalational anthrax is characterized by a widened mediastinum, a clinical finding otherwise seen in few naturally occurring conditions. With botulism, the hallmark presentation is that of a descending, symmetric, flaccid paralysis. Whereas an individual patient with flaccid paralysis might prompt consideration of disorders such as the Guillain-Barre syndrome

TABLE 9-2 Characteristic Clinical Symptoms of Selected Potential BT Agents

Symptom/Finding	Potential Infectious Disease	Differential Diagnoses
Widened mediastinum on chest radiograph	Anthrax	Trauma, cancer (single patients)
Paralysis—symmetric, flaccid	Botulism	Guillain-Barre syndrome (single patients)
Hemoptysis	Pneumonic plague	Tuberculosis, staphylococcal and *Klebsiella* pneumonia, carcinoma, trauma (single patients)
Pox-like rash	Smallpox	Chickenpox, monkey pox, cowpox
Diarrhea (may be bloody)	Cholera Shigellosis	Multiple potential causes exist

and myasthenia gravis, the presentation of multiple patients with flaccid paralysis should point to a diagnosis of botulism. Similarly, individuals with pneumonic plague often present with hemoptysis in the later stages of illness. Such a finding is uncommon among previously healthy individuals but can be caused by tuberculosis, staphylococcal and *Klebsiella* pneumonia, carcinoma, and trauma. The presentation of multiple patients with hemoptysis, however, should prompt consideration of pneumonic plague. Smallpox is characterized by an exanthem, mimicking, to a degree, varicella or syphilis in its earliest stages but readily distinguishable from these entities as it progresses.

The astute clinician should look for a pattern to illnesses and diagnostic clues that might indicate an unusual disease outbreak associated with the intentional release of a biologic agent or a new epidemic source,[17] be mindful of new and emerging diseases such as the recent outbreak of H1N1 influenza, and be aware of trends in current pandemics and epidemics throughout the world. Although commonly ignored in clinical practice, questions about international travel should be included in the routine history and physical examination for any febrile illness.

9.8.1 Public Health Notification

As soon as it is suspected that a case of disease might be the result of exposure to a potentially serious biologic agent, the proper public health authorities must be alerted so that the appropriate warnings may be issued and outbreak control measures implemented. Early involvement of public health officials ensures that an epidemiologic investigation is begun promptly and that potential exposed individuals (beyond the index cases) are identified and treated early, when treatment is most likely to be beneficial. Enhanced surveillance and other emergency public health response actions are discussed in greater detail in Chapter 2, "Public Health Response to Disasters," and in the ADLS® course (v3.0) and supporting course manual.

9.8.2 Transmission-Based Infection Control

Transmission of infections in health facilities can be prevented and controlled through the application of basic infection control precautions, which can be grouped into standard precautions (which must be applied to all patients at all times, regardless of diagnosis or infectious status) and additional (transmission-based) precautions, which are specific to modes of transmission (airborne, droplet, and contact).[18] Three subcategories of more stringent transmission-based precautions exist and should be applied in certain circumstances: droplet precautions, contact precautions, and airborne precautions.

Droplet precautions are used for individuals known or suspected to be infected with microorganisms transmitted by large-particle droplets, generally larger than 5 μm, that can be generated by the infected individuals during coughing, sneezing, talking, or respiratory-care procedures. Health care providers should wear a surgical-type mask when within 3 ft of the infected person. Some health care facilities may require that a mask be worn to enter the room of a patient on droplet precautions.

Contact precautions are used for patients known or suspected to be infected or colonized with epidemiologically important organisms that can be transmitted by direct contact with the patient or indirect contact with potentially contaminated surfaces in the persons' immediate area. Contact precautions require medical providers to:

➤ Wear clean gloves upon entry into a patient room

➤ Wear a gown for all patient contact and all contact with the patient's environment

➤ Remove gowns before leaving a patient's room

➤ Wash hands with an antimicrobial agent; alcohol-based hand washing may not be effective for these patients

Airborne precautions: Airborne precautions are used to limit transmission of airborne droplet nuclei (small particles [5 μm or smaller] of evaporated droplets containing microorganisms that remain suspended in the air for long periods of time) or dust particles that contain an infectious agent. Microorganisms carried by the airborne route can be widely dispersed by air currents and may become inhaled by a susceptible host in the same room or over a long distance from the source patient, depending on environmental factors such as temperature and ventilation. The appropriate precautions for diseases that are spread by airborne transmission include standard precautions plus personal respiratory protection with either:

➤ N95 respirator (fit testing must be repeated annually and fit check/seal check before each use) or

➤ Powered air-purifying respirator (fit testing is required for face mask but not hooded versions)

Airborne infection isolation rooms are required for the care of these patients. At a minimum, these rooms must:

➤ Provide a negative-pressure room with a minimum of six air exchanges per hour

➤ Exhaust directly to the outside or through high-efficiency particulate air filtration

In cases in which diagnosis is uncertain, the use of contact precautions and an N95 or better respirator may be prudent. Although private rooms are generally preferred for patients in isolation, in the event of a massive influx of patients, it may be necessary to consider placing patients together in the same room. However, patients should not be placed in the same room until there is a high degree of certainty regarding the diagnosis to prevent inadvertent disease spread.

9.8.3   Triage

Most mass casualty triage systems in the United States are based on trauma situations and have limited application in large-scale infectious disease outbreaks, in which triage decisions need to be based on infectiousness and duration of illness. The goal of triage in a disease outbreak is to prevent secondary transmission through the implementation of nonmedical strategies (social distancing, sheltering in place, isolation, quarantine, risk communication) and medical interventions (eg, immunization, medication, respiratory support). A population-based triage model called SEIRV has been proposed that is based on five triage categories:[19]

➤ *Susceptible:* Persons who are not yet exposed but are susceptible

➤ *Exposed:* Persons who are susceptible and have been in contact with an infected person; they may be infected but are not yet contagious

➤ *Infectious:* Persons who are symptomatic and contagious

➤ *Removed:* Persons who no longer can transmit the disease to others because they have survived and developed immunity or died of the disease

➤ *Vaccinated* (or medicated): Persons who have received prophylactic medical intervention to protect them from infection

Once self-protective measures are considered and evaluation areas designated, the clinician can begin assessing exposed and infected patients. Biologic casualties may have conventional injuries, so the usual steps of airway, adequate breathing, and circulation (assessment of the ABCs) remain important. Health care systems need to have plans that provide protocols to handle a massive influx of patients seeking care as well as methods to provide prophylaxis to their own health care workers. Population-based triage management is discussed in greater detail in the ADLS® course (v3.0) and supporting course manual.

9.8.4   Clinical Assessment and Diagnosis

The thoroughness and accuracy with which a diagnosis is established will vary according to the circumstances of the event. Where support is readily available, it may be possible, by using polymerase chain reaction (PCR) technology and other sophisticated assays, to arrive at a definitive microbiologic diagnosis fairly promptly. On the other hand, it is equally conceivable that the primary care provider practicing in a remote or rural area may need to intervene promptly on the basis of limited information and without immediate access to subspecialty consultation. Even in such cases, reasonable care can be instituted simply on the basis of a syndromic diagnosis.

A brief but focused physical examination can disclose whether the exposed or infected person exhibits primarily respiratory, neuromuscular, or dermatologic signs, or suffers simply from an undifferentiated febrile illness. By placing individuals into one of these broad syndromic categories, empiric therapy can be initiated; empiric therapy can be refined and tailored once more information becomes available.[20,21] When the situation permits, laboratory studies should be obtained to aid in later definitive diagnosis (see Table 9-3).

TABLE 9-3 Suggested Clinical Laboratory Testing for Biologic Casualties

This is a list of samples to consider obtaining in situations in which the nature of an incident is unclear and empiric therapy must be started before definitive diagnosis. This list is not all-inclusive, nor is it meant to imply that every sample should be obtained from every patient. In general, laboratory sampling should be guided by clinical judgment and the specifics of the situation.

➤ Complete blood cell count (CBC)
➤ Arterial blood gas
➤ Nasal swabs for culture and PCR
➤ Blood for bacterial culture and PCR
➤ Serum for serologic studies
➤ Sputum for bacterial culture
➤ Blood and urine for toxin assay
➤ Throat swab for viral culture, PCR, and enzyme-linked immunosorbent assay
➤ Environmental samples

9.8.5   Therapeutic Interventions

Once a diagnosis (whether definitive or syndromic) is established, prompt therapy must be provided. In the cases of anthrax and plague, in particular, survival is directly linked to the speed with which appropriate therapy is instituted. A delay of more than 24 hours in the treatment of either disease leads to a uniformly grim prognosis. When the identity of a BT agent is known, the provision of proper antimicrobial therapy is warranted. When a clinician is faced with multiple patients and the nature of the illness is not known, empiric therapy must be instituted. Specifically, it is advocated that doxycycline or ciprofloxacin be administered empirically to patients with significant respiratory symptoms when exposure to a biologic attack is considered a possibility.

9.9   BIOLOGIC AGENT–SPECIFIC ISSUES

A Note About Treatment Guidelines for Biologic Agents

Treatment guidelines change over time. All antimicrobials should be checked for current recommended dosages before administration of the medication. The most updated clinical guidelines and dosages are available through various federal agencies and medical specialty societies, such as the:

> ### A Note About Treatment Guidelines for Biologic Agents (continued)

➤ CDC: http://www.bt.cdc.gov

➤ Infectious Diseases Society of America: http://www.idsociety.org/Bioterrorism_Agents/

➤ American College of Physicians: http://www.acponline.org/bioterro/?hp

➤ American Academy of Pediatrics (AAP): http://www.aap.org/disasters/terrorism-biological.cfm

9.9.1 Anthrax (*Bacillus anthracis*)

9.9.1.1 General

Anthrax is a bacterial disease caused by *B anthracis*, a bacterium that forms spores. A spore is a cell that is dormant but may come to life with the right conditions. Anthrax can occur in three forms depending on the site of infection: skin (cutaneous), lungs (inhalation), and digestive (gastrointestinal [GI]). This disease is not known to spread from one person to another. During natural anthrax infection, humans become infected by handling products from infected animals (cutaneous disease), by breathing in anthrax spores from infected animal products such as wool (inhalational anthrax), or by eating undercooked meat from infected animals (GI anthrax). Anthrax also can be used as a biologic weapon, as happened in the United States in 2001, when it was deliberately spread through the postal system. This caused 22 cases of anthrax infection.

9.9.1.2 Clinical Features

Cutaneous anthrax:

➤ Incubation period: 1 to 7 days (may be as long as 12 days).

➤ Presentation: The sore is initially a small itchy papule or vesicle, but by the second day it becomes an ulcer. The sore usually is on an exposed area of the body. Nontender swelling surrounds the ulcer. Other small vesicles may also surround the ulcer (Figure 9-2). Over the next 1 to 2 days a black scab forms, which falls

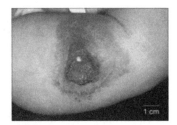

FIGURE 9-2 Lesion of cutaneous anthrax associated with microangiopathic hemolytic anemia and coagulopathy in a 7-month-old infant. By hospital day 12, a 2-cm black eschar was present in the center of the cutaneous lesion.
Reprinted from Henderson DA, Inglesby TV, O'Toole T, eds. *Bioterrorism: Guidelines for Medical and Public Health Management.* Chicago, IL: AMA Press; 2002.

off after about 2 weeks. In about 80% to 90% of patients the lesion completely resolves. Extensive swelling (edema) and tender lymph nodes may occur. Patients will likely have fever.

Inhalational anthrax:

➤ Incubation period: 2 to 43 days (may be longer). In the 2001 anthrax outbreak, the median incubation period was 4 days with a range of 4 to 6 days.

➤ Presentation: Patients present initially with a flu-like illness consisting of fever, not feeling well, fatigue, cough, shortness of breath, headache, anorexia, and chest pain. Upper respiratory symptoms, such as a runny nose or sore throat, can occur but are not typical (10% to 20% of patients). This phase lasts from hours to a few days. If left untreated, patients develop a sudden increase in fever, severe respiratory distress, diaphoresis, and shock. Chest X rays are abnormal, with mediastinal widening (70%), infiltrates (70%), and pleural effusions (80%) (Figure 9-3).

Gastrointestinal (GI) anthrax:

➤ Incubation period: 1 to 7 days.

➤ Presentation: This form of anthrax occurs after the ingestion of undercooked infected meat. It is much less likely than the other forms to occur after a biologic attack. GI anthrax presents as febrile illness with nausea, vomiting, and subsequently bloody diarrhea.

9.9.1.3 Diagnosis

➤ The first clue may be several patients presenting with a severe pulmonary illness as described above.

➤ Blood cultures should be done before administration of antibiotics and are usually positive in less than 24 hours. Gram-positive bacilli with a preliminary

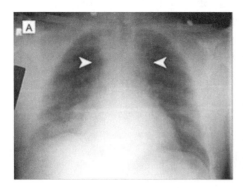 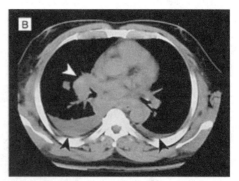

FIGURE 9-3 Chest radiograph and CT of patient with anthrax. A, Portable chest radiograph of 56-year-old man with inhalational anthrax depicts a widened mediastinum (white arrowheads), bilateral hilar fullness, a right pleural effusion, and bilateral perihilar air-space disease. B, Noncontrast spiral CT scan depicts an enlarged and hyperdense right hilar lymph node (white arrowhead), bilateral pleural effusions (black arrowheads), and edema of the mediastinal fat.
Reprinted from Henderson DA, Inglesby TV, O'Toole T, eds. *Bioterrorism: Guidelines for Medical and Public Health Management.* Chicago, IL: AMA Press; 2002.

identification as a *Bacillus* species in the setting of meningitis, pneumonia, or sepsis should be evaluated for anthrax and sent to a public health laboratory that is a part of the Laboratory Response Network (LRN).

➤ Gram stain of pleural fluid or cerebrospinal fluid may also be helpful.

➤ Sputum is usually *not* positive by stain or culture.

➤ Fever and widened mediastinum on chest radiograph or computed tomography (CT) is very suggestive (Figure 9-3).

➤ For cutaneous disease, fluid from under eschar should be cultured.

➤ *Nasal swabs are a poor test to rule out anthrax* and should *not* be used as a clinical test. They cannot rule out infection. One patient with a negative swab died of anthrax during the fall of 2001.

➤ *While sporadic cases of cutaneous disease occur within the United States under natural circumstance, the appearance of pulmonary or GI disease should result in the immediate notification of the proper authorities.*

9.9.1.4 Treatment

Early antibiotic treatment is essential for survival (for pediatric dosing, see Table 9-4). A high-risk individual who is symptomatic needs to be started on appropriate antimicrobial therapy immediately without waiting for confirmatory laboratory tests.

➤ For inhalational and GI disease, and for severely ill patients with cutaneous disease, including pregnant women (for pediatric dosing, see Table 9-4)

  ➤ Ciprofloxacin 400 mg intravenously (IV) every 12 hours (other fluoroquinolones probably also effective) *or* doxycycline IV 100 mg every 12 hours

Plus one or two additional antibiotics (eg, clindamycin, rifampin, vancomycin, penicillin, chloramphenicol, imipenem, clarithromycin)

  ➤ Switch to oral therapy when clinically appropriate (ciprofloxacin 500 mg by mouth [PO] twice daily [BID] *or* doxycycline 100 mg PO BID).

  ➤ Continue therapy for 60 days total.

➤ For localized cutaneous disease (for pediatric dosing, see Table 9-4):

  ➤ Ciprofloxacin 500 mg PO every 12 hours or doxycycline 100 mg PO every 12 hours for 60 days

  ➤ Pregnant women are treated as above.

9.9.1.5 Prophylaxis

(For pediatric dosing, see Table 9-4.)

➤ Ciprofloxacin 500 mg PO BID *or* doxycycline 100 mg PO BID

➤ Continue for 60 days.

➤ Postexposure vaccination may reduce the number of days required for medical prophylaxis.

(This may also be used for cutaneous disease and for inhalational disease in mass casualty setting where IV administration is not feasible.)

9.9.1.6   Infection Control

➤ Standard barrier precautions are needed.

    ➤ Anthrax is not transmitted by person-to-person contact, although some consider cutaneous anthrax to be infectious. Patients do not need to be in airborne isolation.

➤ No need to immunize or to provide prophylaxis to contacts unless they were exposed at time of the BT attack

➤ Need to contact hospital epidemiologist, microbiology laboratory, and state and local public health authorities immediately

9.9.2   Botulism (*Clostridium botulinum* Toxin)

9.9.2.1   General

Botulism is caused by a toxin produced from the bacterium *C botulinum*. As effects are not due to an infection per se but rather a toxin, some describe botulism as more akin to a chemical exposure than a biologic agent. This toxin is one of the most poisonous substances known, producing long-lasting paralysis in affected individuals. Sporadic cases and outbreaks naturally occur because of poor food-handling practices. In a biologic attack, toxin could be delivered as an aerosol or used to contaminate food and water supplies.

9.9.2.2   Clinical Features

➤ Time to symptom onset: 12 to 36 hours (range, 2 hours to 8 days)
➤ Presentation:

    ➤ Patients present with bulbar palsies: blepharoptosis (drooping of the upper eyelid), blurred vision, dry mouth, difficulty speaking, and trouble swallowing. The paralysis is noted for its descending pattern (Figure 9-4).

    ➤ It is not possible to have botulism without the multiple cranial nerve palsies. This fact is helpful in distinguishing botulism from other diseases such as Guillain-Barré syndrome, Miller Fisher syndrome, myasthenia gravis, or a disease of the central nervous system.

    ➤ Patients are not febrile.

    ➤ Patients are not confused or obtunded but may have difficulty speaking.

    ➤ Rapidity of onset and severity are dependent on the amount of toxin absorbed.

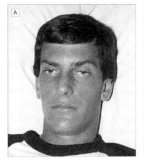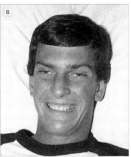

FIGURE 9-4 Seventeen-year-old patient with mild botulism. A, Patient at rest. Note bilateral mild blepharoptosis, dilated pupils, disconjugate gaze, and symmetric facial muscles. B, Patient was requested to perform his maximum smile. Note absent periorbital smile creases, blepharoptosis, disconjugate gaze, dilated pupils, and minimally asymmetric smile. As an indication of the extreme potency of botulinum toxin, the patient had 40×10^{12} g/mL of type A botulinum toxin in his serum (ie, 1.25 mouse units/mL) when these photographs were taken.
Reprinted from Henderson DA, Inglesby TV, O'Toole T, eds. *Bioterrorism: Guidelines for Medical and Public Health Management.* Chicago, IL: AMA Press; 2002.

➤ Patients subsequently develop descending symmetric skeletal muscle paralysis.

➤ Death results from respiratory muscle paralysis.

9.9.2.3   Diagnosis

➤ Diagnosis is based on clinical presentation.

➤ Confirmatory diagnosis is made through toxin assay of blood (may not be positive after inhalation of toxin; stool can also be assayed after ingestion of toxin).

9.9.2.4   Treatment

(For pediatric considerations, see Table 9-5.)

➤ Supportive care includes intensive care with close monitoring of respiratory function, ventilator support for respiratory failure, enteral feeding tubes, and treatment of secondary infections.

➤ Antitoxin is available through state health departments, which will coordinate with the CDC. As the dosing regimens and safety precautions for the antitoxin continue to change over time depending on the type of antitoxin available, clinicians will usually need to consult subject matter experts within the health departments, CDC, manufacturers, or academia before its use.

➤ Recovery takes weeks to months.

9.9.2.5   Prophylaxis

➤ None

9.9.2.6   Infection Control

➤ Standard precautions

➤ Need to contact hospital epidemiologist and public health authority immediately, as this is a public health emergency. Other individuals could be exposed to the contaminated food source if they are not notified.

9.9.3   Pneumonic Plague (*Yersinia pestis*)

9.9.3.1   General

Pneumonic plague is caused by the bacterium *Y pestis*. This organism has a high potential to be used as a BT weapon, as it is endemic in many animals (including prairie dogs in the southwestern United States) throughout the world, is easy to grow and disseminate, has a high fatality rate, and can be spread from person to person. The endemic form is spread to humans via a flea vector, leading to the bubonic form of the disease (Figure 9-5). For a biologic attack, the bacteria would most likely be aerosolized, leading to pneumonic plague, which would create a situation for person-to-person spread of the disease.

9.9.3.2   Clinical Features after a BT Attack

Pneumonic plague following a BT attack would present differently than naturally occurring plague. BT plague would present as follows:

➤ Incubation period: 1 to 6 days

➤ Presentation: Abrupt onset of high fever, chills, malaise, shortness of breath, cough with bloody sputum, sepsis. Patients may also have nausea, vomiting, and diarrhea

➤ Patients subsequently develop a severe, rapidly progressive pneumonia.

9.9.3.3   Diagnosis

➤ Chest radiograph with patchy infiltrates (Figure 9-6)

➤ Culture of blood and sputum. The laboratory needs to be notified of the suspicion of plague, as special culturing techniques may be needed.

➤ Gram stain may show characteristic "safety-pin" bipolar staining.

FIGURE 9-5
Inguinal bubo in patient with bubonic plague.
Source: CDC (http://www.cdc .gov/ncidod/dvbid/plague/ p5.htm).

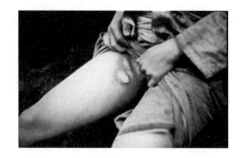

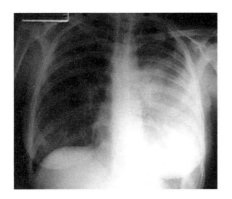

FIGURE 9-6
Chest radiograph of patient with primary pneumonic plague.
Reprinted from Henderson DA, Inglesby TV, O'Toole T, eds. *Bioterrorism: Guidelines for Medical and Public Health Management.* Chicago, IL: AMA Press; 2002.

9.9.3.4   Treatment

(For pediatric dosing, see Table 9-5.)

➤ Preferred choices

➢ Streptomycin 1 g intramuscularly (IM) every 12 hours

➢ Gentamicin 5 mg/kg IM or IV daily

➤ Alternate choices

➢ Doxycycline 100 mg IV every 12 hours

➢ Ciprofloxacin 400 mg IV every 12 hours

➢ Chloramphenicol 25 mg/kg IV every 6 hours

➤ Pregnant women: Gentamicin is the preferred choice, followed by doxycycline and ciprofloxacin at the above doses. *Streptomycin must be avoided.*

9.9.3.5   Prophylaxis

(For pediatric dosing, see Table 9-5.)

➤ Preferred choices

➢ Doxycycline 100 mg PO BID

➢ Ciprofloxacin 500 mg PO BID (other fluoroquinolones probably effective)

➤ Alternative choice

➢ Chloramphenicol 25 mg/kg orally four times a day

➤ Pregnant women: treat as above

➤ Treat for 7 days

9.9.3.6   Infection Control

➤ Patients with pneumonic plague are contagious.

➤ Droplet precautions should be used for the first 48 hours until the patient is clinically improved.

➤ The microbiology laboratory needs to be promptly notified for the staff's protection.

➤ The hospital epidemiologist and public health authorities need to be notified immediately. The appearance of pneumonic plague is highly unusual, and an immediate epidemiologic investigation will need to begin to ascertain those who are exposed and how the outbreak was initiated.

9.9.4   Severe Acute Respiratory Syndrome (SARS)

9.9.4.1   General

SARS is a respiratory infectious disease caused by a novel coronavirus called SARS-associated coronavirus. The disease was first laboratory confirmed in March 2003 in Asia after quickly spreading worldwide. This virus infected numerous health care workers and had a case fatality rate of approximately 10%. Through the use of aggressive infection control, this disease disappeared in July 2003. Many experts, however, believe that SARS or similar diseases will likely reemerge in the near future.

9.9.4.2   Clinical Features

➤ Incubation period: typically 2 to 7 days, but may be up to 10 days

➤ Presentation: The illness begins with a flu-like prodrome consisting of fever and sometimes chills, rigors, headache, muscle aches, and feeling ill. Some patients may have diarrhea. Subsequently, on day 3 to 7 of the illness, the patients develop cough and shortness of breath and may require intubation.

9.9.4.3   Diagnosis

The diagnosis of SARS is currently based on the following CDC case classification, which strongly relies on clinical and epidemiologic criteria to make the diagnosis:

➤ A *probable SARS case* meets the clinical criteria for severe respiratory illness of unknown etiology (as defined below) and epidemiologic criteria for exposure. Laboratory criteria are used to confirm the case.

➤ A *suspected SARS case* meets the clinical criteria for moderate respiratory illness (as defined below) of unknown etiology and epidemiologic criteria for exposure. Again, laboratory criteria are used to confirm the case.

➤ A *moderate respiratory illness* is defined as one in which temperature is greater than 100.4 °F, and one or more findings of respiratory illness (cough, shortness of breath, difficulty breathing, or hypoxia) is present.

➤ A *severe respiratory illness* is one that has the temperature and clinical findings above *and* one of the following:

➢ Radiologic evidence of pneumonia

➢ Respiratory distress syndrome (RDS)

➢ Autopsy findings consistent with pneumonia or RDS without an identifiable cause

The CDC epidemiologic criterion for SARS exposure is travel (including transit in an airport) within 10 days of onset of symptoms to an area with current or previously documented or suspected community transmission of SARS. The last date for illness onset is 10 days (ie, one incubation period) after removal of a CDC travel alert. The patient's travel should have occurred on or before the last date the travel alert was in place.

9.9.4.4 Treatment

Currently there is no proven treatment for SARS. Empiric antibiotic treatment covering community-acquired pneumonia and atypical pathogens should be initially utilized pending the diagnosis.

9.9.4.5 Prophylaxis

➤ Currently there is no known prophylaxis against SARS.

➤ Public health authorities should be contacted to help manage exposed but well individuals.

9.9.4.6 Infection Control

Proper SARS isolation for patients includes the following:

➤ Standard precautions (hand hygiene)

➤ Contact precautions (gowns, gloves)

➤ Airborne precautions (negative-pressure isolation room and N95 or better masks)

➤ Eye protection

Health care workers have been infected after aerosolization of SARS during positive-pressure ventilation, suctioning, and intubation. There is a need for increased personal protective equipment (such as a powered air-purifying respirator) under these and other unpredictable and uncontrolled circumstances.

9.9.5 Smallpox (Variola major)

9.9.5.1 General

Smallpox was once one of the deadliest diseases known, with a mortality rate of 30%. Due to an aggressive and successful multinational vaccination program, infection rates fell during the 1960s and 1970s enabling the World Health Organization to declare the disease eradicated in 1980. With routine vaccination against smallpox ceasing in 1972 in the United States (more than 30 years ago), we now have a large population that would be very susceptible to this disease.

9.9.5.2   Clinical Features

➤ Incubation period: 7 to 17 days (average, 12 days)

➤ Presentation:

    ➤ Prodrome: Smallpox patients have a severe prodrome lasting 2 to 3 days before the development of the rash. This prodrome consists of fever, severe myalgia, prostration, occasional nausea and vomiting, and delirium. This prodrome is one of the key distinguishing features between smallpox and chicken pox. Ten percent of patients will have a light facial erythematous rash.

    ➤ Rash: The smallpox rash is distinctive (Figure 9-7). It develops initially on face and extremities (including palms and soles) and then spreads to trunk. The rash starts as macules and then evolves into papules, vesicles, and finally pustules. All lesions are in the same stage of development. These lesions are firm, deep, and frequently umbilicated. The rash scabs over in 1 to 2 weeks, resulting in scars.

    ➤ Chickenpox vs. smallpox: Key diagnostic clues to help distinguish smallpox from chicken pox include the following:

        • The prodrome of smallpox is much more severe than that seen in chicken pox. Smallpox patients look sick before the rash occurs.

        • The chicken pox rash occurs in crops with lesions in different stages of maturity, while the smallpox lesions are in the same stage of maturity. Chicken pox lesions are also more oval in shape, while smallpox lesions are more rounded. Chicken pox lesions are smaller (2-4 mm vs. 4-6 mm in smallpox) and are centralized on the trunk, while the smallpox lesions occur more on the extremities and face. Smallpox also involves the palms and soles, while this is unusual for chicken pox.

        • The smallpox rash starts peripherally and moves centrally, while the chicken pox rash starts centrally and moves peripherally. Figure 9-7 shows the appearance of the rash at days 3, 5, and 7 of evolution. Note that lesions are more dense on the face and extremities than on the trunk, and that they are similar in appearance to each other. If this were a case

FIGURE 9-7

Typical case of smallpox.
Reprinted from Henderson DA, Inglesby TV, O'Toole T, eds. *Bioterrorism: Guidelines for Medical and Public Health Management.* Chicago, IL: AMA Press; 2002.

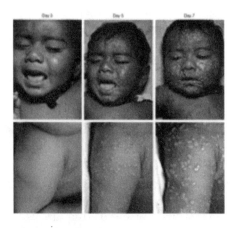

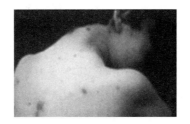

FIGURE 9-8
Typical case of chicken pox

Source: CDC (http://www.cdc.gov/
vaccines/vpd-vac/varicella/photos.htm).

of chickenpox (see Figure 9-8), one would expect to see, in any area, macules, papules, pustules, and lesions with scabs.

9.9.5.3 Diagnosis

➤ Clinical recognition and complete history of the disease is essential to assist in diagnosis.

➤ Confirmatory tests are available at CDC. However, in many states (eg, Texas) public health laboratories have developed screening tests for orthopox virus.

➤ Febrile illness after potential exposure should prompt isolation.

9.9.5.4 Treatment

(For pediatric considerations, see Table 9-5.)

➤ Vaccination against smallpox, especially if in the early stages of disease

➤ Supportive care

➤ Penicillinase-resistant antibiotics if:

    ➤ Smallpox lesions are secondarily infected

    ➤ Bacterial infection endangers the eyes

    ➤ The eruption is very dense and widespread

➤ Daily eye rinsing

➤ Adequate hydration and nutrition

➤ Specific therapy

    ➤ No specific therapy has been approved by the Food and Drug Administration (FDA).

    ➤ Topical idoxuridine (Dendrid, Herplex, or Stoxil) may be useful for the treatment of corneal lesions (efficacy is unproved)

    ➤ Cidofovir:

        • This antiviral medicine is licensed for the treatment of cytomegalovirus.

        • Animal studies suggest that cidofovir may be useful in the treatment of smallpox.

        • Cidofovir could be made available under an investigational-new-drug protocol for smallpox.

9.9.5.5   Prophylaxis

(For pediatric considerations, see Table 9-5.)

➤ Vaccine is effective if given within 3 days of exposure.

9.9.5.6   Infection Control

➤ Airborne *and* contact precautions are required.

➤ Patients should be treated in a negative-pressure room.

9.9.6   Tularemia (*Francisella tularensis*)

9.9.6.1   General

Tularemia is a bacterial infection that is endemic in North America and Eurasia. Sporadic human cases occur after spread by ticks or biting flies and occasionally from direct contact with infected animals (often rabbits). Tularemia has previous been developed as a biologic weapon by several countries. Biologic attack with this agent would most likely occur via aerosolized bacteria, resulting in typhoidal tularemia with or without pneumonia.

9.9.6.2   Clinical Features

➤ Incubation period: 3 to 5 days (range, 1 to 14 days)

➤ Presentation after a BT event:

  ➤ Acute febrile illness with prostration

  ➤ May have associated conjunctivitis or skin ulcer with regional adenopathy (Figure 9-9)

  ➤ Radiographic evidence of pneumonia in one or more lobes in approximately 80% of cases (Figure 9-10)

9.9.6.3   Diagnosis

➤ Culture of blood and sputum (note: isolation and identification of this organism can take several weeks)

➤ Gram-negative coccobacillus—confirmation may require reference laboratory

➤ Laboratory personnel should be notified whenever tularemia is suspected, as special safety precautions and diagnostic procedures are required.

➤ Public health laboratories that are part of the LRN have other diagnostic tools, such as PCR, and antibody tests to help identify this pathogen.

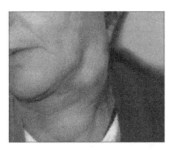

FIGURE 9-9 Cervical lymphadenitis in a patient with pharyngeal tularemia. Patient has marked swelling and fluctuant suppuration of several anterior cervical nodes. Infection was acquired by ingestion of contaminated food or water.
Source: World Health Organization.
Reprinted from Henderson DA, Inglesby TV, O'Toole T, eds. *Bioterrorism: Guidelines for Medical and Public Health Management.* Chicago, IL: AMA Press; 2002.

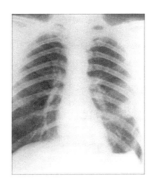

FIGURE 9-10 Chest radiograph of a patient with pulmonary tularemia, showing infiltrates in left lower lung, tenting of diaphragm (probably caused by pleural effusion), and enlargement of left hilum.
Reprinted from Henderson DA, Inglesby TV, O'Toole T, eds. *Bioterrorism: Guidelines for Medical and Public Health Management.* Chicago, IL: AMA Press; 2002.

9.9.6.4 Treatment

(For pediatric dosing, see Table 9-5.)

➤ Preferred choices

  ➢ Streptomycin 1 g IM every 12 hours

  ➢ Gentamicin 5 mg/kg IM or IV daily

➤ Alternative choices

  ➢ Doxycycline 100 mg IV every 12 hours

  ➢ Ciprofloxacin 400 mg IV every 12 hours (other fluoroquinolones probably effective)

  ➢ Chloramphenicol 15 mg/kg every 6 hours

➤ Pregnant women: gentamicin is preferred over streptomycin

9.9.6.5 Prophylaxis

(For pediatric dosing, see Table 9-5.)

➤ Doxycycline 100 mg PO BID

➤ Ciprofloxacin 500 mg PO BID (other fluoroquinolones probably effective)

➤ Treat for 14 days

9.9.6.6 Infection Control

➤ Tularemia is not spread person to person.

➤ Standard precautions should be utilized.

➤ Patients do not need to be in airborne, droplet, or contact isolation.

➤ Microbiology personnel, the hospital epidemiologist, and public health authorities must be immediately notified on suspicion of tularemia.

9.9.7   Viral Hemorrhagic Fevers (VHFs)

9.9.7.1   General

VHFs include filoviruses (ie, Ebola, Marburg) and arenaviruses (eg, Lassa, Machupo). These viruses are transmitted to humans by contact with infected animals or arthropod vectors. In some cases, the arthropod vector has not yet been determined. VHFs have been weaponized by several countries in the past. Sporadic outbreaks of these infections occur in Africa and, rarely, in parts of Asia and Europe. If a VHF were used for a BT attack, it most likely would occur from aerosolized virus. Case fatality rates have been reported to range from 0.5% for Omsk hemorrhagic fever to 90% for Ebola.

9.9.7.2   Clinical Features

➤ Incubation period: 2 to 21 days, depending on the virus

➤ Presentation:

➤ Depending on the virus, a variety of clinical manifestations could occur. Early in the course of the disease, patients develop a nonspecific prodrome with fever, headache, arthralgias, myalgia, abdominal pain, and diarrhea. Initial examination may show only flushing of face and chest, conjunctival injection (Figure 9-11), rash, and petechiae (Figure 9-12).

➤ Patients subsequently develop hypotension, relative bradycardia, rapid breathing, conjunctivitis, and pharyngitis. They develop progressive generalized bleeding problems including mucous membrane hemorrhage, as well as shock. Bleeding problems include a hemorrhagic or purple rash, nosebleeds, vomiting blood, coughing up blood, and blood in stools.

➤ If two of the above hemorrhagic symptoms occurs in a severely ill febrile patient (temperature greater than 101° F) who has been ill less than 3 weeks and has no other obvious cause for bleeding or other alternative diagnosis, a VHF should be suspected.

9.9.7.3   Diagnosis

➤ Diagnosis is based on the above clinical presentation and will require a high index of suspicion.

➤ Thrombocytopenia, leukopenia, and aspartate aminotransferase elevation are common.

➤ Definitive diagnosis requires detection of antigens or antibodies; testing is done at the CDC.

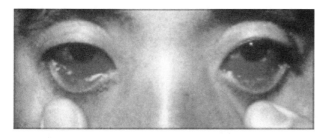

FIGURE 9-11 Ocular manifestations in Bolivian hemorrhagic fever. Ocular manifestations associated with hemorrhagic fever viruses range from conjunctival injection to subconjunctival hemorrhage, as seen in this patient.
Reprinted from Henderson DA, Inglesby TV, O'Toole T, eds. *Bioterrorism: Guidelines for Medical and Public Health Management.* Chicago, IL: AMA Press; 2002.

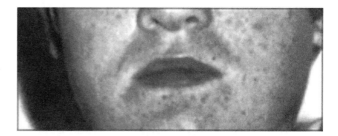

FIGURE 9-12 Maculopapular rash in Marburg disease. A nonpruritic maculopapular rash (resembling the rash of measles) may occur in up to 50% of patients infected with the Ebola or Marburg viruses within the first week of illness. The rash is more common in light-colored skin and desquamates on resolution.
Reprinted from Henderson DA, Inglesby TV, O'Toole T, eds. *Bioterrorism: Guidelines for Medical and Public Health Management.* Chicago, IL: AMA Press; 2002.

➤ Public health authorities should be notified immediately, without waiting to confirm the diagnosis.

9.9.7.4 Treatment

(For pediatric considerations, see Table 9-5.)

➤ Supportive care

➤ Ribavirin may be useful for some of the hemorrhagic fever viruses. If available, it can be started empirically (30 mg/kg IV load [maximum, 2 g] then 16 mg/kg [maximum, 1 g] every 6 hours for 4 days, then 8 mg/kg [maximum, 500 mg] IV every 8 hours for 6 days). An oral dosing regimen is also available.

➤ Pregnant women receive the same treatment as above.

9.9.7.5 Prophylaxis

➤ None

➤ The National Institutes of Health (NIH) is currently evaluating the safety of candidate vaccines.

9.9.7.6 Isolation

➤ Hemorrhagic fever viruses are extremely contagious after contact with blood and bodily fluids. Beyond routine contact precautions, personnel should wear liquid-impervious protective coverings (including leg and shoe coverings) and use double gloves. Although airborne spread has never been demonstrated, the possibility has not been excluded. Personnel should wear N95 or better respirators. In addition, face shields or goggles should be used to protect the eyes from possible contact with infected materials. Patients should be placed in a negative-pressure room if possible. Experts should be contacted for further recommendations.

9.9.8   Clinical Considerations for Pediatric Casualties

Children may be particularly vulnerable to aerosolized biologic agents because they breathe more times per minute than adults. As a result, they would receive a relatively larger dose of the substance than an adult would in the same period of time. Children are more vulnerable to the biologic agents that act through the skin because their skin is thinner, and they will receive a higher exposure because they have a larger surface-to-mass ratio than adults. Children also are more vulnerable to the effects of biologic agents that produce vomiting and diarrhea because they have smaller fluid reserves than adults. This makes them more susceptible to dehydration and shock. They have smaller circulating blood volume reserves than adults and would be potentially at greater risk for hemorrhagic shock than an adult exposed to VHF.

In addition, some of the biologic agents have *shorter incubation periods* in children. As such, they will become symptomatic earlier, but this also presents a window of opportunity for surveillance systems. They can also present with different symptoms than they do in adults.

Many preventive and therapeutic regimens recommended for adults exposed or potentially exposed to biologic agents have not been studied in infants and children and may be contraindicated in children. In addition, pediatric dosages may not be established. For most CDC category A agents, though, there are suggested dosages (see Table 9-4 and Table 9-5).

TABLE 9-4 Recommended Therapy and Prophylaxis of Anthrax in Children[22]
(Note: all antimicrobials should be checked for current recommended dosages before administration of the medication.)

Form of Anthrax	Therapy/Prophylaxis	Antibiotic and Dosage
Inhalation	Therapy[a]	Ciprofloxacin[b] 10-15 mg/kg IV every 12 h (maximum, 400 mg/dose) *or* Doxycycline 2.2 mg/kg IV (maximum, 100 mg) every 12 h *and* Clindamycin[c] 10-15 mg/kg IV every 8 h *and* Penicillin G[e] 400 000-600 000 U/kg/d IV divided every 4 h Patients who are clinically stable after 14 days can be switched to a single oral agent (ciprofloxacin or doxycycline) to complete a 60 d course[d] of therapy.
Inhalation	Postexposure prophylaxis (60 d course[d])	Ciprofloxacin[f] 10-15 mg/kg PO (maximum, 500 mg/dose) every 12 h *or* Doxycycline 2.2 mg/kg (maximum, 100 mg) PO every 12 h

(Continued)

TABLE 9-4 *(Continued)*

Cutaneous, endemic	Therapy[g]	Penicillin V 40-80 mg/kg/d PO divided every 6 h
		or
		Amoxicillin 40-80 mg/kg/d PO divided every 8 h
		or
		Ciprofloxacin 10-15 mg/kg PO (maximum, 1 g/d) every 12 h
		or
		Levofloxacin 10-15 mg/kg IV every 24 h
		or
		Doxycycline 2.2 mg/kg PO (maximum, 100 mg) every 12 h
Cutaneous (in setting of terrorism)	Therapy[a]	Ciprofloxacin 10-15 mg/kg PO (maximum, 1 g/d) every 12 h
		Doxycycline 2.2 mg/kg PO (maximum, 100 mg) every 12 h
GI	Therapy[a]	Same as for inhalational

This table was created from recommendations developed at the Consensus Conference, in part based on reviewed reference materials from the American Academy of Pediatrics (AAP), CDC, FDA, and Infectious Disease Society of America, and was updated in 2008 and 2010. It is reproduced with permission from the Center for Disaster Medicine, New York Medical College.

[a]In a mass casualty setting, in which resources are severely limited, oral therapy may need to be substituted for the preferred parenteral option. Discussion with a pediatric infectious disease specialist may help. Recent literature has suggested that, instead of clindamycin or penicillin, one may use rifampin, vancomycin, ampicillin, chloramphenicol, imipenem, clindamycin, and clarithromycin (Update: Investigation of bioterrorism-related anthrax and interim guidelines for exposure management and antimicrobial therapy. *MMWR.* 2001;50:909-919).
[b]Ofloxacin (and possibly other quinolones) may be acceptable alternatives to ciprofloxacin or levofloxacin.
[c]Rifampin or clarithromycin may be acceptable alternatives to clindamycin as drugs that target bacterial protein synthesis.
[d]On confirmation of antibiotic sensitivities, infants and children may be switched to oral amoxicillin (40-80 mg/kg/d divided every 8 h) to complete a 60-day course. It is recommended, however, that the first 14 days of either therapy or prophylaxis be conducted with the agents listed above, regardless of sensitivities, before making this change.
[e]Ampicillin, imipenem, meropenem, or chloramphenicol may be acceptable alternatives to penicillin as drugs with good central nervous system penetration.
[f]According to most experts, ciprofloxacin is the preferred agent for oral prophylaxis.
[g]Ten days of therapy may be adequate for endemic cutaneous disease. If the mechanism of exposure is unknown, a full 60-day course should be strongly considered because of the possibility of concomitant inhalational exposure, especially in children.

TABLE 9-5 Recommended Therapy and Prophylaxis in Children for Additional Select Diseases Associated with Bioterrorism[22]
(Note: all antibiotics should be checked for current recommended dosages prior to administration of the medication.)

Disease	Therapy/Prophylaxis	Treatment,[a] Antimicrobial Agent, and Dosage
Smallpox	Therapy	Supportive care. While not approved, there may be a potential role for the antiviral medication cidofovir,[b] but this should be discussed with a pediatric infectious disease specialist.
	Prophylaxis	Vaccination[c] may be effective if given within the first several days after exposure and is recommended for patients of any age.

(Continued)

TABLE 9-5 *(Continued)*

Plague	Therapy	Gentamicin 2.5 mg/kg IV every 8 h *or* Streptomycin 15 mg/kg IM every 12 h (maximum, 2 g/d, although only available for compassionate usage and in limited supply) *or* Doxycycline 2.2 mg/kg IV every 12 h (maximum, 200 mg/d) *or* Ciprofloxacin[d] 15 mg/kg IV every 12 h *or* Levofloxacin 10-15 mg/kg IV every 24 h *or* Chloramphenicol[e] 25 mg/kg every 6 h (maximum, 4 g/d)
	Prophylaxis	Doxycycline 2.2 mg/kg PO every 12 h *or* Ciprofloxacin[d] 20 mg/kg PO every 12 h
Tularemia	Therapy	Same as for plague
Disease	**Therapy/Prophylaxis**	**Treatment,[a] Antimicrobial Agent, and Dosage**
Botulism	Therapy	Supportive care, antitoxin and/or botulism immune globulin may halt progression of symptoms but are unlikely to reverse them
VHFs	Therapy	Supportive care, ribavirin may be beneficial in select cases[f]

This table was created from recommendations developed at the Consensus Conference, in part based on reviewed reference materials from the AAP, CDC, FDA, and Infectious Diseases Society of America, and was updated in 2008 and 2010. It is reproduced with permission from the Center for Disaster Medicine, New York Medical College.

[a]In a mass casualty setting, parenteral therapy might not be possible. In such cases, oral therapy (with analogous agents) may need to be used.
[b]Cidofovir is available only through the CDC.
[c]There may be a potential role for cidofovir and/or vaccinia immune globin in the treatment of pediatric adverse reactions to vaccinia administration. This should be done in discussion with a pediatric infectious disease specialist.
[d]Ofloxacin (and possibly other quinolones) may be acceptable alternatives to ciprofloxacin or levofloxacin; however, they are not approved for use in children.
[e]Concentration should be maintained between 5 and 20 µg/mL. Some experts have recommended that chloramphenicol be used to treat patients with plague meningitis because chloramphenicol penetrates the blood-brain barrier. Use in children younger than 2 years may be associated with adverse reactions but might be warranted for serious infections.
[f]Ribavirin is recommended for arenavirus or bunyavirus infections and may be indicated for a viral hemorrhagic fever of an unknown etiology, although not FDA approved for these indications. For intravenous therapy, a loading dose should be used: 30 kg IV once (maximum dose, 2 g), then 16 mg/kg IV every 6 h for 4 days (maximum dose, 1 g) and then 8 mg/kg IV every 8 h for 6 days (maximum dose, 500 mg). In a mass casualty setting, it may be necessary to use oral therapy: a loading dose of 30 mg/kg PO once, then 15 mg/kg/d PO in 2 divided doses for 10 days.

9.10 PUBLIC HEALTH ACTIONS IN A BT ATTACK

If an outbreak proves to be the result of terrorism, or if the scope of the outbreak overwhelms local resources, a regional or national response becomes imperative. Under such circumstances, an extensive number of supporting assets and capabilities may be summoned. The CDC and the US Army Medical Research Institute for Infectious Diseases (USAMRIID; http://www.usamriid.army.mil/) provide national laboratories through the Laboratory Response Network (LRN) (http://www.bt.cdc.gov/lrn/), which are capable of dealing with virtually all potential biologic threat agents.[23] Most state public health laboratories participate as reference laboratories in the LRN. These facilities support hundreds of sentinel laboratories in local hospitals throughout the nation and can provide sophisticated confirmatory diagnosis and typing of biologic agents.[24,25]

Expert consultation and epidemiologic investigative assistance are also available through the CDC; bioweapons threat evaluation and medical consultation is likewise available through USAMRIID. Where there is danger of global spread of human disease, the provisions in the IHR should be considered. The IHR provide a global regulatory framework to prevent the spread of diseases through infection control measures for travelers and cargo and at border crossing points.

9.10.1 Threat Assessment

Law enforcement, in coordination with the Federal Bureau of Investigation (FBI), is responsible for the analysis of threat credibility. If the threat is considered credible, the FBI coordinates laboratory testing with the state public health laboratory. Public health personnel are responsible for assessing the extent of human exposure and for making recommendations for antibiotic prophylaxis or other treatment. Law enforcement personnel classify BT threat assessments into three categories: (1) a covert release of a pathogen into the environment in which the first indication to health care providers occurs when patients present at clinical facilities; (2) a release that is heralded by the receipt of a localized threat, such as a package or piece of mail, perhaps accompanied by a warning letter; and (3) an event that is witnessed or announced as the pathogen is released into the environment, thereby exposing persons who are at the release site.[26]

The timely communication of intelligence with medical professionals at the front line may markedly cut response time for any possible epidemics due to BT. Conversely, if the medical provider is suspicious of a particular pathogen, this information should be rapidly passed to the proper authorities for further investigation and testing.

9.10.2 Medical Countermeasures and Point-of-Distribution Access

In a serious outbreak, health officials will be responsible for distributing medications and vaccines to large numbers of individuals, including at mass vaccination and treatment clinics, and will also be responsible for staffing of such clinics. A basic part of disaster planning is the need to establish dispensing sites for distributing medications or providing vaccinations in various community settings.

Mass vaccination may be considered if the number of cases is high, if outbreaks occur in a number of locations, and/or if the outbreak continues to grow despite the use of more targeted vaccination strategies (eg, "ring" vaccination). Public health agencies have developed vaccination plans for pandemics and BT attacks as part of their preparedness efforts. It is important for health professionals and the public to know about vaccination options that will be available.

In addition to vaccines, public health officials will consider the use of medications to prevent or control the spread of disease. Antibiotics can be effective against the bacteria that cause plague, anthrax, and tularemia, among others. While the anthrax vaccine may have a role in postexposure prophylaxis after an anthrax event, the primary preventive measure will be antibiotic prophylaxis. For viral diseases such as influenza, various antiviral medications will be considered. The urgency and scale of providing medications is significantly increased after a serious disease outbreak or act of BT. To be effective, most medications must be given to exposed people within a very short time frame.

Public health management of large-scale infectious disease outbreaks is discussed in more detail in the ADLS® course (v3.0) and supporting course manual.

9.11   SUMMARY

Human exposure to biologic agents may occur through inhalation, skin (cutaneous) exposure, or ingestion of contaminated food or water. In recent years, global concern has increased about bioterrorism, the deliberate use of certain pathogens or biologic products by terrorists to influence the conduct of government or to intimidate or coerce a civilian population. As was learned in the spring of 2003, epidemics resulting from emerging infectious diseases like SARS can cause widespread civil panic and conditions similar to a BT event. Effective response to a disease outbreak (natural or intended) depends on rapid identification of the causative agent and specific diagnosis. To enhance detection and treatment capabilities, health professionals should be familiar with the clinical manifestations, diagnostic techniques, isolation precautions, treatment, and prophylaxis for likely causative agents (eg, CDC category A agents). For some of these agents, delay in the health system response could result in a potentially devastating number of casualties.

To mitigate such consequences, early identification and intervention are imperative. Front-line health professionals must have an increased level of suspicion regarding the possible intentional use of biologic agents as well as an increased sensitivity to reporting those suspicions to public health authorities, who, in turn, must be willing to evaluate a predictable increase in false-positive reports. Clinicians should report noticeable increases in unusual illnesses, symptom complexes, or disease patterns (even without definitive diagnosis) to public health authorities. Prompt reporting of unusual patterns of illness can allow public health officials to initiate an epidemiologic investigation earlier than would be possible if the report awaited definitive etiologic diagnosis.

Health system response efforts require coordination and planning with emergency management agencies, law enforcement, health care facilities, and social service agencies. Public health agencies should ensure that physicians and other health professionals know who to call with reports of suspicious cases and clusters of infectious diseases and should work to build a good relationship with the local medical community. Resource integration is absolutely necessary to establish adequate capacity to initiate rapid investigation of an outbreak, educate the public, begin mass distribution of medications and vaccines, ensure mass medical care, and control public anger and fear.

9.12 DISCUSSION POINTS

Biologic Disasters: Putting the PRE-DISASTER Paradigm™ into Practice	
P Planning and Practice	A biologic event demands close collaboration and coordination among federal, state, and local officials. Given these special demands, all communities need to develop, implement, and test preparedness plans for biologic events in ways that engage all appropriate response agencies.
R Resilience	The psychological impact of a pandemic or BT event on survivors may be huge. Psychosocial support will be extremely important to restore a sense of calm, reduce public fear, and support the grieving process. Concerns that people have about future outbreaks, about their ability to get life back to normal, or about other worries must be identified, recognized, and dealt with as soon as possible. Resilience is the capacity of individuals and communities to rebound from adversity, become strengthened, and become more resourceful. Gender, age, and previous medical conditions may influence the impact of a biologic disaster on families and individuals and should be taken into account by disaster planners and by those providing psychosocial support.
E Education and Training	To respond appropriately, health personnel must maintain a specified level of proficiency. Education and training of health professional staff in good infection control practices can be carried out at all levels. Heath professionals should maintain an appropriate awareness of biologic agents that can cause human disease, whether naturally occurring or spread by human-caused means.
Biologic Disasters: Putting the DISASTER Paradigm™ into Practice	
D Detection	It is important to maintain a healthy index of suspicion at all times. Initial detection of a potential BT agent or emerging infection may occur days and weeks after initial exposure. Health professionals should know how to alert proper authorities about actual or perceived biologic emergencies.

I	Incident Management	Incident management will involve a unified command involving public health, public safety, and other emergency management entities. A true scene may be absent. Health professionals need to work as members of an integrated disaster team under the structure of the incident command system. They must comply with regulatory and legal as well as accepted moral and ethical principles during management of the event.
S	Safety and Security	Personal protection is paramount. Health professionals should adhere to proper decontamination and infection control policies and procedures to mitigate disease spread.
A	Assess Hazards	Health personnel should be knowledgeable about epidemiologic and clinical investigation strategies to characterize the causative agent and identify the population at risk to break the "chain of infection."
S	Support	Responders and citizens should be aware of local, regional, and national surge capacity and support services that may be available in a biologic disaster.
T	Triage and Treatment	In a biologic disaster, appropriate casualty management includes assessment of and response to both medical and psychological casualties. Therapeutic countermeasures depend on the specific biologic agent. Countermeasures that can be employed include the following:

➤ *Hand washing* will prevent the spread of biologic agents from person to person in many cases. Although not completely effective, it is inexpensive, readily available, and reasonably effective.

➤ Similarly, appropriate *hygiene and sanitation* will generally decrease the spread of the agent from contaminated areas and decrease potential vectors such as rodents from proliferating.

➤ *Vaccines* are available for selected biologic agents such as influenza, smallpox, and, to a lesser extent, anthrax. Generally, these vaccines must be administered in advance of exposure and may require periodic revaccination, although for some viral exposures vaccination after exposure may reduce severity of the disease process.

➤ *Antibiotics and antivirals* can be effective if administered after exposure but before symptoms occur (prophylactic administration). Once the disease process has started, antibiotics are generally given intravenously. Early treatment is essential as some of these diseases progress rapidly. |

		➤ *Antitoxins* are available for selected agents, such as botulinum toxin. Antitoxins do not reverse the course of the illness but can prevent further progression. Rapid administration is essential for enhanced recovery from the effects of the agent.
E	Evacuation	It is unlikely evacuation will be required in a BT or emerging pandemic. However, specific shelter-in-place may be recommended by local public health departments.
R	Recovery	Recovery begins immediately after the event. Pre-event resilience is key to recovery. The medical and mental health impact of pandemic or BT attack can be significant. Recovery involves a long-term commitment to affected communities and may last for years. Mechanisms for long-term public health surveillance must be implemented and maintained.

REFERENCES

1. Waterer GW, Robertson H. Bioterrorism for the respiratory physician. *Respirology*. 2009;14: 5-11.

2. Utrup LJ, Frey AH. Fate of bioterrorism-relevant viruses and bacteria, including spores, aerosolized into an indoor air environment. *Exp Biol Med*. 2004;229:345-350.

3. Ligon BL. Plague: a review of its history and potential as a biological weapon. *Semin Pediatr Infect Dis*. 2006;17:161-170.

4. Tomes N. "Destroyer and teacher"; managing the masses during the 1918–1919 influenza pandemic. *Public Health Rep*. 2010;125(suppl 3):48-62.

5. Cox NJ, Tamblyn SE, Tam T. Influenza pandemic planning. *Vaccine*. 2003;21:1801-1803.

6. Webster RG. Influenza: an emerging disease. *Emerg Infect Dis*. 1998;4:436-441.

7. Steelfisher GK, Blendon RJ, Bekheit MM, Lubell K. The public's response to the 2009 H1N1 influenza pandemic. *N Engl J Med*. 2010;362(22).

8. Wheelis M, Rózsa L, Dando M. *Deadly Cultures: Biological Weapons Since 1945*. Boston, MA: Harvard University Press; 2006.

9. Elmer-Dewitt P. America's first bioterrorism attack. *Time*. 2001. http://www.time.com/time/magazine/article/0,9171,1101011008-176937,00.html. Accessed April 28, 2011.

10. Health experts fear bioterror attack. *Grand Rapids Press*. January 28, 2007;G1.

11. Kahn AS, Swerdlow DL, Juranek DD. Precautions against biological and chemical terrorism directed at food and water supplies. *Public Health Rep*. 2001;116:3-14.

12. Fine A, Layton M. Lessons from the West Nile viral encephalitis outbreak in New York City, 1999: implications for bioterrorism preparedness. *Clin Infect Dis*. 2001;32:277-282.

13. Lampton LM. SARS, biological terrorism, and mother nature. *J Miss State Med Assoc*. 2003;44:151-152.

14. Feldman KA, Enscore RE, Lathrop SL, et al. An outbreak of primary pneumonic tularemia on Martha's Vineyard. *N Engl J Med.* 2001;345(22):1601-1606.

15. Dembek ZF, Buckman RL, Fowler SK, Hadler JL. Missed sentinel case of naturally occurring pneumonic tularemia outbreak: lessons for detection of bioterrorism. *J Am Board Fam Pract.* 2003;16:339-342.

16. Multistate outbreak of monkeypox—Illinois, Indiana, and Wisconsin, 2003. *MMWR Morb Mortal Wkly Rep.* 2003;52:537-540.

17. Pavlin JA. Epidemiology of bioterrorism. *Emerg Infect Dis.* 1999;5:528-530.

18. Siegel JD, Rhinehart E, Jackson M, Chiarello L. Healthcare Infection Control Practices Advisory Committee. 2007 Guideline for Isolation Precautions: Preventing Transmission of Infectious Agents in Healthcare Settings. Washington, DC: US Dept of Health and Human Services; 2007. http://www.cdc.gov/hicpac/pdf/isolation/Isolation2007.pdf. Accessed April 28, 2011

19. Burkle FM. Population-based triage management in response to surge-capacity requirements during a large-scale bioevent disaster. *Acad Emerg Med.* 2006;13:118-129.

20. Henretig FM, Cieslak TJ, Kortepeter MG, Fleisher GR. Medical management of the suspected victim of bioterrorism: an algorithmic approach to the undifferentiated patient. *Emerg Med Clin North Am.* 2002;20:351-364.

21. Cieslak TJ, Henretig FM. Biological and chemical terrorism. In: Berman E, Kliegman, Jenson, eds. *Nelson's Textbook of Pediatrics.* 17th ed. Philadelphia, PA: Saunders; 2003.

22. Markenson D, Redlener I. *Pediatric Preparedness for Disasters and Terrorism: A National Consensus Conference. Executive Summary and Final Report.* New York, NY: National Center for Disaster Preparedness, New York Medical College School of Public Health; 2007. http://www.njcphp.org/legacy/drup/sites/default/files/Pediatric_Preparedness_Conference_Report.pdf. Accessed April 28, 2011.

23. Biological and chemical terrorism: strategic plan for preparedness and response. Recommendations of the CDC Strategic Planning Workgroup. *MMWR Recomm Rep.* 2000;49 (RR-4):1-14.

24. Gilchrist MJ. A national laboratory network for bioterrorism: evolution from a prototype network of laboratories performing routine surveillance. *Mil Med.* 2000;165(suppl 2):28-31.

25. Morse SA, Kellog RB, Perry S, et al. Detecting biothreat agents: the laboratory response network. *ASM News.* 2003;69:433-437.

26. Kortepeter MG, Cieslak TJ. Bioterrorism: plague, anthrax, and smallpox. In: Baddour L, Gorbach SL, eds. *Therapy of Infectious Diseases.* Philadelphia, PA: Saunders; 2003.

CHAPTER TEN

Natural Disasters

CHAPTER CHAIR

Italo Subbarao, DO, MBA

CONTRIBUTING AUTHORS

Jim Lyznicki, MS, MPH

Lauren Walsh, MPH

John Broach, MD, MPH

Alessandra Rossodivita, MD, PhD

Dan Kirkpatrick, RN, MSN

Kelly R. Klein, MD

Alison Hayward, MD

Andrew Milsten, MD, MS

Raymond Swienton, MD

Mary-Elise Manuell, MD, MA

10.1 PURPOSE

This chapter discusses the characteristics and epidemiology of natural disasters that occur throughout the world. Clinical and public health considerations are discussed for several specific natural disasters (eg, earthquakes and tsunamis, floods, extreme heat, hurricanes and cyclones, tornadoes, volcanic eruptions, wildfires, and winter storms).

Common prevention and mitigation strategies are also reviewed. Natural infectious disease outbreaks, such as an influenza pandemic, are not addressed in this chapter. For such information, readers are referred to Chapter 9, "Biologic Disasters," and the Advanced Disaster Life Support™ course (v 3.0) and supporting course manual.

10.2   LEARNING OBJECTIVES

After completing this chapter, readers should be able to:

➤ Provide historical trends and epidemiologic patterns of illnesses and injuries seen in common natural disasters.

➤ Describe appropriate clinical management guidance for injuries and illnesses seen in common natural disasters.

➤ Describe appropriate public health management guidance for injuries and illnesses seen in common natural disasters.

➤ Provide prevention and mitigation strategies for common natural disasters.

Learning objectives for this chapter are competency-based, as delineated in Appendix B.

10.3   BACKGROUND

Worldwide, millions of lives have been lost and millions more people have been injured or had their lives disrupted by natural disasters. Damage caused by earthquakes, tornadoes, floods, wildfires, and volcanic eruptions can leave entire communities completely incapacitated. Depending on the event, a large number of people may be seriously injured; extensive structural damage may occur; and many will seek shelter, food, and other assistance. Casualty care will be challenged not only by the sheer initial volume of ill and injured but also by the degree of disruption to the preexisting health care infrastructure. That combined with the wave-like surges of affected people seeking health care during the aftermath of many natural disasters increases the challenges.

Global trends indicate that the risk of exposure to natural hazards is on the rise, resulting in an increase in the frequency and magnitude of natural disasters. According to the World Health Organization (WHO) Center for Research on the Epidemiology of Disasters (WHO/CRED), the worldwide frequency of natural disasters has doubled since 1995. This is likely due to the combined increase in natural hazard frequency and an increase in population vulnerability. Because fluctuations in global temperature may increase the frequency of natural hazards, climate change has emerged as an important global factor that may influence disaster trends. Factors such as urbanization, overpopulation, and encroachment on regions susceptible to disasters have increased population vulnerability. Globalization, which connects countries through economic interdependencies (eg, increased buying of products in one country subsequently increases productivity in another country), has led to increased travel and commerce around the world. Such activity has resulted in increased urbanization and overpopulation of cities worldwide, as well as increased migration of people to coastal, wildland-urban interface areas and other disaster-prone regions.

In 2010, more than 370 natural disasters occurred, causing more than 290,000 deaths and affecting more than 296 million people.[1] Economic damages were projected at $109 billion. Statistics from past years are presented in Table 10-1. According to the CRED database, more natural disasters occur in Asia than on any other continent; China experiences the most natural disasters of any country. The CRED database also demonstrates that floods are the most common type of disaster throughout the United States and the world.

Center for Research on the Epidemiology of Disasters (CRED)

The CRED was established in 1973 as a nonprofit institution located within the School of Public Health of the University Catholique de Louvain in Brussels, Belgium. The CRED became a WHO Collaborating Center in 1980 and has expanded its support of the WHO Global Program for Emergency Preparedness and Response. The center focuses on health aspects and impacts from disasters and complex emergencies. These include all types of natural and human-caused events, longer-term disasters such as famines and droughts, and situations creating mass displacement of people such as civil strife and conflicts. For more information, refer to the CRED Web site at http://www.cred.be/.

TABLE 10-1 Global Natural Disaster Statistics for the 21st Century[1-3]

Natural Disaster Impact	2010[1]	2009[2]	2008[3]	2007	2000-2006 Average
Number of country-level disasters	373	335	354	414	394.7
Number of countries affected	129	111	Data not found	133	116.3
Number of people killed	296 800	10 655	235 000	16 847	73 946
Number of people affected	207 million	119 million	214 million	211 million	234 million
Economic damage (US dollars)	$109 billion	$41.3 billion	$190 billion	$75 billion	$81.9 billion

10.4 NATURAL DISASTER–SPECIFIC CONSIDERATIONS

Most natural disasters are time-limited and do not become public health emergencies. However, after a primary natural disaster, responders must be prepared for subsequent or secondary emergencies. Special attention must be given to structural collapse, impassible roads and bridges, downed power lines, fuel leaks, ruptured gas lines, and loss of basic services. While a building may sustain no immediately apparent effects after a disaster, it may be structurally damaged or otherwise unstable enough to pose a serious risk for its inhabitants and need to be evacuated. For example, a hospital that suffers structural damage during an earthquake may not exhibit any visible changes but could actually be an impending mass casualty incident with the need for evacuation.

Moreover, natural disasters may create a need for a wide variety of resources. For example, the collapse of a building after an earthquake would require rapid mobilization of construction personnel and heavy equipment, urban search and rescue teams, and mortuary services. The consequences of prolonged power outages, contaminated drinking water supplies, and infectious disease outbreaks must also be considered. Natural disasters pose a substantial risk of communications disruptions, infrastructure destruction, and large numbers of displaced persons who require food, shelter, and medical care.

10.4.1   Situational Awareness

The ability to mitigate the impact of an event is essential to disaster planning. Unfortunately, not all natural disasters are predictable with any degree of accuracy. Earthquakes, for example, usually strike with little or no warning. Storm fronts are also volatile and dynamic and permit limited warning at best. That said, many natural disasters *can* be reliably monitored and tracked before they occur (Table 10-2). The role of detection in natural disasters is intensely focused on pre-event identification. Proper advance warning, timely evacuation orders, and shelter access are important factors in decreasing disaster-related mortality and morbidity.

The National Weather Service (NWS; http://weather.gov) is the primary US agency responsible for providing warnings of threatening conditions or impending problems due to weather-related phenomena. Active alert systems such as local sirens are most effective because they require no initiative by the population being warned, as opposed to passive systems such as the news media, radio stations, and the Internet, which require the target population to access this information to receive the alert.

TABLE 10-2 Early Detection or Warning of Natural Disasters

Type of Warning	Definition	Examples
Early warning	Detected before impact; monitoring allows prediction of impact and permits preparation	Hurricanes, floods, volcanic eruptions
Limited warning	Volatile situations with rapidly changing course or intensity	Severe thunderstorms with damaging winds; tornadoes; impending structural collapse following a natural disaster.
No warning	No ability to detect before impact; monitoring is unpredictable but may play a role in quantifying and qualifying the event after occurrence	Earthquakes, wildfires[a], transportation and industrial incidents after a natural disaster

[a]While there is typically no ability to detect wildfires before impact, they often persist for several days. Therefore, those not in the immediate path of the fire may have ample warning to evacuate.

10.4.2   Health Facility Expansion of Surge Capability

Large-scale natural disasters can cause widespread destruction, power disruptions, and/or water supply contamination. This may render some hospital facilities inoperable and will require directing medical services delivery to external, nontraditional alternate care facilities (ACFs). Additional space and staff needed for patient management of overwhelmed emergency departments may also be met in an ACF. Limited specialty services (such as hemodialysis) may even be accomplished in a well-planned alternate care site.

During Hurricane Katrina (2005), the Pete Maravich Assembly Center, a large sporting arena on the Louisiana State University campus in Baton Rouge, was utilized as an ACF. In 2006, The Joint Commission reported that this was the largest acute care field hospital in the United States since the Civil War. It is estimated that more than 6000 patients were treated or housed and more than 15 000 people were triaged at this site during its operation. The acuity of patients was significant. At times, it was reported that up to 14 ventilator-dependent patients were managed concurrently, as well as approximately 80 patients in cardiac-monitored beds.[4]

The ACF may be large, as just described, or small (ie, a 50-bed portable field hospital). The key is to maintain as near the community standard of care as possible in these surge facilities. This is especially challenging during large-scale natural disasters when supply access, including appropriate personnel, is commonly quite limited. The goal once an ACF is operational is to immediately focus on closing it as soon as possible. This is important, as the focus must always be on returning community health care delivery to the usual standards of care and proper facilities as soon as possible.

10.5   CASUALTY MANAGEMENT

Mass trauma is the term used to describe the multiple injuries, deaths, disabilities, and emotional responses caused by a catastrophic event, such as a natural disaster. Natural disasters often have predictable injury time lines and patterns, regardless of disaster type (Table 10-3). Initial injuries are often trauma-related, and most deaths occur in the early aftermath of the event.

In subsequent days and weeks, the medical community will experience an exacerbation of routine chronic diseases such as asthma, accompanied by orthopedic injuries and lacerations sustained from initial cleanup efforts. These are followed by an increase in infections from untreated wounds received during the initial incident.

In the months and years following the event, the health system will be challenged further in managing the psychological effects of the event. As discussed in Chapter 3 of this manual, mental and behavioral health is a very important component of the disaster recovery process. As such, mental health resources should be part of any natural disaster response plan. Early intervention may allow mental health professionals to identify and offer treatment to people who are at risk for anxiety, depression, stress disorders, and other behavioral health problems (eg, suicide ideation, substance abuse).

TABLE 10-3 Medical Needs Timeline in Natural Disasters

Time Frame (Time After Event)	Injury/Disease Process	Treatment Needs
Immediate (0 to 48 hours)	Trauma	Orthopedics Laceration repair Surgery Burns
Intermediate (2 d to 2 wk)	Trauma	Orthopedics Laceration repair Dialysis Fasciotomy
	Acute medical	Exacerbation of chronic illness (eg, myocardial infarction, acute asthma attack, congestive heart failure) Dialysis Carbon monoxide poisoning
Long term (weeks to years)	Public health, medical	Exacerbation of chronic illness (eg, myocardial infarction, acute asthma attack, congestive heart failure) Communicable disease outbreaks: ➤ Water-borne diseases ➤ Diarrheal (eg, cholera, dysentery) ➤ Person to person (eg, measles, meningitis) ➤ Vector-borne diseases (eg, malaria, West Nile virus)
	Mental and behavioral health	Posttraumatic stress Anxiety Substance abuse Depression

While they may follow a similar time line and pattern of injury, natural disasters do not always cause the same *types* of casualties. Specific health consequences according to natural disaster typology in the United States are summarized further in Table 10-4.

Injuries and medical conditions that can be expected after a natural disaster may be extensive. Trauma, from simple lacerations and fractures to complicated blunt and penetrating injuries, will be present. Structural collapse may result in crush injuries and the need for extremity amputations. A common feature of natural disasters is that injured individuals are covered with dirt and debris, which can impair medical assessment during prehospital and emergency department evaluations. Decontamination showers in both settings are very useful, and this aspect should be taken into account in disaster planning for natural events.

Wound management should be an essential part of hospital disaster planning. With tornadoes, wounds tend to be more contaminated and complex as the majority of casualties present with wounds with embedded foreign bodies from projectile debris.

TABLE 10-4 Natural Hazard Health Consequences and Considerations

Natural Event	Mortality	Morbidity	Other Considerations
Earthquakes, tsunamis	Crush injury Exsanguinations, asphyxiation from building collapse Drowning from tsunamis	Closed fractures Superficial trauma Exacerbation of preexisting conditions	As many as 95% of all deaths occur before extraction One study showed that 93% of casualties extricated within 24 hours survived[a]
Floods	Major cause of death drowning, primarily of people trapped in vehicles	Outbreaks of communicable disease Exacerbation of chronic illnesses Lacerations and punctures Electrocution from downed power lines Exposure to hazardous biological and chemical agents	Increased number of soft-tissue injuries Submersion injuries, hypothermia, and trauma also expected
Extreme heat events	Most deaths due to heat stroke	Heat syncope and heat exhaustion are more common	At-risk populations most susceptible (elderly, those with chronic disease, pregnant women, and children)
Hurricanes, cyclones, typhoons	90% of fatalities are due to storm surge[b] Major cause of death is drowning	Lacerations, blunt trauma, puncture wounds About 80% of these injuries are confined to the feet and lower extremities, most commonly from clean-up phase[c]	Wounds may be prone to secondary infection Hurricane flooding can lead to long-term public health problems such as food and water contamination, mold overgrowth, and injuries due to massive infrastructure damage
Tornadoes	An average of 60-80 people die from tornadoes each year in the United States Fatalities are largely due to head injuries and crush injuries from flying debris	Most injuries caused by flying debris or people getting thrown by high winds Typical injuries include head injury, soft tissue injury, and secondary wound infection	A large number of tornado-related injuries are actually suffered during rescue attempts, cleanup, and other post-tornado activities
Volcanic eruptions	Pyroclastic flow Suffocation from ash, steam scalding, lethal gases	Eye injuries and respiratory illness exacerbation from volcanic ash Burns Dehydration Trauma from building collapse	Potential for increased emergency department visits due to emphysema, asthma, and chronic bronchitis

(Continued)

TABLE 10-4 *(Continued)*

Natural Event	Mortality	Morbidity	Other Considerations
Wildfires	Most deaths due to toxic inhalation (carbon monoxide, cyanide) and significant burn injury	Increased asthma, chronic bronchitis, and emphysema Potential for heat stress, especially among firefighters	Expected increase in emergency department visits No expected increase in hospital admissions
Winter storms	Most deaths indirectly related to storm (eg, due to automobile crashes or heart attack)	Hypothermia Exhaustion and heart attack due to overexertion Injuries attributed to increase in house fires	Elderly are more susceptible to hypothermia Carbon monoxide poisoning may result from improper use of generators

[a]de Bruycker M, Greco D, Annino I, et al. The 1980 earthquake in Southern Italy: rescue of trapped victims and mortality. *Bull World Health Organ*. 1983;27:1130-1135.
[b]Meredith JT, Bradley S. Hurricanes. In: Hogan DE, Burstein JL, eds. *Disaster Medicine*. Philadelphia, PA: Lippincott Williams & Wilkins, 2002:179-186.
[c]Noji EK. Analysis of medical needs during disasters caused by tropical cyclones: anticipated injury patterns. *J Trop Med Hyg*. 1993;96:370-376.

During earthquakes and floods, significant wound contamination also is common. Tetanus prophylaxis is an important part of wound care management for this reason. It may also be prudent to have a "no-close" wound policy as part of emergency department protocols for natural disasters, although this has not been definitively addressed in the literature.

Another common cause of casualty after a natural disaster is the exacerbation of preexisting medical conditions. Dust and fumes can cause acute attacks in people with asthma and chronic obstructive pulmonary disease (COPD). It is also well documented that acute cardiac events including cardiac arrest and myocardial infarction (heart attacks) typically increase after a significant natural disaster, such as an earthquake.

Clinical and Public Health Considerations by Disaster Typology

The preceding sections provided an overview of general concepts and principles for the management of mass casualties in a natural disaster. The following sections discuss clinical and public health considerations for specific natural disasters: earthquakes and tsunamis, floods, heat emergencies, hurricanes and cyclones, tornadoes, volcanic eruptions, wildfires, and winter storms.

10.6   EARTHQUAKES AND TSUNAMIS

Earthquakes are among the most powerful and potentially devastating natural occurrences. Earthquakes that occur in oceans or seas additionally have the potential to cause large displacements of water that result in a series of large waves known as a *tsunami*. Large earthquakes, while always releasing massive amounts of energy, often occur far from population centers and are therefore not disasters, simply impressive geologic events. Every year, there are about 500 000 earthquakes worldwide, of which only about 20% are perceptible.[5] It is only when an earthquake or its resulting tsunami occurs in a place that causes damage or loss of life that the potential for disaster exists.

That said, the number of earthquakes that do cause significant damage is increasing yearly. In 2009, there were 91 earthquakes that affected large populations and had magnitudes greater than 5.9 on the Richter scale. Of these, 28 generated tsunamis. Although earthquake magnitude plays an important role in the extent of resulting damage, it is not the only factor. The 2008 Sichuan earthquake in China, for example, measured 8.0 on the Richter scale, caused more than 50 000 deaths, and left more than 4 million people homeless. Interestingly, the 2010 Haiti earthquake measured 7.0 on the Richter scale but is estimated to have caused more than 200 000 deaths and many more injuries. The 2011 Japan earthquake with an estimated magnitude of 9.0 on the Richter scale and the associated tsunami have caused more than 12 000 deaths, with as many or more people still unaccounted for, and have displaced tens of thousands more. At the time of this writing, final mortality and morbidity calculations are still pending. This highlights the importance of factors other than magnitude (such as earthquake depth, proximity of the epicenter to population centers, and construction and building codes) that may contribute to the effect of the event on human populations.[6]

10.6.1   Causes and Characteristics

While the exact mechanism of earthquake is still largely unknown, the elastic-rebound theory is one commonly cited mechanism to describe the process that creates the energy release of an earthquake. According to this theory, the tectonic plates of the earth's crust are in constant motion and slip along each other tangentially. At the boundary between plates, called *faults*, friction causes the plates to adhere to each other even while the natural movement of the plates creates strain on this interlocked area. Eventually, this strain is enough to overcome the friction holding the two plates in place. The plates suddenly and violently move laterally with respect to each other, releasing the potential energy stored at the interface. The place where this release occurs is known as the *earthquake hypocenter*, or focus. This is the place from which the seismic waves are generated that radiate out in all directions. The epicenter of the earthquake is the location on the earth's surface directly above the underground hypocenter.

Two commonly used scales describe the strength of an earthquake: the Richter scale and the moment magnitude scale (MMS). Both scales gauge the shaking amplitude of an earthquake as measured by displacement of seismographs at various fixed distances from the epicenter. The MMS is a more accurate scale across a wide range of earthquake strengths and has replaced the Richter scale for most official geologic measurements. Both scales, however, range from 0 to 10 and are logarithmic. An increase of one "point" on either scale represents both a 10-fold increase in the shaking amplitude associated with the earthquake and an increase in energy release of 31.6 times.[7]

Earthquakes with magnitudes 6.0 or greater are generally considered significant events and have the potential to cause widespread damage. Each year, 70 to 75 damaging earthquakes occur throughout the world. Geographically, the Asian Pacific Rim (from Japan to Indonesia), also known as the Ring of Fire, is the most seismically active area in the world.

A proportion of earthquakes result in a phenomenon known as a *tsunami*. Tsunamis are created when large volumes of ocean or sea water are displaced, usually by undersea earthquakes. The majority of tsunamis occur after subduction zone earthquakes, in which one plate moves vertically with respect to the other. This upward movement displaces a large volume of water at the epicenter of the earthquake. The resulting waves often go undetected in the open sea as the wavelength of the displacement is long and the amplitude is small. However, as the displacement reaches shallow water, the crest of the wave can build and reach many meters in height. The rise in sea level of a tsunami is often preceded by what is known as a "drawback," or a negative displacement of water, which can expose areas of shoreline that are normally underwater.

The majority of tsunamis occur in the Pacific Ocean, although they can and do occur in all oceans and seas on earth. The destruction caused by tsunamis is related both to the height of the actual tidal wave and to the subsequent rise in sea level, which can cause devastating flooding in heavily populated coastal areas. This was demonstrated dramatically during the 2011 Japan earthquake and tsunami, which at the time of this writing was responsible for an estimated 20 000 deaths, when factoring in the missing.

10.6.2   Early Detection and Warning Systems

Most earthquakes strike with little or no warning, and they can occur at any time of year and at any time of day. Despite constant monitoring of seismic activity and geographic features, the ability to predict or detect a significant earthquake in time to warn communities and to mitigate its effects is limited. With continued improvement in understanding how to predict the timing and location of earthquakes, preventing loss of life may be more feasible in the future. At present, however, updating building codes and improving land use and engineering legislation remains the most viable way to mitigate the impact of earthquakes.

Tsunamis, because they are triggered and preceded by other geologic events, lend themselves more readily to warning and alert systems. Tsunami warning systems use seismographs to detect earthquakes and then use the data to alert populations that a subsequent tsunami may occur. While tsunami waves can travel at up to 1000 km/h, seismic waves travel much faster, at more than 14 000 km/h. Thus, the detection of an earthquake can precede arrival of a tsunami. A complete tsunami warning and response system includes this detection of seismic activity followed by monitoring of conditions at sea using specialized buoy systems, such as the Deep Ocean Assessment and Reporting of Tsunamis (http://nctr.pmel.noaa.gov/Dart/). These buoys have both an ocean surface component that measures sea levels and ocean floor pressure sensors. Unfortunately, it is impossible to predict with 100% accuracy which earthquakes will precipitate tsunamis. Thus, these systems create a large number of false-positive alerts.

Naturally, an effective warning system requires not only the ability to detect earthquakes and tsunamis, but also the ability to communicate the danger to at-risk populations. Several regional and international warning systems exist, most notably the Pacific Tsunami Warning System, Indian Ocean Tsunami Warning System, and Tsunami Early Warning and Mitigation System in the Northeast Atlantic, Mediterranean, and connected seas.

10.6.3 Acute Hazards and Effects

Earthquake forces cause disruption of gas lines, power grids, water supplies, communications, and other components of infrastructure in addition to the physical damage caused to buildings and other structures. These massive geologic energy releases can also trigger other natural events, such as floods, landslides, avalanches, tsunamis, and events related to humanmade structures (eg, fires, leaking of toxic materials, downed electrical wires). These examples of secondary disasters are of real concern after any earthquake that strikes near a human population center.

10.6.4 Clinical Implications: Immediate and Long Term

US Geological Survey
Part of the US Department of the Interior, the US Geological Survey (USGS) collects, monitors, analyzes, and provides scientific understanding about natural resource conditions, issues, and problems. A major goal of the USGS is to reduce the vulnerability of the people and areas most at risk from natural hazards. The USGS Earthquake Hazards program (http://earthquake.usgs.gov/) and Volcano Hazards Program (http://volcanoes.usgs.gov/) provide up-to-date global information about seismic and volcanic activity, respectively. The USGS also provides timely information on wildfires, hurricanes, floods, drought, and tsunamis. For more information about the USGS, refer to the Web site at http://www.usgs.gov/.

Demand for health care is greatest in the period immediately after the earthquake, with studies showing peaks between 12 hours and 3 days after the event. Data from the 1995 earthquake in Nishinomiya, Japan, and the 1999 earthquake in Taiwan suggest that serious injury is most common among the very young and the elderly.[8,9] The data also suggest that people with preexisting disabilities are at higher risk for injury, perhaps because of inability to quickly flee collapsing structures or to free themselves effectively. Another study of the casualties after the Taiwan earthquake indicates that casualties are higher in areas closer to the earthquake epicenter, areas with fewer physicians per 10 000 residents, and areas with fewer hospital beds per 10 000 people.[8]

Not surprisingly, these data suggest that the presence of strong medical infrastructure may be protective. However, in many instances, health care infrastructure has been damaged and therefore cannot be relied on to provide aid for casualties. If local hospitals are still operational after an earthquake, emergency departments are likely to see a surge of patients within the first 24 to 48 hours after the event, highlighting the need for patient surge planning at medical centers that may be involved in disaster response. A study of the patients treated in an academic medical center after the 1999 Marmara, Turkey, earthquake found that 645 patients were seen at the hospital for earthquake-related trauma in the 50 days following the earthquake.[10] A total of 271 (42%) were seen in the first 24 hours. The most common surgical procedures were fasciotomy, tube thoracostomy, and open reduction with internal fixation, but it should be noted that this hospital was a referral hospital and therefore attracted the most critical casualties. In addition to orthopedic injuries, hypothermia and other forms of exposure injury may be prevalent after an earthquake, depending on the climate and season in which the event occurs.

Care for earthquake casualties in the immediate aftermath of an earthquake typically focuses on orthopedic and soft-tissue trauma, including wound care and operative and closed management of fractures. Because of the typical increase in prevalence of head injuries, neurosurgical intervention will also be important. Because of the high demand for surgical intervention, anesthesiology is also an important component of care in the postearthquake environment. Deep sedation for surgical procedures and pain management with narcotic medication are important elements of the response to earthquake injuries.

In the period immediately after an earthquake, crush injuries, long-bone fractures, head trauma, and superficial injuries such as lacerations and contusions predominate.[11,12] Most of these injuries are caused by collapsing structures. Crush injuries are one of the most common types of injury after an earthquake. Crush syndrome is a specific, complicated pathophysiologic condition precipitated by reperfusion of crushed tissue and release of potassium, myoglobin, and other normally intracellular molecules and electrolytes. As described in Chapter 6, "Explosions and Traumatic Disasters," crush syndrome can cause direct cardiac toxicity, renal failure, and rhabdomyolysis and can be fatal without prompt treatment. Recognition of this syndrome and provision of intravenous crystalloid resuscitation before and immediately after rescue is a vital part of disaster medical response to earthquakes. Because concentrations of several serum enzymes, most importantly creatine kinase, are elevated in a large number of earthquake crush syndrome victims, there is a need for laboratory facilities capable of measuring and monitoring these serum enzymes in the medical response to earthquakes.[13] Renal dialysis may also be needed in severe cases or when resuscitation is not instituted promptly. In fact, in the experience following the Marmara earthquake in Turkey, a total of 639 casualties with renal complications were registered, of whom 477 needed dialysis.[14]

Mortality rates after an earthquake are dependent on multiple factors. A study of the Armenian earthquake of 1988 showed that the mortality rate for those inside buildings was 55.1% but was only 8.8% for those outside when the earthquake struck.[15] An analysis of injuries caused by this disaster illustrates that of more than 4800 patients admitted to hospitals throughout Armenia, more than 39% had combined injuries; superficial lacerations, head injuries, lower-extremity injury, crush syndrome, and upper-extremity trauma were the most common conditions.[15]

Asphyxiation from dust and debris created by the collapse of structures has also been hypothesized to be a significant cause of mortality after earthquakes, especially among those trapped in collapsed structures. This is supported by findings of oropharyngeal soot identified in the bodies of many casualties in the Armenian earthquake.[15]

Length of time trapped also affects survival probability. A study of mortality after the 1980 southern Italy earthquake suggests that the probability of live rescue drops from 87.9% on the day of the earthquake to 35.3% 24 hours after the event to nearly 0% at 4 days out.[16] In the 2010 Haiti earthquake, survivors were rescued from rubble in Port-au-Prince several days after the earthquake, and again in the 2011 Japan earthquake and tsunami a few were rescued days later, but these cases were exceptional. Most successful rescues were made immediately after the earthquake, in many cases by ordinary people using unsophisticated means of extrication.

10.6.5 Public Health Considerations

While much attention is paid to the acute phase of the response to earthquakes and other disasters, health effects of the event can last for weeks or months. The displacement of people and destruction of medical infrastructure can create health hazards that extend well beyond the immediate postdisaster time frame. Several studies suggest that exacerbation of chronic disease, often untreated in the immediate aftermath of earthquakes, is an important contributor to morbidity and mortality in displaced populations.[17-19] In a study of patients presenting to a Red Cross hospital in Banda Aceh, Indonesia, after the 2004 tsunami, 21% of cases seen in a 2-week period beginning 22 days after the tsunami were related to respiratory disease, 17% were related to a variety of chronic illnesses, 9.8% were related to trauma, and 9% were related to gastrointestinal complaints.[18] This corroborates that within 1 to 2 weeks after the tsunami or earthquake, infectious disease complaints, health effects of displacement, and conditions related to chronic illness will begin to account for the bulk of new patient consultations and that traumatic injury will remain an important source of illness for some time. For example, the public health issues, threat analysis, and long-term effects of the radiation leaks following the 2011 Japan earthquake and tsunami are still being determined.

The sheltering options available to displaced persons also have an effect on health outcomes of the affected population and should be considered when planning the long-term response. One study suggests that those living in temporary shelters were almost 1.7 times as likely to seek care as those living in permanent shelters.[18] The health needs of people in smaller, less organized temporary camps are generally greater than those of people living in larger, better organized systems of dwellings.[19] The Haiti earthquake of 2010 serves as yet another illustration of the need for more permanent sheltering options.[20] A study of the inhabitants of the large tent camps around Port-au-Prince 1 week after the earthquake found that respiratory infections, gastrointestinal problems, and genitourinary complaints were the most prevalent ailments. The study also demonstrated that children are particularly vulnerable, with 25% of all patients seen being under 5 years old. Malnutrition was an additional problem in the camps and was encountered in a number of the patients seen in this study.

In addition to traumatic injuries and medical problems related to lack of adequate shelter, several studies have shown that morbidity and mortality from cardiovascular disease also increases after earthquakes, presumably from the stress of the event, and potentially from disruption of medical infrastructure or lack of access to cardiac medications. After the Northridge, California, earthquake of 1994, investigators found an increased rate of cardiac mortality on the day of the event with a decline thereafter.[21] This finding has been replicated in a number of other studies showing both immediate and short-term risk of myocardial infarction after earthquakes, which can persist for years after the event.[22-25]

As with many types of natural and human-caused disasters, earthquakes produce significant psychological effects in the populations that experience them. After the 2007 Pisco, Peru, earthquake, more than 25% of one study population exhibited symptoms of posttraumatic stress disorder (PTSD).[26] Not surprisingly, this increased prevalence of acute stress reaction has also been seen after tsunamis, with an increase of symptoms being seen after a number of these events, including the 2004 Indian Ocean tsunami.[27] In a study of the 2004 Niigata-Chuetsu earthquake in Japan, factors including female sex, physical injury as a result of the earthquake, and feeling strong aftershocks were associated with increased psychological stress.[28] Living in temporary shelter and separation from family members and familiar people on the night of the earthquake were associated with delayed recovery at 5 months after the event. These data emphasize the need for psychological first aid (PFA) and other mental health interventions as parts of effective earthquake response.

10.6.6   Prevention and Mitigation of Future Events

Many techniques are employed to make buildings more resistant to earthquake damage. During the violent shaking that occurs during earthquakes, the strength of the building is important. Crucial to building safety is *ductility*, or the ability of a material to deform to a significant degree before failing. The most basic measure to reduce earthquake damage is the use of reinforced concrete, which is building concrete with steel beams embedded throughout the slabs. Lack of building codes in Port-au-Prince and the infrequent use of reinforced concrete to build homes and other structures in this area are thought to be two important contributors to the massive loss of life seen in the 2010 Haiti earthquake.[29]

In the United States, building codes for structures in seismically active areas have strict requirements for the ability to withstand the force of earthquakes. Sophisticated technologies include base isolation, which is the decoupling of the above-ground super-structure of a building and its foundation, and vibration dampening, which helps to decrease building displacement by balancing weight shift of the structure. Base isolation decreases the transmission of ground vibration through the building by allowing flexibility between the building structure and base. One method of vibration dampening uses large pendulums in the interior of the building that move opposite to the motion of the rest of the building in order to decrease the overall displacement of the structure.

Prevention and mitigation steps have limitations, as shown by the devastation caused by the 2011 Japan earthquake, which had a 9.0 magnitude measured on the Richter scale. Damage and structural collapse are still very real threats even in well-prepared countries where such events may occur.

10.7   FLOODS

Flooding is the most common disaster in the world. In 2008, there were more than 166 flooding disasters worldwide. On average, 100 people lose their lives and flood damage exceeds $2 billion each year. In the United States, 90% of all natural disasters involve flooding. According to the Federal Emergency Management Agency (FEMA), from January 2000 to March 2007, there were 62 flooding disasters in the United States that required federal assistance. In 2008, there were 82 flood-related deaths with 54 attributed to flash flooding.[30] Although floods may be more predictable than some other types of natural disasters, they are largely unpreventable and usually prolonged.

10.7.1   Causes and Characteristics

Floods can be categorized as *regional, flash, ice-jam, dam-levee failure, debris or landslides, mudflow,* and *sea-level rise.* The regional geographic conditions that make a particular type of flooding more likely is important for situational awareness, as well as for planning and overall operational preparedness.

Regional floods occur seasonally when winter or spring rains couple with melting snow and fill water basins too quickly with too much water. These types of floods are usually associated with slow-moving, low-pressure or frontal storm systems. The floods that occurred in the Mississippi River Basin in 1993 caused more than $300 million in damage.

Flash floods occur in a matter of minutes to several hours with little to no warning. They can cause flood waves in excess of 30 feet and can occur miles from an actual rainfall area. These types of floods are particularly dangerous because they can produce large and dramatic rises in water levels and have flow velocities capable of propelling large quantities of debris. Even relatively small quantities of water or water rushing at low speeds can be dangerous, as it takes just 2 feet of water to move an automobile.

Flash floods are the leading weather-related killer in the United States. They can occur within a few minutes or hours of excessive rainfall, a dam or levee failure, or a sudden release of water held by an ice jam. Urban areas are also prone to flash flooding because of the high percentage of surface area that it covered by streets and buildings, preventing water from being absorbed into the ground. Desert regions experience a similar phenomenon when heavy rains cannot be absorbed into the ground quickly enough and raging flash floods cascade through seemingly quiet dried river beds and washes miles from the deluged regions. Because underwater debris and road damage increase the potential for injury and death, flash floods are also known as *blind traps*.

Ice-jam floods occur when rivers partially or totally freeze and jammed ice acts as a dam that causes water to back up upstream. Eventually, water overflows river banks and causes flooding.

Dam and levee-failure floods are usually due to excessive water buildup behind a levee or dam. Examples of this are the Johnstown, Pennsylvania, flood of 1889 that killed more than 2200 people and the floods that occurred in New Orleans in 2005 when the levees surrounding New Orleans failed.

Debris and landslide floods are generally caused by the accumulation of debris, mud, rocks, logs or other large objects that converge in a channel or narrowed area and form a temporary dam that prevents the normal flow of water. As water pressure builds up behind the dam, it eventually overwhelms the dam, breaches it, and becomes a flash flood. *Mudflow floods* can occur when volcanic activity melts mountain snows or glaciers, releasing large quantities of water and mud.

Sea-level rise floods are directly tied to a rise in sea level. Sea-level rise is generally caused by a variety of factors including storm-related activities such as hurricanes, typhoons, tsunamis, or the timing of tides. There is a growing concern that climate change may also play a factor in sea levels rising. Floods of this type can destroy shorelines through erosion and cause salinity intrusion, leading to soil and aquifer contamination.

10.7.2 Early Detection and Warning Systems

Monitoring the local and national weather service that is charged with providing warning for floods can save lives, reduce flood damage to property, and decrease community losses. The success of any flood warning system will depend on many things, including the awareness of the exposed population regarding flood hazards, the amount of advance warning given, the availability of trained staff and supplies, and the efficiency and reliability of the warning system. An educated public is better able to respond to a flood advisory. Populations at risk for flooding, especially for flash flooding, should be aware of their risk as well as the relevant terminology. NWS warning terminology includes the following:

➤ *Flood watch*: A flood is possible. Tune in to National Oceanic and Atmospheric Administration (NOAA) weather radio, commercial radio, or television for information.

➤ *Flash flood watch*: Flash flooding is possible. Be prepared to move to higher ground; listen to NOAA weather radio for information.

➤ *Flood warning*: Flooding is occurring or will occur soon. If advised to evacuate, do so immediately.

➤ *Flash flood warning*: A flash flood is occurring; seek higher ground immediately.

10.7.3   Acute Hazards and Effects

Floods can cause massive physical damages, including the destruction of buildings, cars, sewage systems, power grids, bridges, and roadways. They may additionally cause injury, illness, and death in humans and livestock. Because of massive physical damage and loss of human-worker productivity, floods can cause major economic decline in affected areas. Rebuilding costs, increased cost of food due to crop shortages, and a decline in tourism can all contribute to economic hardship. Floods can also be triggered by other natural events such as earthquakes and hurricanes, thereby compounding the effects of those events.

The secondary effects of floods include the contamination and subsequent scarcity of drinking water, a shortage of crops and food supply, and the local extinction of intolerant plant and animal species. Contamination of the water supply can lead to unhygienic conditions, which may increase disease prevalence. Floods are related to an increase in waterborne (typhoid fever, cholera, leptospirosis, and hepatitis A) and vector-borne (malaria, dengue and dengue hemorrhagic fever, yellow fever, and West Nile fever) diseases. Because of massive structural damage, tetanus is also typically prevalent after major floods.

10.7.4   Clinical Implications: Immediate and Long Term

Injuries during floods will vary depending on several factors, including the flood characteristics (eg, depth and velocity of flood waters), the location of people during a flood (eg, indoor, outdoors, in vehicles), and population characteristics (eg, age, health, concentration of people, special needs groups). More densely populated areas in flood-prone locales are more likely to suffer higher numbers of injuries and deaths. Flood warnings with subsequent evacuation become a key factor in averting and reducing death and injuries.

Injury patterns and deaths during flooding frequently involve motor vehicle accidents in which individuals drown after being submerged in roadways or streams. Roadways are particularly dangerous during floods. It only takes 6 inches of water to reach the bottom of most modern automobiles, which can result in sudden loss of control. When water levels reach 1 foot, many vehicles will begin to float. Rushing water only 2 feet deep will carry away many vehicles, including most sport-utility vehicles and small trucks. Serious injuries or deaths are often caused by the force of fast water flow, various forms of debris, and vehicles being swept away by flood waters. In the initial aftermath of the flood, morbidity and mortality are generally attributed to typical soft-tissue and traumatic injuries and drowning.

10.7.5   Public Health Considerations

Health effects of a flood are not limited to the traumatic injuries acquired as a direct result of the flood waters or debris. Secondary contamination of water supplies from sewage and vector overgrowth from pooling of water are issues of concern over the long term. In the days to weeks after a flood, there is potential for increased fecal-oral transmission of disease, especially in areas where the population did not have access to clean water and sanitation before the event. Diarrheal diseases begin just weeks after flooding, especially if the affected individuals stay in their flooded homes or if there is standing water in the yard. This holds true in developed countries as well as underdeveloped nations. Typical diarrheal illnesses seen after flooding include cholera, cryptosporidiosis, nonspecific diarrhea, poliomyelitis, rotavirus, typhoid, and paratyphoid.

With a lack of sanitation and increased prevalence of stagnant water, there are also increased rates of vector-borne diseases (eg, spread by mosquitoes or rodents). In areas with increased chemical loads, especially industrial chemicals, there is an increased opportunity for a chemical exposure and contamination.

Mold exposure is a lasting health hazard following flooding. Mold can develop in as short a time as 24 to 48 hours after water exposure. Although it is a naturally occurring substance, it can be detrimental to human health. It may cause allergic reactions, asthma episodes, infections, and other respiratory problems. Continued exposure to mold may result in nasal or sinus congestion; eye, nose, or throat irritation; and adverse effects on the nervous system.

10.7.6   Prevention and Mitigation of Future Events

Reducing the impact of floods is both a personal and a community responsibility. Individuals must act appropriately before, during, and after a flood event.[31,32] Education is a key factor in understanding the potential impact of floods on people. Communities that engage in activities to reduce the effect of flooding, such as aggressive public information programs, mapping and regulating areas that are flood prone, and having flood damage reduction strategies, experience significantly lower levels of flood-related casualties. Communities also need to plan for the aftermath of flooding. This includes consideration of populations such as the elderly, the mentally ill, those with economic hardships, and others who may have difficulty accessing disaster relief agencies such as FEMA and the American Red Cross.

Personal measures that can be taken before a flood include avoiding building in flood-prone areas; elevating and reinforcing foundations if building in flood-prone areas is unavoidable; elevating electrical panels, furnaces, and ventilation systems; installing check valves in sewer traps to prevent floodwaters from backing up into household drains; sealing basement and foundation walls to prevent or reduce water seepage into homes; knowing and practicing evacuation routes before a flood occurs; and having a family plan in place.

10.8   HEAT EMERGENCIES

Heat emergencies typically occur during prolonged periods of excessively hot, humid weather (heat waves). The Centers for Disease Control and Prevention (CDC) estimated that from 1999 to 2003 there were a total of 3442 deaths attributed to extreme heat, with an average of 688 annually. The incidence of heat-related illness and death appears to be on the rise because of increasing land and sea temperatures in the United States. Heat waves are the leading environmental cause of death in the United States, and the number of deaths from extreme heat events often exceeds that of all other weather-related sources combined.

10.8.1   Causes and Characteristics

As stated, a heat wave is a prolonged period of heat and humidity. Extreme heat events are defined as a temperature/humidity level that remains markedly above the average high values for the region during a comparable period. Extreme heat events are defined not only by looking at the absolute temperature, but also by considering other environmental factors, such as humidity, air circulation, and nighttime temperature fluctuations. Mass outdoor gatherings can result in hundreds or even thousands of people who may need treatment for heat-related illnesses.

10.8.2   Early Detection and Warning Systems

The NWS will initiate an alert if the local heat index is expected to rise above 105°F to 110°F for at least 2 consecutive days. The "heat index" is a measure of how hot it really feels when relative humidity is factored with the actual air temperature. The alert procedures include giving heat index values with zone and city forecasts and issuing special alert notices to the public detailing the heat risk, who is most at risk, and safety tips. The NWS also will assist state and local health officials in preparing civil emergency messages, if needed, and release information on heat-related risks to the media and via its own radio station.

10.8.3   Acute Hazards and Effects

The hazards and effects from a heat-related disaster are the combined effects of environmental temperature, humidity, and the duration of exposure. Contributing factors include hydration status, degree of work-stress effort, and underlying health status. The use of personal protective equipment (PPE), and working in enclosed or poorly ventilated spaces may also be contributing factors.

10.8.4   Clinical Implications: Immediate and Long Term

Illness during heat waves occurs when the body can no longer maintain its temperature regulation homeostasis because of the elevated ambient temperature. Air temperature is the greatest factor affecting the onset of heat-related illness, but the humidity and motion of the air can also contribute. The human body has several mechanisms for cooling: *evaporative heat loss* is cooling though perspiration; *conduction* is heat loss through contact with cooler surfaces; *convection* is heat loss through water or air motion around a person's body; and *radiant heat loss* is thermal radiation being released from the body. When the air temperature approaches normal human body temperature, most heat loss occurs through evaporative cooling. Greater humidity levels slow the body's ability to perspire effectively, so the combination of high humidity levels and high air temperature can result in serious heat illness.

Several factors may contribute significantly to an individual's likelihood of developing heat-related illness. Groups at risk include the elderly; the very young; individuals with comorbid conditions such as cardiovascular illnesses, endocrine disorders, renal dysfunction, and nervous system disorders; those with cognitive impairment or who are taking psychotropic/neuroleptic medication; and those who live in poorly ventilated buildings that do not shelter them from direct sunlight.

Heat illnesses can span a continuum from minor to life-threatening illness. The following is a list of commonly seen heat illnesses.

Heat cramps: Heat cramps are pain and cramping, thought to be an effect of hyponatremia. Results of physical examination are normal, including body temperature in most cases. Blood work may show hyponatremia, hypokalemia, hypomagnesemia, hypophosphatemia, or respiratory alkalosis. Clinicians should be aware that rhabdomyolysis may present after similar exposure and should rule out this condition and its complications through laboratory testing. Treatment includes rest in a comfortably cool area, oral or parenteral fluid, and electrolyte repletion as needed.

Heat edema: Heat edema is heat-related swelling of the hands and feet related to peripheral vasodilation. Physical examination will show extremity edema but should not show other physical findings that would be more consistent with heart failure. Laboratory and other diagnostic testing may be undertaken to rule out heart failure or renal failure, if indicated. Treatment includes avoidance of excessive heat and elevation of the legs.

Heat syncope: Syncope due to exposure to extreme temperature elevation is thought to be secondary to peripheral venous pooling, which results in orthostasis. It can occur after either prolonged standing or quickly rising from a seated or supine position. Treatment includes lowering the individual slowly to the ground followed by rehydration.

Heat exhaustion: Excessive perspiration or diaphoresis in extreme heat can result in heat exhaustion. The symptoms include malaise, copious perspiration, fatigue, nausea and vomiting, lightheadedness, and headache. Physical examination will demonstrate a diaphoretic patient who may also be tachycardic and hypotensive, with an elevated core body temperature less than 104°F. The individual will be alert and oriented. Treatment should include cooling, removal from hot environment, and oral or parenteral rehydration.

Heat stroke: Heat stroke is the most serious form of heat-related illness and can be fatal. If heat exhaustion is untreated, it can progress to heat stroke. The individual typically has a core body temperature of 104.9°F or greater. Physical examination will demonstrate a person with abnormal mental status and tachycardia. Some individuals may cease perspiring by the point at which they develop heat stroke; this should be considered a late finding of concern. Other associated complications can include coagulopathy, thrombocytopenia, hepatic failure, and heart failure. Treatment consists of rapid, aggressive cooling including ice packs to the groin and axilla, spray mist, and fans, as well as parenteral fluids. Other resuscitative measures to support airway, breathing, and circulation should be taken as needed. Core body temperature should be closely monitored. Rapid sequence induction medications should not include paralytics that might induce hyperkalemia, such as succinylcholine.

10.8.5   Public Health Considerations

Heat-related illnesses and deaths are typically preventable. The public health system can mitigate the potential for illness and death secondary to extreme heat events by implementing a number of measures. Alert systems can be activated that provide early warnings of the expected extreme heat to the public and emphasize the potential health risks and how to avoid them. Public cooling centers or air-conditioned shelters can be established, taking care to target their use toward those most at risk in the population.

10.8.6   Prevention and Mitigation of Future Events

Government agencies and municipal authorities may distribute free or subsidized air conditioning units or fans or activate a policy for forgiveness of public utility bill nonpayment or modified bill payment protocols. At a building design level, policies should include comfortable cooling, adequate ventilation, and mechanical aids to assist radiant and convective heat loss.

Individuals can take precautions against heat-related illness by wearing light-colored and lightweight clothing, planning to stay inside a cool environment during the hottest hours of the day, ensuring adequate fluid intake, and avoiding alcohol intake.

For occupational and athletic pursuits that may increase risk of heat-related illness, recommendations include institution of pre-event medical examinations, provision of adequate cool rest areas and fluids, and modification of the work-rest or exercise-rest cycle to adapt to higher outdoor temperatures.

An important point is protecting the disaster workforce from heat-related illness. The austere and challenging environmental conditions and the use of PPE may contribute to the onset of heat-related illness in this group during many typical response scenarios. Continual monitoring and preventive action steps should always be implemented.

10.9 HURRICANES, CYCLONES, AND TYPHOONS

Hurricane is the name given to a subset of storms produced around the equator of the earth. These storms are characterized by a rotating storm core that is fueled by warm, moist air that rises and eventually condenses to produce heavy rainfall. In the Indian Ocean region they are known as *cyclones*, in the Western Pacific they are called *typhoons*, and in the Atlantic and Eastern Pacific Oceans they are *hurricanes*. All these terms refer to essentially the same phenomenon of warm-core/low-pressure, rotating storms with a central area of relative calm known as the "eye" and a surrounding area characterized by high wind speeds and intense precipitation.

Hurricanes are among the most destructive and deadly natural events and are capable of causing significant injury, loss of life, and extensive property and infrastructure damage. Worldwide, between 1900 and 2004, there were 77 hurricanes that resulted in at least 1000 deaths each.[32] The most lethal among these occurred in Bangladesh in 1970 and resulted in more than 300 000 deaths. Developing nations bore the brunt of this loss of life, with 50 of these storms occurring in developing countries in Southeast Asia and another 15 in the Caribbean and Central America. The most lethal hurricane in US history, a category 4 storm that occurred in 1900, killed between 6000 and 12 000 people in Galveston, Texas. Most of these deaths were caused by storm surge and may have been preventable today through the use of hurricane warning systems.[33]

10.9.1 Causes and Characteristics

Hurricane intensity and severity is classified from 1 to 5 according to the Saffir-Simpson scale. The damage caused by a hurricane increases by a factor of about four for each one-point increase on this scale. Hurricane categories based on this scale are determined by wind speed ranging from up to 95 mph for category 1 to greater than 155 mph for category 5. The category 3, 4, and 5 storms are considered major hurricanes. In general, more severe category 5 storms cause more devastation, but even less powerful "tropical depressions" and "tropical storms" can be very destructive, largely because of resultant flooding, landslides, and torrential rain, as opposed to the high wind speeds and storm surge that cause the majority of damage in more powerful storms. The sheer size of the hurricane is also a factor; in 2008, Hurricane Ike, as it approached landfall on the Texas coast, had tropical storm–force winds that extended more than 200 miles across and hurricane-force winds that extended more than 100 miles across. *Storm surge* is the onshore rush of water caused by the powerful winds associated with the landfall of a hurricane. These secondary environmental effects are one of the hallmarks of hurricanes.

10.9.2   Early Detection and Warning Systems

The task of forecasting hurricanes and disseminating warnings about their approach to coastal areas is managed in the United States by the NWS through the National Hurricane Center headquartered in Miami, Florida. This agency tracks hurricanes and provides warnings about hurricanes in the Atlantic and eastern Pacific oceans and provides warning about their approach toward land. The Central Pacific Hurricane Center based in Hawaii monitors storms in the central north Pacific basin, and the Joint Typhoon Warning Center, also based in Hawaii and comanaged by the US Air Force and the US Navy, is responsible for detecting and forecasting storms in the northwest Pacific Ocean, south Pacific Ocean, and Indian Ocean. These services use a variety of detection and monitoring technology to monitor and predict storms, including satellite images, land-based Doppler radar, and direct measurements made by reconnaissance flights undertaken by the US government to measure and forecast storms as they develop. These prediction systems have drastically reduced morbidity and mortality caused by hurricanes in the United States, although their inconsistent application in developing countries still leaves millions of people at risk around the world.

10.9.3   Acute Hazards and Effects

Before the use of early warning systems, the bulk of the mortality from hurricanes and typhoons resulted from storm surge and other causes of acute trauma as the storms made landfall.[34] Because modern systems can now predict the place and time of hurricane landfall with some accuracy, much of the morbidity and mortality associated with these events has shifted from the acute phase of the event to the days and weeks following it. It should be noted that in developing nations without successfully implemented early warning systems, storm surge and trauma directly related to storms still account for the majority of injury and death.[32] In fact, a study of the risk factors for injury from Typhoon Saomei, which struck southern China in 2006, noted that failure to institute simple protective measures such as reinforcing doors and windows was among the most important risk factors for injury.[35] This study also found that because evacuations were not performed effectively before this storm, living in a home directly facing the ocean increased risk by 18 times compared to living in houses farther from the shore.

Despite the effectiveness of modern early warning systems, hurricanes still represent a significant natural hazard. In general, the effects of hurricanes are not limited to the morbidity and mortality directly attributable to the storm itself. In the days and weeks afterward, flooding can cause large standing pools of water, which contribute to the spread of waterborne and vector-borne illnesses. Crowding in shelters can lead to a poor standard of health and increased transmission of disease. Massive damage to infrastructure and widespread displacement of people from their homes and jobs can make it difficult to rebuild, greatly affecting the recovery process of the community, families, and individuals.

10.9.4   Clinical Implications: Immediate and Long Term

Studies of hurricane morbidity and mortality in the United States since the implementation of early warning systems and improvement to building codes note that, increasingly, injuries are associated with structural hazards such as downed power lines and with motor vehicle accidents.[32] A study of cause of death during the 2004 and 2005 hurricane seasons in Florida showed that, despite the violent winds and storm surge associated with the landfall of hurricanes, only 31% of deaths occurred during the actual impact phase of storms, while the postimpact phase accounted for 60%.[36] In addition, the majority of deaths were not due directly to trauma caused by winds or flooding from the storm but were indirectly caused by trauma sustained during preparations for, or cleanup and recovery after, the storm.

While the trend toward more indirect deaths and fewer drownings is clear in the United States, Hurricane Katrina proved an exception to this rule and deserves special consideration. Indeed, in Louisiana in 2005, some 40% of deaths related to Katrina were due to drowning, with other types of trauma accounting for 25% of deaths.[37] The greatest proportion of these drowning deaths were centered in the lower Ninth Ward of New Orleans, where residents faced not only the direct storm surge but catastrophic failure of levees resulting in large-scale flooding. Importantly, elderly people, especially those 75 years and older, were more likely to be storm victims, underscoring the importance of focused evacuation and warning efforts aimed at vulnerable populations.

Clinical management of casualties in the acutely affected communities is the initial concern. In preparing to care for these individuals, it is vital to understand injury and mortality patterns to design interventions and plan response. Analysis of presentations to emergency departments and Disaster Medical Assistance Team (DMAT) service locations in Mississippi after Hurricane Katrina found that the greatest proportion of presentations were for traumatic injuries, accounting for 21.8% of visits. Of these, most (91.6%) were for minor injuries such as lacerations and contusions. The most common illnesses identified in this study were skin and wound infections, upper and lower respiratory infections, rashes, and gastrointestinal complaints.[38] The most common specific types of injuries encountered included lacerations, contusions, and fractures, especially of the extremities. These injuries occur not only during the impact phase of the hurricane but during the pre-impact and postimpact phases as well. This underscores that care for orthopedic and soft-tissue injuries must be included in disaster response planning.

Clinical management of sheltered populations is an important consideration after evacuation for hurricanes. Because of the potential for massive infrastructure damage, individuals may be displaced for long periods of time, and the local health care infrastructure may be too badly damaged to continue caring for them. Both the sheltering site and the clinical services demands will likely be placed on distant communities not affected by the hurricane. Two of the most significant sheltering and medical care operations in US history were the establishment of the "Katrina Clinic" at the Houston Astrodome and the Dallas Convention Center Medical Unit, both following Hurricane Katrina.[39] The Houston operation provided care for more than 25 000 evacuees and provided more than 15 000 clinical patient encounters in the wake of the storm. Analysis of the diagnoses made in the various treatment areas of the Katrina Clinic operation indicates that, while musculoskeletal complaints and injury were important reasons for visits, circulatory, digestive and respiratory complaints accounted for more visits at all levels of care, from shelters to catastrophic medical treatment areas.[39]

The Dallas Convention Center Medical Unit operated for a 16-day period during the aftermath of Hurricanes Katrina and Rita.[40] As reported in the *Journal of Trauma*, this medical unit provided a total of 10 367 emergent or urgent care visits, which averaged 619 care visits per day of operation. Only 236 patients (2.9%) were transported to area emergency departments, and there were no deaths reported. The most common complaint during the first 3 days was wound management; however, also seen were acute gastrointestinal illness and acute exacerbations of chronic illness, notably from asthma, diabetes mellitus, and cardiovascular disorders. This population had already been evacuated from the storm impact area hundreds of miles away and showed an expected shift away from traumatic and toward more medical complaints. This serves to highlight the need for a wide array of medical services in response to hurricanes.

In this setting, management of chronic disease was also an important part of the medical response in many locations. A study of people arriving at American Red Cross shelters in Louisiana in the 2 weeks after Hurricane Katrina's landfall found that 56% of people had chronic medical conditions, 48% lacked medications that they needed to treat their conditions, and the presence of preexisting comorbidity was significantly associated with the likelihood of needing emergency medical treatment on arrival.[41] Several studies have shown that the most commonly encountered preexisting medical conditions were hypertension, high cholesterol level, diabetes, psychiatric illness, and lung disease, including asthma.[41] In fact, analysis of patient presentations in New Orleans after Hurricane Katrina showed that 24.3% of all presentations were related to chronic medical conditions and 7.2% were for medication refills.[42] This suggests not only a need for practitioners familiar with the treatment of common chronic medical conditions in the area affected by a disaster but also the possible utility of point-of-distribution sites in responding to the medication refill needs of affected communities, allowing full treatment facilities to focus on the management of acute illness or exacerbations of chronic disease.

Interestingly, as many deaths were due to carbon monoxide (CO) poisoning as to drowning during the 2005 hurricane season in Florida, each accounting for 13% of the total mortality. The most common cause of death from CO poisoning was improper use of gasoline generators in the aftermath of storms. This important source of potential injury was again noted by researchers who analyzed poison center calls in the postimpact phase of Hurricane Ike in Texas in 2008 and found an increase in calls related to gasoline and CO exposure.[43]

Hypothermia and exposure-related illness is another important consideration after hurricanes. In 1999 in North Carolina, 19 cases of hypothermia were observed, resulting in at least one death. This is an especially important consideration when planning for the care of infants, who may be more susceptible to hypothermia and exposure-related illness.

10.9.5   Public Health Considerations

While disaster responders may be overwhelmed with the need for acute and subacute care after a hurricane, excess morbidity and mortality from these events has been shown to persist for some time after the initial response phase. A study of postdisaster excess mortality in the first half of 2006 found a 47% increase in deaths compared to the baseline population mortality rate. This was measured over a period of 6 months beginning in January 2006, 4 months after the landfall of Katrina in August 2005.[43] Other studies have demonstrated even higher rates of mortality up to 1 year after this disaster, suggesting that the true impact of a hurricane is often a long-term public health emergency.[44,45]

As with other disasters, excess morbidity and mortality due to cardiovascular disease has been observed after hurricanes and likely contributes to long-term increased mortality. Analysis of the incidence of acute myocardial infarction showed a threefold increase in incidence 2 years after Hurricane Katrina at one acute care hospital.[46] While only from a single-center study, this finding is consistent with the proposed effect of psychological stress after disasters and its effect on the incidence of cardiovascular disease.[47] The need for medical intervention for this type of illness is another important component of disaster medical response.

While physical injuries and illness are often the focus of disaster medical response, a growing body of literature supports the inclusion of and focus on care of psychological and mental health illness after disasters. Studies of people living in the Gulf Coast region of the United States after Hurricane Katrina have found that more than half of those surveyed reported mental health distress as long as 2 years after the disaster.[48] Another analysis of a small group of young people in this region found that 79% of the sample reported new onset of mental health symptoms in the year after the storm.[49] These figures suggest that disaster responders will benefit from familiarity with psychological first aid (PFA) or other acute counseling and mental health care techniques.

A long-held myth in disaster response, especially with regard to hydrometeorologic events, is that epidemic diseases naturally follow in their wake. This has been shown in large part to be false; in fact, most hurricanes and other disasters involving displacement of water do not result in large-scale infectious disease outbreaks. However, in certain circumstances, consideration of disease, especially endemic vector-borne disease, may be an important part of disaster response. Specifically, in tropical areas where diseases such as malaria and dengue fever are already endemic, several studies have shown that hurricanes can increase the burden of these diseases dramatically. One such example was Hurricane Flora, which is estimated to have contributed to 75 000 additional cases of malaria above baseline in Haiti in 1963 and 1964. Responders to disaster localities with endemic malaria and dengue fever should be prepared to treat these illnesses at higher than usual rates for several weeks after the event and should investigate local drug resistance patterns for *Plasmodium falciparum* parasites that cause malaria.

10.9.6 Prevention and Mitigation of Future Events

While early warning systems can effectively predict hurricane landfall and intensity, destruction from these events will continue to be significant as long as large population centers exist in hurricane paths in the Caribbean, US Gulf Coast, Southeast Asia, and other locales. Proper planning for evacuation and response are critical to minimize injury and loss of life. Clearly marked evacuation routes, evacuation drills, and awareness of the general public of routes, warning sirens, and emergency shelter locations will help to mitigate morbidity and mortality associated with these storms.

Municipalities can also map floodplains and other areas prone to flooding. This information can be used to promote proper land use planning and to build and operate flood control structures like dams and dykes. Municipalities can also ensure the appropriate precautions are taken to protect the community watershed so that sources of drinking water are not contaminated, as is common in hurricane and flooding events.

> **The National Hurricane Center**
>
> Located within the National Oceanic and Atmospheric Administration (NOAA), the National Hurricane Center (NHC) seeks to save lives, mitigate property loss, and improve economic efficiency by issuing tropical storm watches, warnings, and forecasts through analysis of hazardous weather patterns and by increasing understanding of these hazards through global outreach. For additional information, visit the NHC Web site at http://www.nhc.noaa.gov/.

10.10 TORNADOES

Tornadoes are among nature's most violent storms. While they can and do occur in most parts of the world, in the United States they occur most frequently in the midsection of the country ("tornado alley"). In the United States alone, 40 000 tornadoes occurred between 1950 and 2000. Forty-five of these tornadoes each killed more than 18 people.[50] In an average year, about 1000 tornadoes are reported across the United States, resulting in 87 deaths and more than 1500 injuries.[50]

On April 28, 2011, the NWS estimated 150 tornadoes tore across six southern states, resulting in more than 290 deaths and likely more than 1700 injuries (from preliminary reports available at the time of this writing). At least two-thirds of these deaths occurred in Alabama alone. Early reports also indicated that some of the tornadoes had wind speeds exceeding 200 mph. Less than one month later, on May 22, 2011, another series of tornadoes hit the Midwest, the largest of which struck the town of Joplin, Missouri. The tornado proved to be the most devastating in recent history, with more than 150 deaths and an estimated 3 billion dollars in damage. It also destroyed the community's medical center, severely limiting medical response capacity in the immediate aftermath of the tornado. The Joplin experience brought to the forefront the importance of patient evacuation and transport and mass casualty planning.

Tornadoes are common events throughout the United States. It is important that every responder and the general public understand the significant threat and basics of situational awareness regarding tornadoes. The following are some relevant key facts about tornadoes:

➤ Tornadoes can occur in a wide variety of sizes and shapes, from a few yards wide to more than a mile wide.

➤ Tornadoes can move very slowly or up to 60 mph.

➤ The vertical winds in tornadoes are capable of temporarily lifting heavy objects such as cars and people up to 100 feet into the air.

➤ Tornadoes can be very unpredictable and can change speed and direction very quickly.

➤ Many tornado deaths occur when motorists try to "outrun" a tornado.

➤ The safest place to be if a tornado approaches is in a permanent structure on the lowest level in an interior or basement room with no windows.

➤ Mobile homes and vehicles are the worst places to be if a tornado approaches. Both can be easily picked up and tossed by a tornado.

10.10.1 Causes and Characteristics

Tornadoes are severe windstorms that are characterized by a rapidly rotating column of air extending from a thunderstorm to the ground. The air column converges into a funnel-shaped vortex and develops out of powerful thunderstorms. Tornadoes are very dangerous and can destroy entire communities while causing widespread injuries and fatalities.

Tornado wind speed and the damage inflicted was traditionally assessed and graded by means of the Fujita scale. Developed in 1971, the Fujita scale categorizes the intensity of tornadoes by the damage they cause. To better clarify and understand the destructive nature of tornadoes, the NWS and the NOAA in February 2007 developed an enhanced Fujita (EF) scale. First utilized for an EF-5 tornado in May 2007 that destroyed an estimated 95% of homes and businesses in a small town of 1500 residents,[51] the EF scale provides a more accurate assessment of tornado damage by aligning wind speeds more closely with associated storm damage (see Table 10-5). The scale uses three-second gusts estimated at the point of damage. A review of the EF scale damage indicators is available at http://www.spc.noaa.gov/efscale/ef-scale.html.

TABLE 10-5 Wind Speed Estimates for the Original and Enhanced Fujita (EF) Scales for Tornado Damage (as implemented in the United States, February 2007)*

Fujita Scale			Derived EF Scale		Operational EF Scale	
F No.	Fastest ¼ mi, mph	3-s Gust, mph	EF No.	3-s Gust, mph	EF No.	3-s Gust, mph
0	40–72	45–78	0	65–85	0	65–85
1	73–112	79–117	1	86–109	1	86–110
2	113–157	118–161	2	110–137	2	111–135
3	158–207	162–209	3	138–167	3	136–165
4	208–260	210–261	4	168–199	4	166–200
5	261–318	262–317	5	200–234	5	>200

*The EF Scale, derived from the Fujita Scale, is a set of wind estimates (not measurements) based on 3-second gusts at the point of damage caused by the tornado. The operational EF Scale (which is a slight modification of the derived EF Scale) is used by the NWS to rate the strength of tornadoes in the United States.

10.10.2   Early Detection and Warning Systems

While fatalities from tornadoes have declined dramatically during the past 100 years,[52] tornadoes still pose a significant threat to life and property. The decrease in fatality rates has been attributed to several factors, including improved quality of tornado warnings from the NWS, new and improved technologies to disseminate tornado warnings, and improved public response to tornado warnings.[53] Tornado sirens have been shown to be an effective tool in preventing injuries if blasted at least 20 minutes before the presence of the tornado.

The fact remains, however, that tornadoes can be deadly. Educating the public about the danger of tornadoes is critical. Particularly important is the public understanding of tornado terms:

➤ *Tornado watch*: Tornadoes are possible. Remain alert for approaching storms. Watch the sky and stay tuned to NOAA weather radio, commercial radio, or television for information.

➤ *Tornado warning*: A tornado has been sighted or indicated by weather radar. Take shelter immediately.

Most tornado warnings (and watches) are preceded by severe thunderstorm warnings, which are preceded by severe thunderstorm watches. In areas where tornadoes are common, these signals may indicate potential for tornado formation. It is important to understand that tornado warnings rarely occur without such a progression.

Understanding and having appropriate access to early warning devices is the first key step to mitigating the fatalities and injuries associated with a tornado. The second key is proper home-based or office- or work-based disaster plans that include appropriate sheltering steps taken when warnings are issued. Self- (and family) protection through proper sheltering during an impending tornado is attributed with saving countless lives.

10.10.3   Acute Hazards and Effects

While it is possible to forecast the potential for tornado formation, it is not possible to forecast that it will occur or where it will strike. Most tornadoes are unpredictable and move erratically. The damage from a tornado is a result of the high wind velocity and wind-blown debris. People who are outdoors during a tornado are at increased injury risk. The destruction caused by tornadoes may range from light to severe depending on the path of travel. Typically, structures of light construction, such as residential homes (and particularly mobile homes), suffer the greatest damage from tornadoes. Principal damage is likely to include structural damage to homes and businesses, power and other utility failures, and falling trees.

10.10.4   Clinical Implications: Immediate and Long Term

Studies have demonstrated that tornado-related injuries tend to be soft-tissue injuries in the forms of contusions, complex lacerations, and multiple extremity fractures. Wound infections can also commonly be seen secondary to the wound contamination. Tetanus vaccination, wound debridement, and antibiotics can be considered.

It is important to recognize that a large number of tornado-related injuries are actually suffered during rescue attempts, cleanup, and other post-tornado activities.[54] Rescue workers need to be aware of these post-tornado dangers, which include falling objects; risk of fire, electrocution, and explosions from damage to buildings, gas, and electrical lines; and the potential for lacerations and puncture wounds from broken glass and exposed nails. It should be noted that rescue workers can themselves be direct casualties of tornadoes along with local hospitals and treatment facilities.

10.10.5   Public Health Considerations

The widespread destruction and disruption to any community that has sustained damage from a tornado may likely create public health services demands. The disruption in public works and services (eg, electrical and gas services, roadways) can be significant. The need for general population sheltering may require public health oversight and surveillance. Tetanus immunization distribution may be needed because of the multitude of wounds sustained.

What to Do During a Tornado[55]	
IF YOU ARE:	**THEN:**
In a structure (eg, residence, small building, school, nursing home, hospital, factory, shopping center, high-rise building)	Go to a predesignated shelter area such as a safe room, basement, storm cellar, or the lowest building level. If there is no basement, go to the center of an interior room on the lowest level (closet, interior hallway) away from corners, windows, doors, and outside walls. Put as many walls as possible between you and the outside. Get under a sturdy table and use your arms to protect your head and neck. Do not open windows.
In a vehicle, trailer, or mobile home	Get out immediately, and go to the lowest floor of a sturdy, nearby building or a storm shelter. Mobile homes, even if tied down, offer little protection from tornadoes.
Outside with no shelter	Lie flat in a nearby ditch or depression, and cover your head with your hands. Be aware of the potential for flooding. Do not get under an overpass or bridge. You are safer in a low, flat location. Never try to "outrun" a tornado in urban or congested areas in a car or truck. Instead, leave the vehicle immediately for safe shelter. Watch out for flying debris. Flying debris from tornadoes causes most fatalities and injuries.

10.10.6   Prevention and Mitigation of Future Events

While much has been learned about the violent nature of tornadoes in the past 50 years, they continue to be a challenging problem for municipalities and rescue workers. To minimize morbidity and mortality related to the event, it is important to know what to do during a tornado. The following instructions apply to tornado warnings. If under a tornado warning, people should seek shelter immediately. Education and diligence in following safety guidelines are key to survival.

10.11   VOLCANIC ERUPTIONS

Volcanoes throughout the world are distributed primarily along the edges of continents, as well as along island chains and undersea mountain ranges. This ring of volcanoes correlates roughly with the intersections of the Earth's tectonic plates. Fifty percent of the known active volcanoes on Earth are along a circular region around the Pacific Ocean known as the "Ring of Fire."

Notable Volcanic Eruptions

Eruption	Year	Approximate Casualties	Major Cause of Morbidity/Mortality
Lakagigar (Laki), Iceland	1783	9000	Starvation
Unzen, Japan	1792	15 000	Volcano collapse, tsunami
Tambora, Indonesia	1815	92 000	Starvation
Krakatau, Indonesia	1883	36 000	Tsunami
Mont Pelée, Martinique	1902	30 000	Pyroclastic flows
Mount Saint Helens, Washington	1980	57	Asphyxiation from ash
Nevado del Ruiz, Colombia	1985	25 000	Mudflows

The number of people killed in volcanic eruptions over past centuries is estimated at 300 000. In recent decades, there have been an average of two to four fatal eruptions per year. An analysis of mortality showed that many deaths occurred in the first 24 hours.[56]

10.11.1   Causes and Characteristics

A simplified way to classify volcanoes is according to whether they are effusive or explosive. The most common type is *effusive*. With effusive volcanoes, molten rock (magma) flows down the slopes, covering great areas of land and creating a volcano type known as a *shield* (eg, Mauna Loa volcano in Hawaii). Such volcanoes eject large volumes of relatively viscous magma that flows slowly enough to allow the evacuation of the affected area; this causes a slowly expanding area of burned property.

Volcanoes categorized as *explosive* erupt less frequently but are characterized by greater violence. Air shock waves and shrapnel-like rock projectiles may affect distant communities. Mount Saint Helens is an example of an explosive volcano.

Some volcanoes can have features of both. Mount Etna, in Italy, is an example of a mainly effusive volcano, but it demonstrated explosive behavior in 2001 and 2002.

10.11.2   Early Detection and Warning Systems

Early warning systems vary by location, but they typically denote the probability of an eruption by either color codes or numeric alert levels. The US Geological Survey (USGS), for example, uses a four-tiered alert system with green, yellow, orange, and red denoting normal, advisory, watch, and warning levels, respectively. Communities in the proximity of volcanoes should be aware of the local risk of eruption.

10.11.3   Acute Hazards and Effects

Pyroclastic flows and mudslides are the most common direct cause of death associated with volcanic eruptions. Pyroclastic flows are associated with volcanoes producing viscous magma; they are extremely hot mixtures of gas, ash, pumice, and rocks. These flows may travel for great distances at more than 60 mph. Pyroclastic flows have been associated with the majority of volcano-related deaths over the past 400 years. Death from pyroclastic effects is due to intense heat and asphyxiation. In 1908, between 28 000 and 30 000 people were killed within minutes after the eruption of Mount Pele. The Mount Saint Helens eruption of 1980 saw similar effects as people were killed by intense heat and asphyxiation due to the intense pyroclastic flows.[57]

Mudflows and debris flows associated with volcanoes, known as *lahars*, are deadly volcanic phenomena. These are composed of water from rain, crater lakes, melted snow, or steam that mixes with volcanic debris to form mudflow. The mudflows are heavy and gravity-dependent and may travel rapidly for kilometers. Casualties may be overcome and buried under tons of fluid mud. These flows may also quite hot and can result in fatal thermal injury even if the victim is not totally buried. A large number of casualties could simply be trapped in mud and can require a long process of extrication and rescue. Crush syndrome is an important clinical consideration for these individuals.

The release of ash represents one of the most significant hazards associated with volcanic eruptions. Ash and dust may cause substantial visibility problems for many days after an eruption. Air filters in motor vehicles, electrical generators, and other critical machinery may quickly become clogged and inoperable. Ground accumulations of ash can cause stopping or vehicular damage. Small amounts of wet or dry pumice, ash, or dust make road surfaces extremely hazardous. Ash may settle on buildings and may lead to roof collapse. Buildings are at high risk of collapse due to ash deposits. Ash may be distributed over an extensive region and contribute to significant deterioration in air quality.

Electrical storms can often accompany volcanic eruptions. Electrical storms can cause fires, may damage electrical equipment, and may result in death or injury by lightning strike. In large volcanic eruptions, storm effects could involve communications, information technology, telemetry transmission, and emergency medical services (EMS) radio services.

Volcanic eruptions can cause interruption of electricity, fresh water, and sewage facilities because of the release of carbon dioxide, sulfur dioxide, hydrogen chloride, hydrogen sulfide, hydrogen fluoride, and CO. Sulfur dioxide mixed with steam from volcano or atmospheric water has resulted in acid rain with a pH as low as 2.0, and this acid rain could contaminate ground or fresh water and agricultural lands, resulting in long-term crop failure and possibly famine in the affected population.

10.11.4   Clinical Implications: Immediate and Long Term

Volcanoes and their eruptions can result in a wide range of health effects and kill people in a remarkably large number of ways.[58,59] Volcanic activity and eruption could involve areas hundreds of miles away, as a result of airborne dispersion of gases and ash, or even on a hemispheric to global scale because of impacts on climate.[60]

Thermal injury is as important as asphyxia in causing immediate deaths. The high temperature of the gases and entrained particles readily causes severe burns to skin and air passages, and the presence of both types of injury in an individual may combine to increase the delayed mortality risk from respiratory complications or infection of burns. Trauma from missiles or body displacement is also common, but the role of asphyxiant or irritant gases, as well as steam, remains unclear.

The hot mixture of particles and gases associated with eruptive and explosive phenomena presents a hazard due to the unsurvivable high temperatures (<200°C) and high overpressures (higher than hydrostatic pressures), as well as from the dense and irrespirable concentration of ash and dust causing laryngeal obstruction and asphyxia.

Carbon dioxide, sulfur dioxide, hydrogen chloride, hydrogen sulfide, hydrogen fluoride, and CO are among the more important gases emitted; however, few primary studies of the health effects of volcanic gases have been conducted. Those that exist are limited in terms of exposure assessment, so a clear picture of all health effects due to volcanic gas emission is still not available. Carbon dioxide and hydrogen sulfide pool in low-lying areas and represent a serious threat to individuals located within those regions. Hydrogen fluoride and hydrogen chloride become extremely corrosive when they make contact with water. As mentioned in the previous section, sulfur dioxide mixed with steam from volcano or atmospheric water can result in acid rain with a pH as low as 2.0. Sulfur dioxide is related to the incidence of acute respiratory symptoms due to volcanic emission.[61]

Table 10-6 summarizes the major toxic gases from volcanic eruption and the associated risks and therapy.[58]

The most common cause of death from a volcanic eruption is asphyxiation and laryngeal obstruction. Short- and long-term respiratory symptoms are described as resulting from the inhalation of volcanic ash, but they depend on several factors such as the concentration of total suspended particles in the air, the proportion of respirable particles (<10 μm in diameter) in the ash, frequency and duration of exposure, meteorologic conditions, host factors (existing health conditions and the propensity of those exposed to incur respiratory problems,) and the use of respiratory protective equipment.[62]

The acute respiratory effects might include the classic clinical signs and symptoms of acute respiratory distress, bronchial irritation, and acute exacerbation of underlying preexisting lung disease (eg, asthma, chronic obstructive pulmonary disease [COPD], (emphysema). Often these short-term effects are manageable and resolve with appropriate care in people who do not have preexisting respiratory conditions.

Hot ash that is in direct contact with skin can cause partial- or full-thickness burns. The exposure to hot ash may result in serious burns to the respiratory tract from inhalation. Clothing may offer a little protection.[63] More than a small number of

TABLE 10-6 Major Hazardous Gases From Volcanic Eruptions[58]

Substance	Risk	Therapy
Carbon dioxide	10 ppm/8 h TLV allowed 20-30 ppm: loss of consciousness, seizures CNS stimulant, vasodilation	Oxygen supplementation Supportive therapy
Sulfur dioxide	40 ppm: severe symptoms Respiratory irritant Inflammation, edema, bronchospasm, and hypoxia	Oxygen and respiratory support Beta agonists Corticosteroids
Hydrogen chloride	Respiratory irritant Inflammation, edema, bronchospasm, and hypoxia	Beta agonists
Hydrogen sulfide	<10 ppm/10 min allowed 50 ppm: evacuation of area 200 ppm: respiratory irritant >1000 ppm: lethal Respiratory irritant Inflammation, edema, bronchospasm, and hypoxia	Hyperbaric oxygen therapy
Hydrogen fluoride	Topical and respiratory irritant Airway inflammation, edema, bronchospasm, and hypoxia	Hydrofluoric acid burns treated with calcium gluconate therapy Supportive care for airway problems
Carbon monoxide	35 ppm TLV/8 h 100 ppm × 1 h causes hypoxia, loss of consciousness, seizures, chest pain	Oxygen therapy Hyperbaric oxygen

Abbreviations: TLV, threshold limit value; CNS, central nervous system.

casualties with 20% to 40% total body surface area burns would exceed the national burn unit capacity of most countries. A national and international network of burn centers would need to be available to receive patients when local facilities were overwhelmed.[63]

Eye injuries and irritation are a common medical issue. Because volcanic ash is abrasive, many people experience eye discomfort or eye irritation during and after ash fall, especially those who wear contact lenses. Signs and symptoms include foreign-particle sensation; conjunctivitis; painful, itchy, or bloodshot eyes; mucous discharge or tearing; and corneal abrasions or scratches. Individuals with existing dry-eye syndrome might also experience ailments due to the presence of ash. Chronic ocular effects have been noted.

Other injuries expected include lacerations and smoke inhalation from fires ignited by the hot ash. Fractures and crush injury, as well as secondary infections, are also common.

Late health consequences or chronic consequences related to the lung involvement are potentially silicosis, asthma, bronchitis, and development of chronic obstructive pulmonary diseases (COPDs).[64-66]

10.11.5   Public Health Considerations

Evacuation routes and methods, as well as communications, will be disrupted. Mudflows, lava flows, and floods can destroy roads and railways; often driving through suspended ash is almost impossible. Evacuation of large populations through specific routes will be essential. Darkness is a feature of ash falls and can last for several days. Fixed-wing aircraft and helicopters may be unable to fly because of poor visibility and the risk of engine damage from the ash. Elaborate precautions may be needed to protect engines.

Water supplies and sewage systems can be significantly affected by volcanic eruptions. Water intakes at rivers and reservoirs can be destroyed. Power outages may close down pumping stations. Water supplies can be severely depleted by cleanup activities (eg, washing ash off sidewalks, streets, and rooftops). Sewage and water treatments plants can break down in heavy ash falls. Water supplies may be contaminated by sewage. Adequate chlorination of water must be reinstituted. Epidemic diseases, malaria, and leptospirosis could be promoted by devastation and flooding of water resources.

Population displacement may become significant in a large-scale volcanic eruption. Providing adequate sheltering, food, water, safety, security, sanitation, and access to medical care will be paramount.

Psychological stress and long-term behavioral effects are important public health considerations.[67,68] Issues such as anxiety, depression, and posttraumatic stress are concerns that are discussed in greater detail in Chapter 3, "Population Health and Mental Health in Disasters."

10.11.6   Prevention and Mitigation of Future Events

Increasing population density around active volcanoes worldwide has increased the probability of significant volcano-related disasters. All such communities must be prepared and should have response plans integrated into their overall community disaster plan. Plans for large-scale population displacement and sheltering must also be considered.

10.12   WILDFIRES

Wildland fires are increasing in activity and affect most regions of the United States. During the 2009 wildfire fire season, there were 78,792 individual fires in the United States. These consumed more than 5.9 million acres of land and cost billions of dollars.[69]

10.12.1   Causes and Characteristics

Wildfires occur because of either human actions or natural events. Human causes are more common and include faulty machinery releasing sparks, discarded cigarettes, burning of leaves, children playing with matches, loss of control of intentionally lit fires, golf ball hits causing sparks, downed power lines, arson, and destruction of forested lands. Furthermore, fire suppression can lead to more severe fires because of buildup of fuel (vegetation). Natural causes include lighting strikes (most common), volcanic activity, falling rocks (causing sparks), spontaneous combustion, and coal steam fires. US Fire Administration data show that, of 116 573 fires from 1988 through 1997, humans caused 88%; 12% were due to lightening strikes. In the Amazon region of South America, wildfires are mostly caused by drought, logging, cattle ranching practices, and slash-and-burn practices.[70] Wildfires are important to the ecological long-term health of forest and grassland systems.

Wildfires can have several secondary effects on the natural ecology. After a wildfire, there is an increased potential for flooding, debris flows, landslides, introduction of invasive species, and changes in water quality. Floods and debris flows can occur 2 years later, after a high-intensity rainfall, but can also be due to root damage and loss of soil strength. Flash floods occur when the precipitation amount meets or exceeds the threshold value of a drainage basin. Debris flows and landslides can occur with little or no warning and are caused by either postfire surface erosion caused by rainfall runoff and/or rainfall infiltration into the ground. Debris flows can be quite large, ranging from 600 m^3 to 300 000 m^3 (which would cover a football field with debris to depth of 65 m).

10.12.2   Early Detection and Warning Systems

Early warning systems can mitigate fire-related problems and escalating fire suppression costs.[70] Fire danger rating based on daily weather information is commonly used to provide early warning of the potential for serious wildfires. The rating is often determined on the basis of satellite data, such as hot spots for early fire detection, with spectral data on land cover and fuel conditions. Fire danger rating systems can provide a 4- to 6-hour warning of the highest fire danger for any day for which the weather data are supplied. However, by using forecasted conditions from advanced numerical weather models, extended early warning (ie, 1 to 2 weeks) can be provided.

10.12.3   Acute Hazards and Effects

Wildland firefighters work at enormous risk to personal safety, and there has been much research indicating their high rates of morbidity and mortality, with volunteers being at greater risk than those specially trained by the Forest Service. As with all firefighters, physical fitness and comorbid conditions are factors.

The threat of fatal and severe thermal burn injury is ever present. The environmental issues (eg, wind-direction changes, continued dry ambient conditions) remain prominent in hazard risk assessment. Smoke inhalation and asphyxia are issues, as many firefighters may not use a self-contained breathing apparatus. Some will use particulate masks (or just a wet bandana over their mouths), and there is a risk of longer exposure periods for firefighters who work 12-hour shifts for several days and spend rest periods in smoke-filled base camps.

10.12.4   Clinical Implications: Immediate and Long Term

A variety of injury patterns are seen by health care providers when humans come in contact with wildland fires.[72] Civilians and wildfire firefighters are both at risk of smoke and dust exposure with subsequent respiratory complaints, exposure to toxic combustion products (CO, cyanide, and hydrochloride acid), thermal injuries (burns), bites and stings from wild animal contact, heat and cold stresses, psychological stressors, exhaustion, eye complaints, dehydration, musculoskeletal injuries, lacerations, electrocution, and trauma from many sources including falls and automobile/traffic-related incidents. Emergency department visits during the 1991 Oakland, California, wildfires were analyzed. This was a big fire, with 790 homes burned within the first hour; there were 25 fatalities, 150 injured, and 227 emergency department visits (19% were admitted). Half of the emergency department cases were due to smoke exposure; most were minor, and a quarter of the cases were work-related.[72]

From 1990 to 1998, there were 133 wildfire firefighter fatalities in total, occurring during 94 events in 33 different states; California was the highest, followed by Colorado.[72] A study of fatal work injuries with data from 1992 to 2006 analyzed 307 fatalities. Most fatal occupational injuries were due to wildfires, followed by hurricanes and floods. Causes of wildfire-related death included burnover (29%), aircraft/crashes (23%), acute coronary syndrome (21%), motor vehicle crashes (19%), miscellaneous (4%), and snags (fallen branches) (4%).[73] During the 1988 Yellowstone fires (1.2 million acres burned), there were 30 000 first aid station visits by firefighters over 4 months. Of these visits, 40% were for respiratory issues, and 660 firefighters required a higher level of care.[73,74]

Civilians are more prone to other injury patterns as well, depending on whether they evacuated or attempted to fight fires while protecting their homes. One specific respiratory issue to contend with is contact with superheated air. This can lead to facial burns, nasal hair singing, facial edema, stridor, and respiratory distress. If a person was trapped in a burning area, injuries could be more severe. Also, morbidity can be delayed for up to 24 hours. Direct visualization of larynx and early intubation are advised in patients with respiratory distress. Heat stress and thermal injuries are also common sources of morbidity and mortality. Heat stress can occur because of environmental issues, less water consumed than lost, and exertion of physical stress. Heat cramps and heat exhaustion are common; symptoms include fatigue, dizziness, weakness, vomiting, headache, and cramps. As core temperature rises and central nervous system (CNS) involvement occurs, heat stroke, rhabdomyolysis, and acute renal failure become problems. Treatment consists of cooling and correcting water deficits.

10.12.5   Public Health Considerations

Injury patterns are not limited to the period directly following exposure. Long-term implications can include exacerbation of chronic illnesses and issues with medical infrastructure disruptions (eg, dialysis clinic closed). Smoke contains CO, aldehydes, and other compounds that cause local airway irritation. Prolonged exposure can be a health issue, particularly at higher altitudes. A study of the 2007 California wildfires, which surveyed 161 people at shelters and local assistance centers, found that prescription medications and mental health services were the most frequently identified health care needs that were lacking.[75,76] A study of the 2003 California wildfires found an increase in respiratory admissions, especially related to asthma and bronchitis.[77]

10.12.6   Prevention and Mitigation of Future Events

Wildfire management consists of multiple activities existing at the urban-wildland interface. Behind-the-scenes activities include jurisdictional barriers, mutual aid agreements, zoning, legal mandates, building codes, insurance, environmental actions, and public education. These strategies can roughly be divided into three categories (which have varied over the years): prevention (including controlled burns), detection, and suppression. Controlled burns reduce fuel levels and create buffer strips or firebreaks. Other actions individuals and local communities can take include individual citizens and local communities setting firebreaks around houses/buildings, prohibiting vegetation from growing up to edges of structures, not storing potential fire fuels (farm machine fuel, dry firewood) next to housing, cleaning gutters and leaves, developing personal fire plans and home disaster kits, involvement of local emergency managers, evacuation and traffic management planning, and preparing for continuation of normal EMS and health care services as people are displaced.

Multiple agencies are involved in wildfire management. The lead federal agency is the Forest Service, which is part of the US Department of Agriculture. The Forest Service publishes regular fire danger forecasts, collects data, conducts fire suppression (billions of dollars are spent annually on this function), and maintains MODIS (Moderate Resolution Imaging Spectroradiometer), in collaboration with the National Aeronautics and Space Administration (NASA), an active fire mapping program. The National Fire Protection Association has a wildfire training course, which includes essentials such as entrapment procedures, wildfire behavior, communications, and escape protocols.

10.13   WINTER STORMS

Winter storms include blizzards, heavy snowfall, and extreme cold. These storms can immobilize an entire region and result in flooding, storm surge, closed highways, blocked roads, downed power lines, and hypothermia. Blizzards and other severe winter storms frequently cause extensive damage, injuries, and deaths in the United States. From 1949 to 2003, 202 severe winter storms caused more than $35 billion dollars in damage while killing on average 30 to 40 persons each year. In 1978, the states of Massachusetts and Rhode Island experienced a total of 99 deaths and more than 4500 injuries and illnesses directly attributed to a massive blizzard.[78] In addition to deaths and damage to property, severe winter storms can cause or contribute to a variety of injuries and illnesses.

10.13.1 Causes and Characteristics

A blizzard is generally defined as a dangerous combination of blowing wind and snow, and low temperatures with poor visibility of less than 1/4 mile for an extended period lasting at least 3 hours. In addition, fog is common in about 50% of blizzards. Blizzards develop when high wind speed causes existing snow on the ground or new snowfall to lift into suspension in the atmosphere near the earth's surface, severely reducing visibility. Due to the potential for whiteout conditions, traveling during blizzards can also create dangerous and life-threatening situations. It has been estimated that 70% of deaths in blizzards actually occur when individuals become stranded in automobiles.[79] When these conditions are forecasted or exist, the NWS or other weather organizations will issue alerts and warnings.

Winter storms, including blizzards, have a list of defining typology. This characterization has merit in situational awareness, as well as to advance planning and overall operational preparedness. A brief description of each type follows:

Freezing rain/drizzle or sleet: Widespread, dangerous, and damaging accumulations of ice or sleet.

Frost or freeze warning: Issued when temperatures are critical for crops and sensitive plants. Criteria are season dependent, but usually a freeze warning is appropriate when temperatures are expected to fall below freezing for at least 2 hours.

In addition to blizzards, severe winter storms can be characterized in several additional ways:

Ice storms: These result when freezing rain accumulates to at least 1/4 inch. Freezing rain is caused by rain droplets that freeze on contact with the ground or objects near the surface. Freezing rain frequently causes extremely hazardous driving or walking conditions.

Lake effect: Lake effect snow occurs when a mass of sufficiently cold air moves over a body of warmer water, creating an unstable temperature profile in the atmosphere. This can result in extremely heavy snowfall. The term generally applies to areas downwind of the North American Great Lakes but has also been applied to the Great Salt Lake in Utah.

Nor'easter: Among winter's most ferocious storms, nor'easters get their name from continuous strong northeasterly winds blowing in from the ocean ahead of a storm and over a coastal area. They are known for producing heavy snow or rain and oversized waves that crash onto Atlantic beaches, often causing extensive erosion and structural damage. Wind gusts associated with these storms can exceed hurricane force in intensity.

10.13.2 Early Detection and Warning Systems

Accurate prediction of blizzards and other winter storms is still an imprecise science. While satellites track blizzards, their paths are predicted on the basis of computer modeling. According to the NWS, these models have the ability to correctly predict the path of the storm about 85% of the time. However, models rely on the data they are given, and there is always an opportunity for introduction of inaccurate measurements. Nevertheless, it is important to monitor weather patterns and provide the public advance notice of potential winter storm conditions.

In the United States, the NWS broadcasts winter storm advisories. Many local weather offices will also activate their emergency alert systems and broadcast the alarm tone on relevant NOAA weather radio stations.

10.13.3   Acute Hazards and Effects

Protective actions should be taken whenever a winter storm warning is issued. A blizzard warning refers to a severe winter storm with significant snow and high winds that will lead to deep snow drifts, poor visibility, and life-threatening cold. People should avoid going outdoors unless absolutely necessary. If one must go outside, it is important to wear well-insulated boots; multiple layers of loose-fitting, dry clothing; a hat to minimize heat loss through the head; and gloves or mittens and a scarf. When shoveling snow, overexertion should be avoided to minimize the risk of a heart attack.

People need to be cautious of structural damage to homes and buildings due to snow and ice buildup. Unintentional CO poisoning may occur when motor vehicle exhaust systems are obstructed with snow; when kerosene or propane heaters and gasoline-powered generators are used indoors; or when charcoal briquettes are used to cook food indoors. Structure fires also may result from faulty or careless use of space heaters and from faulty electrical wiring.

10.13.4   Clinical Implications: Immediate and Long Term

Injuries during blizzards generally are caused by frostbite and/or hypothermia. Frostbite is simply damage to body tissue caused by freezing of the tissue. Damage may be temporary but can be permanent if not promptly treated and can lead to loss of body parts such as toes, fingers, ears, and noses. Pets are susceptible to frostbite and can suffer from similar loss of ears, toes, tails, legs, and, in male dogs, genitalia.

Hypothermia occurs when body temperatures drop below 96°F. Extreme cold is not required for this to occur. Even in milder temperatures as high as 60°F, individuals can suffer from hypothermia. Some of the warning signs of hypothermia include uncontrollable shivering, disorientation, memory loss, slurred speech, stumbling and uncoordinated walk, failing eyesight, drowsiness, and exhaustion.

Managing injuries and preventing death from severe cold and hypothermia involves first removing the individual from the source of cold, followed by slow rewarming of body parts and the entire body. If removing a person from the cold source is not possible, removing wet clothing is essential. Slowly rewarming the body, chest, shoulders, and stomach areas are critically important. The heat source should be kept warm, not hot. Elevating the feet and lowering the head can speed rewarming of the chest area. If the person is conscious, he or she should be given warm (not hot) liquids. Alcohol and sedatives should be avoided. Appropriate medical care should be obtained as soon as possible.

10.13.5 Public Health Considerations

At-risk populations, including those of lower socioeconomic status and the homeless, are at disproportionate risk for injury or death in blizzards because of inadequate sheltering (lack of heat or water). Providing risk communication messaging about locations for public shelters is critical.

Public health along with local media can educate and train the community on safe and proper heating methods, venting of stoves, fireplace use, etc. Information about exposure and duration to freezing temperatures or cold and wet environments is also important.

10.13.6 Prevention and Mitigation of Future Events

To prepare homes for a winter storm, it is important to have rock salt, sand, and snow shovels on hand; rock salt will melt ice, sand will improve traction, and shovels can be used for snow removal. People may also winterize homes by insulating walls and attics, caulking and weather stripping doors and windows, and installing storm windows or covering windows with plastic. It is important to prepare for possible isolation at home by having sufficient heating fuel and keeping a good supply of food and water on hand. Residents should learn how to shut off water valves in case a pipe bursts and be instructed to allow faucets to drip during very cold weather to avoid freezing.

10.14 SUMMARY

Global trends indicate that the risk of exposure to natural hazards is on the rise, resulting in an increase in the frequency and magnitude of natural disasters. In the United States, intensive monitoring by government agencies such as the US GS, NWS, and NOAA can provide early warning for some of these events. This allows for the early implementation of emergency communication and evacuation plans. Although some natural disasters are predictable according to season and geographic location and through the use of tracking systems, many others (eg, wildfires, flash floods) can occur with little or no warning.

Factors such as urbanization, overpopulation, and encroachment on regions susceptible to disasters have increased population vulnerability to natural disasters. Globalization, which connects countries through economic interdependencies, has led to increased travel and commerce around the world. Such activity has resulted in increased urbanization and overpopulation of cities worldwide, as well as increased migration of people to coastal, wildland-urban interface areas and other disaster-prone regions.

After a disaster occurs, local authorities will watch the situation and decide what protective actions citizens should take. The most appropriate action will depend on the situation. Natural disasters and weather-related events can disrupt communication systems; destroy roads, homes, and businesses; and create large numbers of displaced persons who require food, shelter, and medical care. Special attention must be given to damaged buildings, downed power lines, ruptured gas lines, contaminated drinking water, and infectious disease outbreaks. Natural disasters often have predictable injury timelines and patterns, regardless of disaster type. Initial injuries are often trauma-related, and most deaths occur in the early aftermath of the event. In subsequent days and weeks, the medical community will experience an exacerbation of routine chronic diseases such as asthma, accompanied by orthopedic injuries and lacerations sustained from initial cleanup efforts. These are followed by an increase in infections from untreated wounds received during the initial incident.

10.15   DISCUSSION POINTS

Natural Disasters: Putting the PRE-DISASTER Paradigm™ into Practice	
P Planning and Practice	Not all natural disasters can be predicted, but certain measures can be addressed now to mitigate the ill effects of most events. Participation in drills and exercises and understanding local and professional response plans will help maintain order in potentially chaotic situations. Medical facilities, public health departments, civic organizations, and humanitarian agencies can also organize memoranda of understanding for personnel and resource sharing.
R Resilience	Cohesive, healthy communities will likely be more resilient in times of disaster. Increasing situational awareness and general all-hazards preparedness is paramount to increasing community resilience. At the legislative level, policies and procedures can be put in place to expedite political decision making in times of disaster or public health emergency. Considerations for improved infrastructure and land use planning can also be addressed.
E Education and Training	Education and training can be acquired at all levels to improve outcomes. The general population can be trained in all-hazards preparedness and disaster-specific techniques. They can additionally be trained in first response and cardiopulmonary resuscitation. Responders can be further trained, and a volunteer base can be established.
Natural Disasters: Putting the DISASTER Paradigm™ into Practice	
D Detection	Close monitoring of weather and seismologic activity can help to provide extra warning time before a major disaster—time that is potentially lifesaving. However, not all localities are equipped with early warning systems; efforts should be made to provide disaster-vulnerable areas with the appropriate means of surveillance and warning. The citizenry should also have a base-level awareness of indicators of disaster and the knowledge of where to report such information.

I	Incident Management	Incident management includes the appropriate reporting of hazard detection to incident managers and the lay public. It also encompasses the assessment and response to a natural disaster. While management decisions will differ by event, the decision structure and chain of command should be consistent. All personnel involved in emergency response should be aware of the incident management structure under which they are expected to perform. Personnel should also be aware of agreements for resource and staff sharing that may affect their traditional work role.
S	Safety and Security	Natural disasters often cause extensive damage to both humanmade and natural landscape. It is important to protect oneself from both the primary effects of the hazard (ie, flying debris, flowing floodwater, or very strong winds) and the secondary effects (ie, building collapse, downed power lines, water source contamination). Responders should mark potentially dangerous sites, wear appropriate personal protective equipment (PPE), and proceed with caution into disaster sites. Securing the scene will help to prevent injury and/or illness of responders and citizens alike.
A	Assess Hazards	In addition to securing the scene, it is important to do a thorough assessment of potential health and safety hazards after a disaster. Because no disaster is the same, there is no cut-and-dried hazard assessment checklist. Attention should be paid to readily apparent hazards as well as less obvious possibilities.
S	Support	Both responders and citizens should be aware of the local, regional, and national support services that may be offered in an emergency or disaster setting. Trained responders and medical personnel should also be prepared to help nearby localities, ideally through a predetermined affiliation with a humanitarian group or through a mutual aid agreement.
T	Triage and Treatment	Appropriate clinical casualty management will include assessment and response to both medical and psychological casualties. Personnel should be trained with an all-hazard approach and understand appropriate use of medical and mental health assessments, applicable emergent and ongoing intervention opportunities, and the local protocols for information sharing and reporting of all casualties triaged and treated. Legal and ethical considerations for triage and treatment should also be considered.
E	Evacuation	Some natural disasters will necessitate evacuation, while others will require specific shelter-in-place methods. It will also be important to consider the impact of the natural disaster on existing health care infrastructure, as migration of the affected population will influence surge capacity management and continuity of operations in local and neighboring health care facilities.

(Continued)

Natural Disasters: Putting the DISASTER Paradigm™ into Practice	
R Recovery	Physical, psychological, social, and familial effects can last long after the disaster has passed and homes, buildings, and other infrastructure have been restored. Knowing what resources are available, understanding evacuation routes and response plans, and creating professional and personal plans will help expedite the recovery process.

REFERENCES

1. Guha-Sapir D, Vos F, Below R. *Annual Disaster Statistical Review 2010: The Numbers and Trends.* Brussels, Belgium: Centre for Research on the Epidemiology of Disasters; 2011. http://www.cred.be/sites/default/files/ADSR_2010.pdf. Accessed May 13, 2010.

2. Vos F, Rodriguex J, Below R, Guha-Sapir D. *Annual Disaster Statistical Review 2009: The Numbers and Trends.* Brussels, Belgium: Centre for Research on the Epidemiology of Disasters; 2010. http://cred.be/sites/default/files/ADSR_2009.pdf. Accessed May 13, 2010.

3. Rodriguez J, Vos F, Below R, Guha-Sapir D. *Annual Disaster Statistical Review 2008: The Numbers and Trends.* Brussels, Belgium: Center for Research on the Epidemiology of Disasters; 2009. http://www.cred.be/sites/default/files/ADSR_2008.pdf. August 31, 2009.

4. Franco C, Toner R, Waldhorn B, et al. Systematic collapse: medical care in the aftermath of Katrina. *Biosecurity Bioterrorism Biodefense Strategy Pract Sci.* 2006;4(2):135-146.

5. US Geological Survey (USGS). Earthquake facts. http://earthquake.usgs.gov/learn/facts.php. Accessed May 13, 2010.

6. Rosenberg M. Haiti death toll could reach 300,000: Preval. Reuters; February 22, 2010.

7. Emergency Preparedness Innovations Corporation (EPIC). Facts About Earthquakes. 2007. http://epicicorp.com/EARTHQUAKE__Facts__Edition_1_Final.pdf. Accessed May 13, 2010.

8. Liang N-J, Shih Y-T, Shih F-Y, et al. Disaster epidemiology and medical response in the Chi-Chi earthquake in Taiwan. *Ann Emerg Med.* 2001;38:549-555.

9. Yoneatsu Osaki Y, Minowa M. Factors associated with earthquake deaths in the Great Hanshin-Awaji Earthquake. *Am J Epidemiol.* 1995;153:153-156.

10. Bulut M. Medical experience of a university hospital in Turkey after the 1999 Marmara Earthquake. *Emerg Med J.* 2005;22:494-498.

11. Naghii M. Public health impact and medical consequences of earthquakes. *Rev Panam Salud Publica/Pan Am J Public Health.* 2005;18:216-221.

12. Mohebbi H, Mehrvarz S, Saghafinia M, et al. Earthquake related injuries: assessment of 854 victims of the 2003 Bam disaster transported to tertiary referral hospitals. *Prehosp Disaster Med.* 2008;23:510-515.

13. Feng J, Zen P, Liu Y, et al. Serum enzyme profile characteristics of victims following the Wenchuan earthquake in China. *Clin Chem Lab Med.* 2009;47:590-595.

14. Sever M, Erek E, Vanholder R, Yurugen B, et al. Renal replacement therapies in the aftermath of the catastrophic Marmara earthquake. *Kidney International.* 2002; 62: 2264-2271.

15. Noji E, Kelen GD, Armenian HK, Oganessian A, Jones NP, Sivertson KT. The 1988 earthquake in Soviet Armenia: a case study. *Ann Emergen Med.* 1990;19:891-897.

16. de Bruycker M, Greco D, Annino I, et al. The 1980 earthquake in Southern Italy: rescue of trapped victims and mortality. *Bull World Health Organ.* 1983;61:1021-1025.

17. Daniels A, Chapin E, Aspilcueta D, Doocy S. Access to health services and care-seeking behaviors after the 2007 Ica earthquake in Peru. *Disaster Med Public Health Prep.* 2009;3:97-103.

18. Guha-Sapir D, van Panhuis WG, Lagoutte J. Short communication: patterns of chronic and acute diseases after natural disasters – a study from the International Committee of the Red Cross field hospital in Banda Aceh after the 2004 Indian Ocean tsunami. *Trop Med Int Health.* 2007;12:1338-1341.

19. Chan EYY, Kim JJ. Characteristics and health outcomes of internally-displaced populations in unofficial rural self-settled camps after the 2005 Kashmir, Pakistan earthquake. *Eur J Emerg Med.* 2010;17:136-141.

20. Broach J, McNamara M, Harrison K. Ambulatory care by disaster responders in the tent camps of Port-au-Prince Haiti, January 2010. *Disaster Med Public Health Prep.* 2010;4:16-121.

21. Kloner RA, Leor J, Poole WK, Perritt R. Population-based analysis of the effect of the Northridge earthquake on cardiac death in Los Angeles County, California. *J Am Coll Cardiol.* 1997; 30:1174-1180.

22. Katsouyanni K, Kogevinas M, Trichopoulos D. Earthquake-related stress and cardiac mortality. *Int J Epidemiol.* 1986;5:326-330.

23. Suzuki S, Sakamoto S, Miki T, et al. Hanshin-Awaji earthquake and acute myocardial infarction. *Lancet.* 1995;345:981.

24. Ogawa K, Tsuji I, Shiono K, et al. Increased acute myocardial infarction mortality following the 1995 Great Hanshin-Awaji earthquake in Japan. *Int J Epidemiol.* 2000;29:449-455.

25. Nakagawa, Nakamura K, Oyama M, et al. Long-term effects of the Niigata-Chuetsu earthquake in Japan on acute myocardial infarction mortality: an analysis of death certificate data. *Heart.* 2009;95:2009-2013.

26. Cairo JB, Dutta S, Nawaz H, Hashmi S, Kasl S, Bellido E. The prevalence of posttraumatic stress disorder among adult earthquake survivors in Peru. *Disaster Med Public Health Prep.* 2010;4:39-46.

27. Frankenberg E, Friedman J, Gillespie T, et al. Mental health in Sumatra after the tsunami. *Am J Public Health.* 2008;8:1671-1677.

28. Kuwabara H, Shioiri T, Toyabe S-I, et al. Factors impacting on psychological distress and recovery after the 2004 Niigata-Chuetsu earthquake, Japan: community-based study. *Psychiatry Clini Neurosci.* 2008;62:503-507.

29. Blham R. Lessons from the Haiti earthquake. *Nature.* 2010;463:878-879.

30. FEMA. Significant flood events. http://www.fema.gov/business/nfip/statistics/sign1000.shtm. Accessed April 7, 2011.

31. Subbarao I, Bostick NA, James JJ. Applying yesterday's lessons to today's crisis: improving the utilization of recovery services following catastrophic flooding. *Disaster Med Public Health Prep.* 2008;2:132-133.

32. Stimpson JP, Fernando A, Wilson FA, Shawn K, Jeffries SK. Seeking help for disaster services after a flood. *Disaster Med Public Health Prep.* 2008;2:139-141.

33. Schultz J, Russell J, Espinel Z. Epidemiology of tropical cyclones: the dynamics of disaster, disease, and development. *Epidemiol Rev.* 2005;27:21-35.

34. National Hurricane Center, National Oceanographic and Atmospheric Association. Hurricane History: Galveston, TX, 1900. http://www.nhc.noaa.gov/HAW2/english/history.shtml#galveston. Accessed May 24, 2010.

35. Malilay J. *Tropical Cyclones*. In: Noji EK, ed. *The Public Health Consequences of Disasters*. New York, NY: Oxford University Press; 1997.

36. Beven JL II, Avila LA, Blake ES, Brown DP, Franklin JL, Knabb RD. Annual summary: Atlantic hurricane season of 2005. *Monthly Weather Rev.* 2008;136(3):1131-1141. doi:10.1175/2007MWR2074.1. http://www.aoml.noaa.gov/general/lib/lib1/nhclib/mwreviews/2005.pdf. Accessed May 23, 2010.

37. Ragan P, Schulte J, Nelson S, Jones K. Mortality surveillance 2004 to 2005 Florida Hurricane related deaths. *Am J Forensic Med Pathol.* 2008;29:148-153.

38. Brunkar J, Namulnada G, Ratard R. Hurricane Katrina deaths, Louisiana. *Disaster Med Public Health Prep.* 2005;2:215-223.

39. McNeill K, Byers P, Kittle T, et al. Surveillance for illness and injury after Hurricane Katrina – three counties, Mississippi, September 5 – October 11, 2005. *JAMA.* 2006;295:1994-1996.

40. Hamilton D, Gavagan T, Smart K, Upton L, Havron D, Weller N. Houston's medical disaster response to Hurricane Katrina, part 2: transitioning from emergency evacuee care to community health care. *Ann Emerg Med.* 2009;53:515-527.

41. Eastman AL, Rinnert KJ, Nemeth IR, Fowler RL, Minei JP. Alternate site surge capacity in times of public health disaster maintains trauma center and emergency department integrity: Hurricane Katrina. *J Trauma.* 2007;63:253-257.

42. Greenough G, Lappi M, Hsu E, et al. Burden of disease and health status among Hurricane Katrina-displaced persons in shelters: a population-based cluster sample. *Ann Emerg Med.* 2007;51:426-432.

43. Sharma A, Weiss E, Young S, et al. Chronic disease and related conditions at emergency treatment facilities in the New Orleans area after Hurricane Katrina. *Disaster Med Public Health Prep.* 2008;2:27-32.

44. Stephens K, Grew D, Chin K, et al. Excess mortality in the aftermath of Hurricane Katrina: a preliminary report. *Disaster Med Public Health Prep.* 2007;1:15-20.

45. Lawry L, Burkle F. Measuring the true cost of natural disasters. *Disaster Med Public Health Prep.* 2008;2:208-210.

46. Larrance R, Anastario M, Lawry L. Health status among internally displaced persons in Louisiana and Mississippi travel trailer parks: a global perspective. *Ann Emerg Med.* 2007;49:590-601.

47. Gautam S, Menachem J, Srivastav S, Delafontaine M, Irimpen A. Effect of Hurricane Katrina on the incidence of acute coronary syndrome at a primary angioplasty center in New Orleans. *Disaster Med Public Health Prep.* 2009;3:144-150.

48. Lavie C, Gerber T, Lanier W. The infarcts beyond the storm. *Disaster Med Public Health Prep.* 2009;3:131-135.

49. Abramson D, Stehling-Arzia T, Garfield R, Redlener I. Prevalence and predictors of mental health distress post-Katrina: findings from the Gulf Coast child and family health study. *Disaster Med Public Health Prep.* 2008;2:77-86.

50. Roberts Y, Witman M, Mitchell M, Taffaro C. Mental health symptoms in youth affected by Hurricane Katrina. *Professional Psychol Res Pract.* 2010;41:10-18.

51. Hammond J. Tornadoes and disaster management: not just in Kansas, Dorothy. *Disaster Med Public Health Prep.* 2007;1:67-68.

52. Ablah E, Tinius AM, Konda K, Synovitz C, Subbarao I. Regional health system response to the 2007 Greensburg, Kansas EF5 tornado. *Disaster Med Public Health Prep.* 2007;1:90-95.

53. Simmons KM, Sutter D. Tornado warnings, lead times, and tornado casualties: an empirical investigation. *Weather Forecasting.* 2008;246-258.

54. Doswell CA III, Moller AR, Brooks HE. Storm spotting and public awareness since the first tornado forecasts of 1948. *Weather Forecasting.* 1999;544-557.

55. Centers for Disease Control and Prevention (CDC). Emergency preparedness and response: after a tornado. http://www.bt.cdc.gov/disasters/tornadoes/after.asp. Accessed May 18, 2010.

56. FEMA. What to do during a tornado. http://www.fema.gov/hazard/tornado/to_during.shtm. Assessed May 18, 2010.

57. Baxter PJ, Aspinall WP, Neri A, et al. Emergency planning and mitigation at Vesuvius: A new evidence-based approach. *J Volcanol Geotherm Res*. 2008;178:454-473.

58. Ford R, Hogan DE. Volcanic eruptions. In Hogan DE, Burnstein JL, eds. *Disaster Medicine*. Philadelphia, PA: Lippincott Williams & Wilkins; 2002.

59. Sigurdsson H, Houghton BF, McNutt SR, Rymer H, Stix J, eds. *Encyclopedia of Volcanoes*. San Diego: Academic Press; 2000.

60. Baxter PJ. Medical effects of volcanic eruptions. I. Main causes of death and injury. *Bull Vulcanol*.1990; 52: 532-544.

61. National Disaster Education Coalition: American Red Cross, FEMA, IAEM, IBHS, NFPA, NWS, USDA/CSREES, and USGS. Talking about disaster: Guide for standard messages. Volcano. http://www.disastercenter.com/guide/volcano.pdf. Accessed May 18, 2010.

62. Ishigami A, Kikuchi Y, Nishiwaki Y, Takebayashi T, Tanaka S, Omae K. Volcanic sulfur dioxide and acute respiratory symptoms on Miyakejima island. *Occup Environ Med*. 2008;65:701-707.

63. Volcanic ash: effects on health and mitigation strategies. volcanoes.usgs.gov/ash/health/. Accessed July 2010.

64. Baxter PJ. Volcanoes. In: Koenig K, Schultz CH, eds. *Disaster Medicine*. Cambridge: Cambridge University Press; 2010.

65. Hansell AL, Horwell CJ, Oppenheimer C. The health hazards of volcanoes and geothermal areas. *Occup Environ Med*. 2006; 63:149-156.

66. *Ibid*[62]

67. Health Effects Associated With Volcanic Eruptions. State of Alaska Epidemiology Bulletin 5 2006. http://www.epi.Alaska.gov/bulletins/docs/b2006_05.pdf. Accessed June 2010.

68. Aghababian RV. *Emergency Medicine: The Core Curriculum*. Philadelphia, PA: Lippincott-Raven; 1998.

69. US Fire Administration. Total Wildland Fires and Acres. http://www.usfa.fema.gov/statistics/estimates/wildfire.shtm. Accessed April 8, 2011.

70. Hogan D, Burstein J. *Disaster Medicine*. Philadelphia, PA: Lippincott Williams & Wilkins, 2007:226-228.

71. Nepstad DC. *The Amazon's Vicious Cycles: Drought and Fire in the Greenhouse*. Gland, Switzerland: World Wide Fund for Nature; 2007. http://www.worldwildlife.org/climate/Publications/WWFBinaryitem7658.pdf. Accessed April 8, 2011.

72. A Global Early Warning System for Wildland Fires. GOFC-GOLD, International Strategy for Disaster Reduction. http://www.fire.uni-freiburg.de/gwfews/index.html. Accessed April 8, 2011.

73. Frantz R. Firestorms and wildfires. In: Hogan DE, Burnstein JL, eds. *Disaster Medicine*. Philadelphia, PA: Lippincott Williams & Wilkins; 2007.

74. Fayard GM. Fatal work injuries involving natural disasters, 1992–2006. *Disaster Med Public Health Prep*. 2009;3:201-209.

75. US Geological Survey. *Wildfire Hazards – A National Threat*. 2006. http://pubs.usgs.gov/fs/2006/3015/2006–3015.pdf. Accessed April 8, 2011.

76. Jenkins JL, Hsu EB, Sauer LM, Hsieh YH, Kirsch TD. Prevalence of unmet health care needs and description of health care-seeking behavior among displaced people after the 2007 California wildfires. *Disaster Med Public Health Prep*. 2009;3(suppl 2):S24-S28.

77. Delfino RJ, Brummel S, Wu J, et al. The relationship of respiratory and cardiovascular hospital admissions to the southern California wildfires of 2003. *Occup Environ Med.* 2009;66:189-197.

78. Changnon SA. Space and time distributions of major winter storms in the United States. *Natural Hazards.* 2008;45:1-9.

79. The great northeast blizzard of 1978 remembered 30 years later in Southern New England. http://www.erh.noaa.gov/box/papers/blizzard78/mainblizzardof78.htm. Accessed June 7, 2010.

80. US Search and Rescue Task Force: Blizzards. http://www.ussartf.org/blizzards.htm. Accessed June 7, 2010.

Appendices

Appendix A: PRE-DISASTER Paradigm™ and DISASTER Paradigm™

Appendix B: BDLS® (v3.0) Competency, Chapter, and Course Objective Linkage

Appendix C: List of Acronyms and Abbreviations

PRE-DISASTER Paradigm™ and DISASTER Paradigm™

PRE-DISASTER Paradigm™

P	Planning and Practice	Do your community and workplace have disaster plans? Do you have a personal or family plan? Are these plans practiced and updated regularly?
R	Resilience	What measures are in place to help individuals, organizations, and communities cope with the environmental and psychological consequences of disaster?
E	Education	What can you do to prepare for disaster through competency-based, inter-professional education and training in disaster medicine and public health preparedness?

DISASTER Paradigm™

D	Detect	Do needs exceed resources? Who is notified that a disaster is happening?
I	Incident Management	What is your role? Who is the incident commander?
S	Safety and Security	Is the scene secure? Is it safe to enter?
A	Assess Hazards	Fire? Hazardous materials? Radiation? Building collapse? Downed power lines? Secondary devices? Contaminated casualties?
S	Support	What outside assistance is needed (eg, police, fire, emergency medical services [EMS], government, other)? Can adequate surge capability and capacity be established to meet local public safety and health needs and priorities?
T	Triage and Treatment	Are protocols, procedures, and resources in place for the rapid triage and immediate treatment of casualties? What public health interventions are needed?
E	Evacuation	Are enough transport units en route to the scene? Should affected people evacuate or shelter in place?
R	Recovery	Has critical infrastructure been damaged? What are the short- and long-term health needs of casualties and affected populations?

BDLS® (v3.0) Competency, Chapter, and Course Objective Linkage

Source document: Subbarao I, Lyznicki J, Hsu E, et al. A consensus-based educational framework and competency set for the discipline of disaster medicine and public health preparedness. *Disaster Med Public Health Prep.* 2008;2:57-68.

Competencies for Health Professionals in Disaster Medicine and Public Health Preparedness Addressed in the BDLS® (v3.0) Course Manual*

Competencies and Subcompetencies	Course Manual Chapter	Course Objective
Domain 1.0: Preparation and Planning		
1.1 Demonstrate proficiency in the use of an all-hazards framework for disaster planning and mitigation.	1,4	▶ Describe deployment readiness components for health professionals in a disaster or public health emergency.
1.1.1 Describe the all-hazards framework for disaster planning and mitigation.	1,4	
1.1.4 Explain the purpose of disaster exercises and drills in regional, community, and institutional disaster preparation and planning.	1,4	
1.2 Demonstrate proficiency in addressing the health-related needs, values, and perspectives of all ages and populations in regional, community, and institutional disaster plans.	1,3	▶ Identify the potential casualty population in a disaster or public health emergency, including persons with acute injuries or illnesses; those with pre-existing disease, injuries, or disabilities; those with age-related vulnerabilities or other functional and access needs; and their family/caregiver support network.
1.2.1 Identify individuals (of all ages) and populations with special needs who may be more vulnerable to adverse health effects in a disaster.	3	
1.2.2 Delineate health care and public health issues that need to be addressed in regional, community, and institutional disaster plans to accommodate the needs, values, and perspectives of all ages and populations.	1,3	
1.2.3 Identify psychological reactions that may be exhibited by victims of all ages, their families, and responders in a disaster or public health emergency.	3	▶ Describe an all-hazards, standardized, scalable casualty management approach for use in disasters and public health emergencies, including lifesaving interventions and medical decision making in an altered care environment. ▶ Describe the clinical assessment and management of injuries, illnesses, and mental health conditions manifested by all ages and populations in a disaster or public health emergency.

Domain 2.0: Detection and Communication

2.1 Demonstrate proficiency in the detection of and immediate response to a disaster or public health emergency.

1,2,4,6-10 ➤ Describe an all-hazards standardized, scalable workforce protection approach for use in disasters and public health emergencies, including detection, safety, security, hazard assessment, support, and evacuation.

2.1.1 Recognize general indicators and epidemiological clues of a disaster or public health emergency (including natural, unintentional, and terrorist events).

1,6-10

➤ Describe an all-hazards standardized, scalable casualty management approach for use in disasters and public health emergencies, including lifesaving interventions and medical decision making in an altered care environment.

2.1.2 Describe immediate actions and precautions to protect yourself and others from harm in a disaster or public health emergency.

1,4,6-10

2.1.3 Characterize signs and symptoms, as well as disease and injury patterns, likely to be associated with exposure to natural disasters or to conventional and nuclear explosives and/or release of biologic, chemical, and radiologic agents.

6-10

➤ Describe the clinical assessment and management of injuries, illnesses, and mental health conditions manifested by all ages and populations in a disaster or public health emergency

2.1.4 Explain the purpose and role of surveillance systems that can be used to detect and monitor a disaster or public health emergency.

2

2.2 Demonstrate proficiency in the use of information and communication systems in a disaster or public health emergency.

1-4,6-10 ➤ Describe information sharing, resource access, communication, and reporting methods useful for health professionals during disasters and public health emergencies.

2.2.1 Describe emergency communication and reporting systems and procedures for contacting family members, relatives, coworkers, and local authorities in a disaster or public health emergency.

2

➤ Identify the potential casualty population in a disaster or public health emergency, including persons with acute injuries or illnesses; those with pre-existing disease, injuries, or disabilities; those with age-related vulnerabilities or other functional and access needs; and their family/caregiver support network.

2.2.2 Describe informational resources that are available for health professionals and the public to prepare for, respond to, and recover from disasters.

1-4,6-10

2.2.4 Access timely and credible health and safety information for all ages and populations affected by natural disasters, industrial- or transportation-related catastrophes (eg, hazardous material spill, explosion), epidemics, and acts of terrorism (eg, involving conventional and nuclear explosives and/or release of biologic, chemical, and radiologic agents).

4,6-10

(continued)

2.3 Demonstrate proficiency in addressing cultural, ethnic, religious, linguistic, socioeconomic, and special health-related needs of all ages and populations in regional, community, and institutional emergency communication systems.

1-3

2.3.1 Describe strategies for and barriers to communicating and disseminating health information to all ages and populations affected by a disaster or public health emergency.

2,3

2.3.2 Delineate cultural, ethnic, religious, linguistic, and health-related issues that need to be addressed in regional, community, and institutional emergency communication systems for all ages and populations affected by a disaster or public health emergency.

1,3

Domain 3.0: Incident Management and Support Systems

3.1 Demonstrate proficiency in the initiation, deployment, and coordination of national, regional, state, local, and institutional incident command and emergency operations systems.

1,2

▲ Describe information sharing, resource access, communication, and reporting methods useful for health professionals during disasters and public health emergencies.

3.1.1 Describe the purpose and relevance of the National Response Framework, National Incident Management System, Hospital Incident Command System, and Emergency Support Function 8 to organizational and community disaster response.

1,2

▲ Describe the purpose and importance of the incident management system for providing health and medical support services in a disaster or public health emergency.

3.2 Demonstrate proficiency in the mobilization and coordination of disaster support services.

1,2

3.2.1 Describe global, federal, regional, state, local, institutional, organizational, and private industry disaster support services, including the rationale for the integration and coordination of these systems.

1,2

3.3 Demonstrate proficiency in the provision of health system surge capacity for the management of mass casualties in a disaster or public health emergency.

1,2,5

▲ Describe field, facility, community, and regional surge capacity assets for the management and support of mass casualties in a disaster or public health emergency.

3.3.1 Describe the potential impact of mass casualties on access to and availability of clinical and public health resources in a disaster or public health emergency.

1,2,5

3.3.2 Characterize institutional, community, and regional surge capacity assets in the public and private health response sectors and the extent of their potential assistance in a disaster or public health emergency.

1,2

Domain 4.0: Safety and Security

4.1 Demonstrate proficiency in the prevention and mitigation of health, safety, and security risks to yourself and others in a disaster.

1-4, 6-10

▶ Describe an all-hazards standardized, scalable workforce protection approach for use in disasters and public health emergencies, including detection, safety, security, hazard assessment, support, and evacuation.

4.1.1 Using an all-hazards framework, explain general health, safety, and security risks associated with disasters and public health emergencies.

1,3,4

4.1.2 Describe infection control precautions to protect health care workers, other responders, and the public from exposure to communicable diseases, such as pandemic influenza.

2,9

▶ Describe an all-hazards, standardized, scalable casualty management approach for use in disasters and public health emergencies, including lifesaving interventions and medical decision making in an altered care environment.

4.1.3 Characterize unique health, safety, and security risks associated with natural disasters, industrial- or transportation-related catastrophes (eg, hazardous material spill, explosion), epidemics, and acts of terrorism (eg, involving conventional and nuclear explosives and/or release of biologic, chemical, and radiologic agents).

4, 6-10

▶ Describe the clinical assessment and management of injuries, illnesses, and mental health conditions manifested by all ages and populations in a disaster or public health emergency.

4.2 Demonstrate proficiency in the selection and use of personal protective equipment at a disaster scene or receiving facility.

4

4.2.1 Describe the rationale, function, and limitations of personal protective equipment that may be used in a disaster or public health emergency.

4

4.3 Demonstrate proficiency in victim decontamination at a disaster scene or receiving facility.

4

4.3.1 Explain the purpose of victim decontamination in a disaster.

4

Domain 5.0: Clinical/Public Health Assessment and Intervention

5.1 Demonstrate proficiency in the use of triage systems in a disaster or public health emergency.

1,5

▶ Describe actions that facilitate mass casualty field triage utilizing a standardized step-wise approach and uniform triage categories.

5.1.1 Explain the role of triage as a basis for prioritizing or rationing health care services for victims and communities affected by a disaster or public health emergency.

1,5

(continued)

Objective	Ref	Notes
5.1.2 Explain the strengths and limitations of various triage systems that have been developed for the management of mass casualties at a disaster scene or receiving facility.	1,5	
5.2 Demonstrate proficiency in the clinical assessment and management of injuries, illnesses, and mental health conditions manifested by all ages and populations in a disaster or public health emergency.	3,4-10	▲ Describe an all-hazards, standardized, scalable casualty management approach for use in disasters and public health emergencies, including lifesaving interventions and medical decision making in an altered care environment.
5.2.1 Describe possible medical and mental health consequences for all ages and populations affected by a disaster or public health emergency.	3,4-10	▲ Describe the clinical assessment and management of injuries, illnesses, and mental health conditions manifested by all ages and populations in a disaster or public health emergency.
5.2.2 Explain basic lifesaving and support principles and procedures that can be used at a disaster scene.	4-10	
5.2.3 Demonstrate the ability to apply and adapt clinical knowledge and skills for the assessment and management of injuries and illnesses in victims of all ages under various exposure scenarios (eg, natural disasters; industrial- or transportation-related catastrophes; epidemics; and acts of terrorism involving conventional and nuclear explosives and/or release of biologic, chemical, and radiologic agents), in accordance with professional scope of practice.	5-10	
5.2.4 Identify strategies to manage fear, panic, stress, and other psychological responses that may be displayed by victims, families, and responders in a disaster or public health emergency.	3	
5.3 Demonstrate proficiency in the management of mass fatalities in a disaster or public health emergency.	1,3,5	▲ Describe the concepts and principles of mass fatality management for health professionals in a disaster or public health emergency.
5.3.1 Describe psychological, emotional, cultural, religious, and forensic considerations for the management of mass fatalities in a disaster or public health emergency.	3,5	
5.3.2 Explain the implications and specialized support services required for the management of mass fatalities from natural disasters, epidemics, and acts of terrorism (eg, involving conventional and nuclear explosives and/or release of biologic, chemical, and radiologic agents).	5	

5.3.3 Explain the significance of (and the need to collect and preserve) forensic evidence from living and deceased humans and animals at a disaster scene or receiving facility.

1,5

5.4 Demonstrate proficiency in public health interventions to protect the health of all ages, populations, and communities affected by a disaster or public health emergency.

2,3,7

► Describe public health interventions appropriate for all ages, populations, and communities affected by a disaster or public health emergency.

5.4.1 Describe short- and long-term public health interventions appropriate for all ages, populations, and communities affected by a disaster or public health emergency.

2,3,7

5.4.2 Apply knowledge and skills for the public health management of all ages, populations, and communities affected by natural disasters, industrial- or transportation-related catastrophes, epidemics, and acts of terrorism, in accordance with professional scope of practice. This includes active/passive surveillance, movement restriction, vector control, mass immunization and prophylaxis, rapid needs assessment, environmental monitoring, safety of food and water, and sanitation.

2

Domain 6.0: Contingency, Continuity, and Recovery

6.1 Demonstrate proficiency in the application of contingency interventions for all ages, populations, institutions, and communities affected by a disaster or public health emergency.

1,3–5

► Describe an all-hazards, standardized, scalable casualty management approach for use in disasters and public health emergencies, including lifesaving interventions and medical decision making in an altered care environment.

6.1.1 Describe solutions for ensuring the continuity of supplies and services to meet the medical and mental health needs of yourself, your family, office practice, institution, and community in a disaster, under various contingency situations (eg, mass evacuation, mass sheltering, prolonged shelter-in-place).

1,3,4

6.1.3 Describe community and institutional protocols and procedures for the evacuation and transport of individuals and populations (of all ages) affected by a disaster or public health emergency.

3,5

(continued)

6.2 Demonstrate proficiency in the application of recovery solutions for all ages, populations, institutions, and communities affected by a disaster or public health emergency. — 1-3,5 — ▲ Describe considerations and solutions to ensure continuity of and access to health-related information and services to meet the medical and mental health needs of all ages, populations, and communities affected by a disaster or public health emergency.

6.2.1 Describe short- and long-term medical and mental health considerations for the recovery of all ages, populations, and communities affected by a disaster or public health emergency. — 1

6.2.2 Describe solutions for ensuring the recovery of clinical records, supplies, and services to meet the physical and mental health needs of you, your family, institution, and community in a disaster or public health emergency. — 1,5

Domain 7.0: Public Health Law and Ethics

7.1 Demonstrate proficiency in the application of moral and ethical principles and policies for ensuring access to and availability of health services for all ages, populations, and communities affected by a disaster or public health emergency. — 1,3,5 — ▲ Describe moral, ethical, legal, and regulatory issues relevant to the health-related management of individuals of all ages, populations, and communities affected by a disaster or public health emergency.

7.1.1 Describe moral and ethical issues relevant to the management of individuals of all ages, populations, and communities affected by a disaster or public health emergency. — 1,3,5

7.2 Demonstrate proficiency in the application of laws and regulations to protect the health and safety of all ages, populations, and communities affected by a disaster or public health emergency. — 2,4

7.2.1 Describe legal and regulatory issues relevant to disasters and public health emergencies, including the basic legal framework for public health. — 2,4

Abbreviations and Acronyms

ABBREVIATIONS AND ACRONYMS

AAP	American Academy of Pediatrics
AAR	After-action review
ABLS	Advanced Burn Life Support
ACE	Alternative care environment
ACF	Alternate care facility
ADA	Americans with Disabilities Act
ADLS®	Advanced Disaster Life Support™
ALI	Annual limit of intake
ARS	Acute radiation sickness
ASPR	Assistant Secretary for Preparedness and Response
ATCN®	Advanced Trauma Care for Nurses®
ATLS®	Advanced Trauma Life Support®
BAL	British antilewisite [agent]
BDLS®	Basic Disaster Life Support™
BLEVE	Boiling liquid expanding vapor explosion
BLS	Basic life support
BSA	Body surface area
BT	Bioterrorism
C-A-T®	Combat Application Tourniquet®
CDC	Centers for Disease Control and Prevention
COPD	Chronic obstructive pulmonary disease
CDLS®	Core Disaster Life Support®
CPA	Cardiopulmonary arrest
CRED	Center for Research on the Epidemiology of Disasters
CRS	Cutaneous radiation syndrome
CSTE	Council of State and Territorial Epidemiologists
DHHS	Department of Health and Human Services
DHS	Department of Homeland Security
DISASTER	Detect; Incident command; Security and safety; Assess hazards; Support; Triage and treatment; Evacuation; Recovery [DISASTER Paradigm™]
DMAT	Disaster medical assistance team
DMORT	Disaster mortuary operational response team
DOD	Department of Defense
DOE	Department of Energy

DOT	Department of Transportation
DPMU	Disaster portable morgue unit
DTPA	Diethylentriamene penta-acetate
EF	Enhanced Fujita scale
EIS	Epidemic Intelligence Service
EM	Emergency management
EMAC	Emergency Management Assistance Compact
EMS	Emergency medical services
EOC	Emergency operations center
EOP	Emergency operations plan
EPA	Environmental Protection Agency
ESAR-VHP	Emergency System for Advance Registration of Volunteer Health Professionals
ESF	Emergency support function
ETT	Endotracheal tube
FAC	Family Assistance Center
FBI	Federal Bureau of Investigation
FDA	US Food and Drug Administration
FEMA	Federal Emergency Management Agency
GCS	Glasgow Coma Scale
GI	Gastrointestinal
GIS	Geographic information system
GPS	Global positioning system
HAN	Health Alert Network
HAZMAT	Hazardous materials
HAZWOPER	Hazardous Waste Operations and Emergency Response
HEOC	Health emergency operations center
HHS	US Department of Health and Human Services
HICS	Hospital Incident Command System
HIPAA	Health Insurance Portability and Accountability Act
HSPD	Homeland Security Presidential Directive
HVA	Hazard vulnerability analysis
ICS	Incident command system
IM	Intramuscularly
IDLH	Immediately dangerous to life or health
IED	Improvised explosive device

IOM	Institute of Medicine
LRN	Laboratory Response Network
MERCS	Mortuary enhanced remains cooling system
MRC	Medical Reserve Corps
NDLS™	National Disaster Life Support™
NDMS	National Disaster Medical System
NGO	Nongovernmental organization
NHC	National Hurricane Center
NHSS	National Health Security Strategy
NIH	National Institutes of Health
NIMS	National Incident Management System
NIOSH	National Institutes for Occupational Safety and Health
MMS	Moment magnitude scale
NNDSS	National Notifiable Disease Surveillance
NOAA	National Oceanic and Atmospheric Administration
NPI	Negative phase impulse
NRC	Nuclear Regulatory Commission
NRF	National Response Framework
NWS	National Weather Service
OSHA	Occupational Health and Safety Administration
PAHO	Pan American Health Organization
PAPR	Powered air purifying respirator
PBI	Pulmonary blast injury or primary blast injury
PCR	Polymerase chain reaction
PFA	Psychological first aid
PGO	Private Governmental Organization
PHTLS	Pre-hospital trauma life support
PIO	Public information officer
POA-F	Power of attorney for finance
POA-HC	Power of attorney for health care
PPE	Personal protective equipment
PRE-DISASTER	Planning and practice; Resilience, and Education and training DISASTER [PRE-DISASTER Paradigm™]
PTSD	Posttraumatic stress disorder
PTT	Pediatric triage tape
RDD	Radiation dispersal device

RDS	Respiratory distress syndrome
RED	Radiation emission device
RNA	Rapid needs assessment
RS	Remote sensing
SALT	Sort, assess, lifesaving interventions, and treatment/transport
SAMHSA	Substance Abuse and Mental Health Services Administration
SAMPLE	Symptoms, Allergies, Medications, Past illnesses, Last meal, Events and environment
SARS	Severe acute respiratory syndrome
SBI	Secondary blast injury
SCBA	Self-contained breathing apparatus
SEIRV	Susceptible, exposed, infectious, removed by death or illness recovery, or vaccine protected
SNS	Strategic National Stockpile
START	Simple Triage and Rapid Treatment
STP	Standard temperature and pressure
TBI	Traumatic brain injury
TBSA	Total body surface area
TNCC	Trauma Nursing Core Course
TJC	The Joint Commission
USAMRIID	US Army Medical Research Institute for Infectious Diseases
USGS	US Geological Survey
USPHS	US Public Health Service Commissioned Corps
VHF	Viral hemorrhagic fever
VOC	Volatile organic compound
WHO	World Health Organization
WHO/CRED	World Health Organization Center for Research on the Epidemiology of Disasters

GLOSSARY

All-hazards preparedness: Planning that considers all potential hazards to a community and takes steps to mitigate, practice, and respond to any potential hazard that may affect the community

Alternative care sites: Facilities that can be used in a disaster to care for casualties transported or directed from a disaster scene or for "overflow" of patients transferred from large hospitals and trauma centers to make room in these facilities for more acutely injured casualties

Capacity assessment: Identifying available resources that can be used to reduce risk, enhance survival, and help affected individuals and populations cope with severe trauma

Conflict-based disaster: An intentional, human-caused disaster event such as those related to war, terrorism, or civil unrest

Containment: Defining and containing an infectious disease outbreak in specific geographic regions for the purpose of reducing or preventing further transmission of the disease

Decontamination ("Dry or Wet"): "Dry" decontamination is the act of removing garments or items that are superficially contaminated or have retained vapor within them, and "wet" decontamination is the process of washing a grossly contaminated, likely exposed to dangerous chemical or substance, or symptomatic casualty from head to toe with soap and tepid water once "dry" decontamination has been completed.

DISASTER Paradigm™: A mnemonic device that organizes the providers' response and planning of a disaster: D, detect; I, incident management; S, security and safety; A, assess hazards; S, support; T, triage and treatment; E, evacuation; R, recovery

Disaster: A serious disruption of the functioning of society, causing widespread human, material, or environmental losses that exceed the ability of affected society to cope by using only its own resources (World Association of Disaster and Emergency Medicine); an occurrence of a natural catastrophe, technological accident, or human-caused event that has resulted in severe property damage, deaths, and/or multiple injuries (FEMA); an event and its consequences that results in a serious disruption of the functioning of a community and causing widespread human, material, economic, or environmental losses that exceed the capacity of the affected area to respond without external assistance to save lives, preserve property, and maintain the stability and integrity of the affected area (NDLS Education Consortium)

Disaster (Operational): A situation in which the imbalance of the need (logistical supply of personnel, equipment, medications, space, etc) exceeds the resources that are immediately available. Need > Resources = Disaster

Emergency management: Coordination and integration of all activities necessary to build, sustain, and improve the capability to prepare for, protect against, respond to, recover from, or mitigate against threatened or actual natural disasters, acts of terrorism, or other humanmade disasters

Emergency operations center (EOC): Physical location where the leaders of a region or organization come together during an emergency or disaster to analyze response and recovery options, coordinate actions, and allocate resources

Hazard assessment: Analyzing various hazards for a particular geographic area and the magnitude of impact given local resources, allowing for prioritization of response and mitigation options

ID-ME: Mnemonic device for remembering the categories of live casualty triage under the SALT method: immediate, delayed, minimal, and expectant. The phrase "identify (eg, ID) me" is implied in the ID-ME mnemonic.

Incident management: The way in which incidents are managed across all Homeland Security activities, including prevention, protection, response, mitigation, and recovery

Isolation: Placement of persons known to have a communicable disease in a separate area where they will not expose others

Mass fatality event: An event that produces fatalities that overwhelm available fatality management resources

Mitigation: Lessening the severity and impact of a potential or ongoing disaster or public health emergency

National Incident Management System (NIMS): A comprehensive, national approach to incident management that is applicable at all jurisdictional levels and across functional disciplines

Natural disaster: Term used for a naturally (ie, not technological-based, nor human systems failure) occurring event or hazard that results in a disaster or public health emergency

Pandemic: A global epidemic from a new or modified infectious disease that emerges to which the population has little or no immunity

PRE-DISASTER Paradigm™: Steps to take before a disaster occurs: P, planning and practice; R, resilience; E, education

Preparedness planning: Development of resources and organizational capacity to prevent or manage the effects of a disaster on the basis of local risk assessments

Public health: A complex network of people, systems, and organizations that work together to ensure the conditions necessary to live healthy lives

Quarantine: Placement of persons exposed to a contagious disease, but currently asymptomatic, in a separate area where they will not expose others and can be monitored for the development of the disease.

Recovery planning: Planning for continuity of operations, restoration of essential services and infrastructure, and resumption of normal social and economic activities with minimal delay after a disaster

Response planning: Planning how local agencies and organizations will be engaged and mobilized when a disaster occurs

SALT: A mnemonic device for mass casualty triage; stands for sort, assess, lifesaving interventions, and treatment and/or transport

SEIRV: Population-based triage method for infectious illness; stands for susceptible, exposed, infectious, removed, and vaccinated.

Social distancing: A disease prevention strategy in which a community imposes limitations on social (face-to-face) interactions to reduce exposure to and transmission of a virus

Surge capacity: The ability of a health care system to rapidly expand beyond normal services to meet the increased demand for care of patients, which may include physical space/hospital beds, qualified personnel, medical care, and public health services

Technological disaster: An event resulting from a human systems failure, such as poorly designed buildings or flawed equipment, and human errors due to inadequate training, worker distraction, or fatigue

Terrorism: Use of any weapon, threatening act, or dangerous substance (eg, chemical, biologic, radiologic, nuclear, and explosive agents) to coerce, intimidate, or cause panic.

Toxidrome: A typical, specific set of signs and symptoms caused by a given chemical class

Triage: Prioritization of care for patients based on the severity of their illness or injury, their ability to survive, and the resources available

INDEX

Page numbers in italics indicate figures and tables.

A

Abdomen
  blast belly, 6-7
  gastrointestinal anthrax, 9-16
  gastrointestinal blast injuries, 6-17
  gastrointestinal syndrome (radiation sickness), 7-28, *7-29*
  gastrointestinal system in identification of chemical agent exposures, *8-11*
Accessible facilities, *See* Disabilities
Acetylcholinesterase, 8-26
ACFs (Alternative care facilities), *See* Health facilities
Acute coronary syndrome, 6-8
Acute radiation sickness (ARS), *See* Radiation
Acute stress disorder, *See* Stress
Adolescents, *See also* Children;
  communicating with, 3-7
  mental health in disasters, 3-35–3-36
After-action review, *See* Health facilities
Aging
  chronic illness, 3-16
  Hurricane Katrina victims, 10-23
  shelter for elderly, 3-22
  vulnerabilities in nuclear and radiation disasters, 7-39
Agitation, depression symptoms, 3-29
Air purification, *See* Respirators
Airborne disease transmission, 9-3–9-4, 9-12
Alcohol drinking, abuse, 3-30–3-31
All-hazards approach, 1-1–1-34
  disaster preparedness and, 1-5

environmental hazard dangers for children, 3-11
  preparedness, 1-29–1-32
  preparedness, glossary term, G-1
Alpha particles, *See* Radiation
Alternative care environment, *See* Health facilities
Aluminum hydroxide, radioisotope decorporation therapies, countermeasures, *7-36*
American Red Cross, 2-6
  mass care services, 2-24
Americans with Disabilities Act, 3-22
Americium 241, radioisotope decorporation therapies, countermeasures, *7-36*
Ammonium nitrate fertilizer, 6-5
Ammonium nitrate-fuel oil, 6-4
Amputation, traumatic, 6-8, 6-14–6-15
ANFO (ammonium nitrate-fuel oil), 6-4
Anhedonia, depression symptoms, 3-29
Animal bites, 4-14
Anthrax, 9-15–9-18
  cutaneous, 9-15–9-16
  cutaneous, in children, *9-31*
  gastrointestinal, in children, *9-31*
  inhalational, 9-16
  inhalational, in children, *9-31*
  potential bioterrorism agents (symptoms, differential diagnoses), *9-11*
  speedy therapy necessary, 9-14
  therapy for children, *9-30–9-31*
Antibiotics, 9-14
Anxiety disorder, generalized, *See* Mental health

Appetite, depression symptoms, 3-29
Arms, *See* Extremity injuries
ARS (acute radiation sickness), *See* Radiation
Arterial gas embolism, 6-12–6-13
Asphyxiation, traumatic, 6-13–6-14
Assessment of hazards, *See* Hazard assessment
Asphyxiation, 10-12, 10-33
Asthma, 6-8
At-risk populations, *See* Vulnerable populations
Atropine, 8-30, 8-31, *8-32*
Auditory system injuries, blast injuries, 6-11, 6-17
Autoinjectors, *See* Atropine; Pralidoxime chloride

B

Bacillus anthracis, *See* Anthrax
BAL, *See* British antilewisite
Ballistic injuries
  blunt, 6-18
  penetrating, 6-18
  wound contamination, 6-19
Banda Aceh, *See* Indonesia
Bangladesh hurricane/cyclone (1970), 10-21
Behavioral emergencies, 6-8
Behavioral health, 7-38
Benzodiazepines, 8-31
Beta particles, *See* Radiation
Bhopal, India, chemical disaster, 8-35
Bicarbonate, radioisotope decorporation therapies, countermeasures, *7-36*

Biologic disasters, 2-16, 9-1–9-38, *See also* Bioterrorism; Communicable diseases;
  agent-specific issues, 9-14–9-32
  basics of infectious disease exposure and transmission, 9-2–9-5
  biologic agent risk categories, characteristics, examples, *9-8*
  clinical decision making, 9-10–9-14
  types of, 9-5–9-7
Bioterrorism, 9-2, 9-6–9-7
  biologic agent risk categories, characteristics, examples, *9-8*
  epidemiologic clues of attacks, 9-9
  food contamination, 9-7
  potential agents (symptoms, differential diagnoses), *9-11*
  public health actions, 9-32–9-35
BioWatch, 9-10
Bites and stings, 4-14
Blast, definition, 6-4
Blast belly, 6-7, 6-17
Blast brain, 6-7
Blast ear, 6-6, 6-7
Blast eye, 6-7
Blast injuries, 6-6–6-9
  common explosion-related injuries, *6-11*
  crush injuries and crush syndrome, 6-15–6-16
  mechanisms of, 6-6–6-9
  primary, traumatic injuries from, *6-7*
  quaternary, *6-8*
  secondary, 6-7–6-8
  tertiary (bodies propelled or structure collapse), 6-8
Blast lung, 6-7, 6-11–6-12
Blast terror, 6-21
Blast waves, 6-5, 6-6–6-9
Blast wind, 6-4, 6-8
BLEVE (boiling liquid expanding vapor explosion), 6-3
Blindness, 3-20
  flash, temporary and permanent, following nuclear detonation, 7-7
Blistering agents, 8-13–8-16

diagnostic, clinical and treatment aspects, *8-15–8-16*
Blood, hematopoietic syndrome (radiation sickness), 7-28, *7-29*
Bloodborne pathogens, 4-15
Blunt trauma, *See* Trauma management
Bodies (corpses), *See* Mass casualty incidents
Boiling liquid expanding vapor explosion (BLEVE), 6-3
Boots, *See* Personal protective equipment
Botulinum antitoxin, 9-19
Botulism, 9-18–9-20
  potential bioterrorism agents (symptoms, differential diagnoses), *9-11*
Brain, blast injuries, 6-7
Breastfeeding, 3-12
Brief psychotic disorder, *See* Mental health
Brisance, description of effect, 6-4
British antilewisite, 8-16
British Petroleum oil spill, 8-36–8-37
Bubonic plague, *See* Plague
Building collapses, 6-8, 6-10, 10-6, 10-12, 10-14, 10-33
Building codes, 10-14, 10-23
Bullets, *See* Ballistic injuries
Burnout, disaster responders, 4-2
Burns
  altered care environment following nuclear and radiologic disasters, 7-27–7-28
  blast injuries, 6-8
  chemical, from mustard, 8-14
  flash (blast injuries), 6-18
  retinal, 7-7
  thermal, 7-6–7-7, 10-33
  volcanic eruptions, 10-33–10-34
  wildfires, 10-36, 10-37
Butyrylcholinesterase (nerve agent exposure), 8-28

C

CAGE questionnaire, 3-30–3-31
Calcium gluconate, radioisotope

decorporation therapies, countermeasures, *7-36*
California wildfires, 10-37–10-38
Cancer, post-nuclear and post-radiologic disaster monitoring, 7-40–7-41
Capacity assessment, *See* Surge capacity
Carbon dioxide, from volcanic eruptions, *10-34*
Carbon monoxide
  poisoning (gas generators), 10-24, 10-25
  volcanic eruptions, *10-34*
Cardiovascular system, *See* Circulatory system
CareFlight (triage system), 5-6
Casualties, *See* Mass casualty incidents
Cataracts, post-nuclear and post-radiologic disaster monitoring, 7-40–7-41
CDC, *See* US Centers for Disease Control and Prevention
Center for Research on the Epidemiology of Disasters, 10-3
Central nervous system injuries, *See* Nervous system injuries
CESIRA (triage system), 5-6
Cesium 137, radioisotope decorporation therapies, countermeasures, *7-36*
Chemical disasters, 8-1–8-41
  Bhopal, India, 8-35
  blister agents, 8-13–8-16
  British Petroleum oil spill, Gulf of Mexico, 8-36–8-37
  casualty assessment, 8-4–8-6, 8-8–8-12
  choking agents, 8-16–8-19
  classes of chemicals, 8-5
  clues to type of chemical agent exposure, *8-11*
  cyanide agents, 8-19–8-26
  decontamination, 8-9–8-10
  detection devices, 8-6–8-7
  emergencies described and compared to disasters, 8-2–8-3
  explosions, 6-4–6-5
  exposure clues, 8-4–8-6, 8-9

incident management and work-force protection, 8-7–8-8

learning from specific events, 8-35–8-37

nerve agents, 8-26–8-33

pediatric treatment, *8-32*, 8-33–8-34

pulmonary agents, 8-16–8-19

size of release, distance of danger zones, 8-7

Tokyo sarin subway attack, 8-35–8-36

toxidromes, 6-8, 8-6

vesicants, 8-13–8-16

Chemical explosions, 6-4–6-5

definitions and descriptions of terms, 6-4

Chest tubes, 6-12, 6-13

Chicago, heat-wave deaths, 1-16

Children, 3-2–3-13

abuse, maltreatment, 3-13

anatomy, 3-3–3-4

anthrax in, *9-30*

body surface area, 3-4

central nervous system risks, 3-4

chemical disaster treatment, *8-32*, 8-33–8-34

circulatory system risks, 3-4, 3-5

communication with, 3-6, 3-7

decontamination, 3-8, 4-24–4-25

developmental considerations, regression, 3-6

environmental hazards, 3-11

explosion disasters, 6-21

family identification and reunification, 3-9–3-10

Glasgow Coma Scale, modified, *5-18*

hypothermia, 3-4, 3-5

immunologic considerations, 3-5

infectious diseases, 3-5, 3-11

lodging and shelter, 3-11

medications, equipment, supplies, 3-9

mental health in disasters, 3-35–3-36

respiratory system risks, 3-4, 3-5

shock and, 3-4, 3-5

skeletal system, 3-4

vulnerabilities in disasters, 3-2–3-6

Chlorine

choking/pulmonary chemical agent, 8-17, 8-18

pediatric management of chemical agents, *8-34*

Choking agents, 8-16–8-19

Cholera, potential bioterrorism agents (symptoms, differential diagnoses), *9-11*

Cholinesterase testing (nerve agent exposure), 8-28

Chronic diseases

children with, 3-12

disaster responders with, 4-7

Hurricane Katrina aftermath, 10-24

records, care and access in disasters, 3-16–3-18

Chronic obstructive pulmonary disease, *See* Pulmonary disease, chronic obstructive

Ciprofloxacin, 9-17

Circulatory system

cardiovascular syndrome (radiation sickness), 7-28, *7-30*

earthquake aftermath, 10-13

hurricane aftermath, 10-25

identification of chemical agent exposures, *8-11*

disseminated intravascular coagulation (DIC), 6-15

explosion-related injuries, 6-11

Clinical competencies, *See* Competencies

Clostridium botulinum, *See* Botulism

Clothing, protective, *See* Personal protective equipment

Coagulation, disseminated intravascular (DIC), *See* Circulatory system

Cobalt 60, radioisotope decorporation therapies, countermeasures, *7-36*

Cold exposure, 4-14

winter storms, 10-38–10-41

Cold zones (disaster scenes), 4-18

Coma, Glasgow Coma Scale, *5-17–5-18*

Commissioned Corps, *See* US Public Health Service

Communicable diseases, *See also* names of specific diseases, *eg*, Anthrax;

basics of exposure and transmission, 9-2–9-5

biologic agent risk categories, characteristics, examples, *9-8*

blood and body fluid dangers, 4-15

CDC's Epidemic Intelligence Service, 2-21–2-22

chain of infection, 9-3–9-5

child susceptibility, 3-5, 3-11

clinical features, diagnosis, treatment, prophylaxis, infection control for specific diseases, 9-14–9-32

epidemics and pandemics, 9-6

epidemiologic surveillance and investigation, 2-11–2-14

hurricane aftermath, 10-25–10-26

incubation periods and recognition of outbreaks, 9-9

infection control, 9-12–9-13

infectious agents, 9-3

modes of transmission described, 9-3–9-4

notable epidemics and pandemics, 9-6

nuclear and radiation disaster infection control, 7-31

pandemic (glossary term), G-2

prevention and control, 2-22–2-23

public health emergencies, 2-9–2-11

risks for children, 3-11

susceptible host, 9-5

treatment guidelines, 9-14–9-15

triage, 9-13

universal precautions (viral transmission), 4-21

Communications

health-related considerations, 1-18–1-19

impaired individuals, 3-20–3-21, 3-22–3-23

infants, toddlers, children, teenagers, 3-6, 3-7

information sharing and media following nuclear or radiologic events, 7-13–7-14 interoperable systems, 1-19

non-English speakers and those with limited English proficiency, 3-20

parents, 3-8

post-crisis mental health recovery, 3-33

risk communication principles, 2-17–2-18

unwarranted and inaccurate information from mass media following nuclear and radiologic events, 7-14

vulnerable and special needs populations, 3-19

Community disaster response, *See also* DISASTER Paradigm™

after-action review and planning, 1-27–1-28

communal events as part of recovery process, 3-33

emergency operations plans, 1-9

evacuation, special needs populations, 3-21–3-22

preparedness, 1-29–1-32

readiness and resilience, 1-28, 1-30

recovery and beyond, 2-25–2-26

registries for special needs populations, 3-24

surge capacity, 1-12–1-13

Compartment syndrome, 6-16–6-17

Competencies

Basic Disaster Life Support, A-B1–A-B8

clinical/public health assessment and intervention, related BDLS® course chapters and objectives, A-B5–A-B7

contingency, continuity and recovery, related BDLS® course chapters and objectives, A-B7–A-B8

incident management and support systems, related BDLS® course chapters and objectives, A-B4–A-B5

preparation and planning, related BDLS® course chapters and objectives, A-B2–A-B4

public health law and ethics, related BDLS® course chapters and objectives, A-B8

safety and security, related BDLS® course chapters and objectives, A-B5

Concentration, depression symptoms, 3-29

Conflicts, *See* War

Contact

direct and indirect, in disease transmission, 9-4

precautions, 9-12, 9-13

Containment, glossary term, G-1

Contamination, *See also* Decontamination; Radiation;

disaster scene exclusion zones, 4-17–4-18

radioisotope, internal, 7-33–7-36

Contingency, continuity and recovery, *See* Competencies

COPD, *See* Pulmonary disease, chronic obstructive

Core Disaster Life Support, 1-5

Corpses (fatalities), *See* Mass casualty incidents

CRED, *See* Center for Research on the Epidemiology of Disasters

Crisis capacity, *See* Surge capacity

Crisis intervention, 3-34

CRS (cutaneous radiation syndrome), *See* Radiation; Skin

Crush injuries, 6-15–6-16

compartment syndrome and, 6-16–6-17

Crush syndrome, 6-15–6-16, 10-12

Cultural issues, 5-26

Cyanide agents, 8-19–8-26

diagnostic, clinical and treatment aspects, *8-25*

pediatric management of chemical agents, *8-34*

Cyanide agents, 8-19–8-26

Cyanide salts, 8-21

Cyanogen chloride, *8-25*

Cyclones, *See* Hurricanes

Cytochrome oxidase, 8-22, 8-23

Cytokine therapy, 7-31

D

Dam failures, 10-15

Deaths, disaster-related, 1-2

Debris floods, 10-15

Decontamination

casualties, 4-22–4-26

chemical disasters, 8-9–8-10

children, 3-8

dry, 4-23, G-1

glossary term, G-1

natural disasters, 10-6

non-ambulatory casualties, 4-23

nuclear and radiologic casualties, 7-18–7-19

separation of sexes, 5-26

wet, 4-23, G-1

zones, 4-18

zones, following nuclear or radiologic disasters, 7-15

Decorporation, *See* Radiation

Definitions, 1-4–1-5

cyclones, 10-21

deployment, 4-2

disasters (NDLS definition), 1-4

glossary of terms, G-1–G-2

hazard, 1-10

hurricanes, 10-21

isolation, 2-11

mass fatality event, 5-22

public health system, infrastructure, 2-2–2-3

quarantine, 2-11

risk, 1-10

special needs populations, 3-19–3-20

surge capacity and surge capability, 1-12

typhoons, 10-21

Deflagration, 6-4

Demobilization, *See* Disaster responders

Dengue fever, 10-25–10-26

Deployment, *See* Disaster responders; Health personnel

Deployment planning, *See* Disaster responders; Planning and practice;

Depression, 3-29–3-30

Detection (DISASTER Paradigm™)
  all-hazards disaster casualty management (discussion points),
    1-30
  biologic disaster situational awareness and, 9-9–9-10
  biologic disasters, 9-35
  chemical disaster discussion points,
    8-38
  chemical disaster situational awareness and, 8-3–8-7
  earthquake and tsunami warnings,
    10-10
  elements of DISASTER Paradigm™ described, A–A3
  explosion disasters (discussion points), 6-23
  floods, 10-15–10-16
  health-related considerations,
    1-14–1-16
  heat emergencies, 10-18
  hurricanes, 10-22
  key elements of DISASTER Paradigm™, 1-6, 1-30
  natural disaster warnings, 10-4
  natural disasters (discussion points), 10-42
  nuclear detonation and radiologic disasters, 7-8–7-9
  public health response (discussion points), 2-28
  radiologic and nuclear disaster discussion points, 7-43
  situational awareness and, 1-14–1-16
  situational awareness, explosion disasters, 6-9–6-10
  tornado watches and warnings,
    10-28
  volcanic eruptions, 10-31
  wildfires, 10-36
  winter storms, 10-39–10-40
Diarrhea, radiation sickness, 7-30
Diazepam, 8-31
DIC (disseminated intravascular coagulation), See Circulatory system
2,2-dichlorodiethyl sulfide, See Sulfur mustard
Diethylenetriamine penta-acetate (DTPA), 7-34–7-36

Digestive system injuries, explosion-related injuries, 6-11
Disabilities, 3-18–3-19
  accessible shelters, 3-22
  casualty assessment, 5-17
  communication with individuals having, 3-20–3-21
  decontamination of casualties with functional and access needs,
    4-25
  special needs populations, 3-19–3-20
Disaster, glossary term, G-1
Disaster exercises, See Disaster response
Disaster management, all-hazards, for casualties, 1-1–1-34
Disaster Medical Assistance Teams,
    2-21
Disaster Mortuary Operational Response Team, 5-23
Disaster (operational), glossary term,
    G-1
DISASTER Paradigm™, 1-1, 1-2, 1-6–1-8, 1-30–1-32
  biologic disasters, 9-35–9-37
  description of elements of, A–A3
  explosion disaster discussion points, 6-23
  glossary term, G-1
  key elements of, 1-6
  preparedness, 1-29–1-32
Disaster plans, See Emergency operations plans
Disaster responders, 4-1–4-27; See also Health personnel; Volunteers;
  activation and mobilization,
    4-15–4-16
  dangers of "second hit" (ie, collapse of World Trade Center towers, etc.), 6-10
  demobilization and deployment-related stress, 4-25–4-26, 4-27
  family concerns of, during nuclear and radiologic disasters,
    7-39
  firefighter injuries, 10-37
  fitness, stress and burnout, 4-2, 4-26, 4-27
  mental health, 3-34–3-35

personal equipment and packing ("go kits"), 4-8–4-9
  personal health and wellness,
    4-7–4-8
  personal protective equipment (PPE), 4-18–4-22
  personnel shortages following nuclear or radiologic events,
    7-13
  plans for handling personal/business affairs, 4-5–4-7
  pre-approvals for work leave, 4-5
  predeployment checklist, 4-3
  predeployment education and training, 4-9–4-11
  predeployment preparation and planning, 4-3–4-13
  professional credentials and equipment (pre-disaster readiness),
    4-9
  protection following nuclear and radiologic disasters,
    7-14–7-19
  protection in chemical disasters,
    8-7–8-8
  protective issues, 4-16–4-22
  radiation field determination,
    7-11–7-12
  radiation hazard awareness, 7-16
  risk awareness and mitigation,
    4-13–4-15
  self-deployment problems, 4-4
  shortages in nuclear and radiologic disasters, 7-38
  targeting of, in explosion disasters,
    6-9
  volunteers, 4-4
Disaster response, See also Community disaster response; DISASTER Paradigm™;
Disaster responders;
  emergency public health powers,
    2-9–2-11
  exercises and drills, 1-13–1-14
  health considerations, 1-14–1-24
  initial local responses, 1-19–1-20
  integration of public health and clinical services in disasters,
    2-15–2-16

multiagency coordination in large-scale disasters, 2-16–2-17

National Health Security Strategy, 1-3

National Voluntary Organizations Active in Disaster, 2-6

preparedness and PRE-DISASTER Paradigm™, 1-5–1-6

public health principles and practices, 2-1–2-30

situational awareness and detection, 1-14–1-16

specific aspects of public health's role, 2-8–2-25

Disaster response, community, *See* Community disaster response

Disaster warnings, *See* Detection (DISASTER Paradigm™)

Disasters, *(For detailed index entries, see also* All-hazards approach; Biologic disasters; Chemical disasters; Disaster responders; Explosion disasters; Mass casualty incidents; Mental Health; Natural disasters; Nuclear disasters; Public health; Radiologic disasters; Trauma management; Vulnerable populations*)*

biologic, 8-1–8-41

chemical, 9-1–9-38

classification systems, 1-4

defined as needs exceeding immediately available resources, 1-4

exclusion zones, 4-17–4-18

explosions and traumatic disasters, 6-1–6-27

glossary terms, G-1–G-2

human systems failures, 1-4

human-caused, deaths from, 1-2

localized, 1-4

mental disorders associated with, 3-28–3-31

natural, 1-2, 1-4, 10-1–10-48, G-2

nuclear and radiologic, 7-1–7-47

population health and mental health, 3-1–3-40

psychosocial effects, 3-26–3-27

recent doubling in frequency of, 1-2

risk communication, 1-18–1-19

technological, glossary term, G-2

time dimensions of, 1-4

war- and conflict-related, 1-4

Disease transmission, *See* Communicable diseases

Disseminated intravascular coagulation (DIC), *See* Circulatory system

Distilled mustard, *8-15*

pediatric management of chemical agents, *8-34*

DMATs, *See* Disaster Medical Assistance Teams

DMSA, radioisotope decorporation therapies, countermeasures, *7-36*

DNA damage, radiation exposure and, 7-5–7-6

Drills, *See* Disaster response

Drinking water, 2-23

Droplets (disease transmission), 9-4

precautions, 9-12

Drugs, *See* Medications

DTPA (diethylenetriamene penta-acetate), 7-34–7-36

DUMBELS (nerve agent mnemonic), 8-28

Dynamite, 6-4

Dysphoria, depression symptoms, 3-29

E

Ear injuries (blast injuries), 6-6, 6-7

Earthquakes and tsunamis, 10-8–10-14

aftermath/public health concerns, 10-12–10-14

types and causes of deaths, injuries, *10-7*

EDTA, radioisotope decorporation therapies, countermeasures, *7-36*

Education and training (PRE-DISASTER Paradigm™)

all-hazards disaster casualty management (discussion points), 1-30

biologic disasters, 9-35

chemical disaster discussion points, 8-38

elements of PRE-DISASTER Paradigm™ described, A-A3

explosion disasters (discussion points), 6-22–6-23

natural disasters (discussion points), 10-42

predeployment, 4-9–4-11

public health response (discussion points), 2-27

radiologic and nuclear disaster discussion points, 7-43

EF, *See* Enhanced Fujita scale

Electrical storms, 10-32

Electromagnetic pulse, 7-8

Electron transport chain, 8-22

Emergency care, 4-12–4-13, *See also* Disaster responders; Triage and treatment (DISASTER Paradigm™);

chemical disasters, 8-2–8-3

mass casualty incidents, 5-1–5-29

psychological first aid, 3-32–3-33

public health response, 2-2

Emergency management, glossary term, G-1

Emergency operations centers, 1-18, 2-17, G-1

Emergency operations plans, 1-8–1-9

coordination of local, state and federal authorities, 1-9

Emergency responders, *See* Disaster responders

Emergency services, *See* Emergency care

Emergency Support Functions, 1-20

ESF 6 (mass care), 1-20

ESF 8 (health and medical services), 1-20

ESF 8 and mental health services, 3-33

nuclear events, 7-12

surge management, 2-20

Emergency System for Advance Registration of Volunteer Health Professionals, 4-4

Emesis, radiation sickness, 7-30

English-language proficiency, 3-20

Enhanced Fujita scale, 10-27, *10-28*

Environmental disasters, *See* Chemical disasters; Nuclear disasters; Radiologic disasters

Environmental hazards, *See* All-hazards approach

Environmental health services, 2-24–2-25

Epidemic Intelligence Service, *See* US Centers for Disease Control and Prevention

Epidemics, *See* Communicable diseases

Epidemiologic surveillance, *See* Communicable diseases; Public health

Equipment, *See also* Personal protective equipment;

pediatric, 3-9

Strategic National Stockpile, 2-22

Erythrocyte cholinesterase (nerve agent exposure), 8-28

ESFs, *See* Emergency Support Functions

Esteem, depression symptoms, 3-29

Ethics, 5-26, 5-27

disaster planning framework, 1-13

Ethics, group decision making, 5-27

Evacuation, 2-18–2-19 (DISASTER Paradigm™)

all-hazards disaster casualty management (discussion points), 1-32

biologic disasters, 9-37

casualties, 5-19–5-20

chemical disaster discussion points, 8-39

elements of DISASTER Paradigm™ described, A-A3

explosion disasters (discussion points), 6-23

key elements of DISASTER Paradigm™, 1-6, 1-8, 1-32

natural disasters (discussion points), 10-43

nuclear and radiologic casualties, 7-20–7-21

public health response (discussion points), 2-29

radioactivity fear and, 7-11

radiologic and nuclear disaster discussion points, 7-45

special needs populations, 3-21–3-22

Explosion disasters, 6-1–6-27

blast injury types described, 6-6–6-9

blast wind and blast waves, 6-4, 6-5

clinical decision making, 6-10–6-20

distance from blast, 6-4–6-5

effects of detonation in open vs. enclosed spaces, 6-5

flash burns, 6-18

hazard assessment checklist, *6-9*

implanted metal fragments to cause secondary blast injuries, 6-7–6-8

increasing numbers of US criminal bombings, 6-3

increasing potential of terrorist attacks, 6-3

injury mechanisms, 6-6–6-9

lifesaving skills, 6-11

magnitude of (positive phase impulse, or "peak overpressure," 6-4–6-5, *6-5*

negative phase impulse, *6-5*

pediatric considerations, 6-21

pre-existing conditions and other risk factors, 6-20

public health considerations, 6-20

secondary devices, 6-21

situational awareness and detection, 6-9–6-10

size of explosive charge, 6-4

surrounding medium (air or water), 6-5

types, 6-3–6-6

types of common injuries in, *6-11*

Extreme heat, *See* Heat emergencies

Extremity injuries

explosion-related injuries, 6-11

traumatic amputation, 6-14–6-15

Eye injuries

blast injuries, 6-7, 6-17–6-18

explosion-related injuries, 6-11

volcanic eruptions, 10-34

F

Facial injuries, explosion-related injuries, 6-11

Fallout, nuclear, *See* Radiation

Families

identification and reunification, 3-9–3-10

survivors in mass casualty incidents, 5-23

Fatalities, *See* Mass casualty incidents

Fatigue, depression symptoms, 3-29

Fecal-oral disease transmission, 9-4

Federal agencies, *See* US government; names of specific agencies, *eg,* US Centers for Disease Control and Prevention

Fetuses, *See* Pregnancy

Firefighter fatalities, 10-37

Fires, *See* Wildfires

First responders, *See* Disaster responders

Flash blindness, 7-7

Flash floods, 10-15

Floods, 10-14–10-18

regional, 10-15

roadway dangers, 10-17

types and causes of deaths, injuries, *10-7*

types of, 10-14–10-15

wildfire aftermath, 10-36

Food chain, radioactive iodine contamination, 7-8

Forensics, 1-20

Forest fires, *See* Wildfires

Fractures, blast injuries, 6-8

Frail elderly, nerve agent therapy, *8-31*

Francisella tularensis, See Tularemia

Frostbite, 4-14–4-15, 10-40

Fujita scale, 10-27, *10-28*

G

G-agents, *See* Nerve agents

Galveston, Texas, hurricane (1900), 10-21

Gamma radiation, *See* Radiation

Gas embolism, 6-12–6-13

Gas generator dangers (carbon monoxide poisoning), 10-24–10-25

Gases, toxic, 10-33, *10-34*

Gastrointestinal injuries, *See* Abdomen

Gastrointestinal syndrome (radiation sickness), 7-28, *7-29*, 7-30

Generalized anxiety disorder, *See* Mental health

Geographic information system, 1-11

Geospatial technology, 1-11

GIS, *See* Geographic information system

Glasgow Coma Scale, responses and scores listed, *5-17–5-18*

Global health, *See* International health

Gloves, *See* Personal protective equipment

Go-kits, *See* Volunteers

Good Samaritan doctrine, 4-12

Gray (Gy; absorbed radiation dose), *See* Radiation

Grief, 3-29

Ground zero, *See* Nuclear disasters; Radiologic disasters

Guilt, depression symptoms, 3-29

Gulf of Mexico/BP oil spill, 8-36–8-37

Gy (absorbed radiation dose), *See* Radiation

H

Haiti earthquake (2010), 10-9, 10-13

Hazard assessment (DISASTER Paradigm™)

all-hazards disaster casualty management (discussion points), 1-31

biologic disasters, 9-36

chemical disaster discussion points, 8-39

disaster scene exclusion zones, 4-17–4-18

earthquakes and tsunamis, 10-11

elements of DISASTER Paradigm™ described, A-A3

explosion checklist, *6-9*

explosion disasters (discussion points), 6-23

floods, 10-16

glossary term, G-1

hazard vulnerability analysis, 1-10

health-related considerations, 1-16

heat emergencies, 10-19

hurricanes, 10-22–10-23

IDLH area (immediately dangerous to life or health), 4-19

key elements of DISASTER Paradigm™, 1-6, 1-7

natural disasters (by type), *10-7–10-8*

natural disasters (discussion points), 10-43

nuclear detonation and radiologic disasters, 7-8–7-11

public health response (discussion points), 2-28

radiation perimeters and control zones, 7-16

radiologic and nuclear disaster discussion points, 7-44

risk analysis, 1-10

risk and, 1-10

risk awareness by disaster responders, 4-26

tornadoes, 10-29

volcanic eruptions, 10-32

wildfires, 10-36

winter storms, 10-40

Hazard vulnerability analysis, 1-10

HAZMAT incidents, *See* Chemical disasters

Health and Human Services Department, *See* US Health and Human Services Department

Health departments, state, *See* State government

Health emergency operations centers (HEOCs), *See* Emergency operations centers

Health facilities

access for children, 3-12–3-13

after-action reviews, 1-26–1-27, 4-25

alternative care environment, 1-23, 1-24, 10-5

alternative care sites, glossary term, G-1

care for special needs populations, 3-23–3-24

decontamination zones, 4-18

emergency operations plans, 1-9

Houston Astrodome (Hurricane Katrina), 10-5

incident command system and, 1-18

mass casualty incidents, 1-21

NIMS Implementation Plan for Hospitals and Healthcare, 4-10–4-11

recovery and continuity of operations, 1-25–1-28

surge capacity and mass casualty incidents, 1-22

surge capacity continuum, 1-23

surge management, 1-20–1-24, 10-5

transfers of pre-disaster patients, 5-5

Health personnel, *See also* Disaster responders; Volunteers;

dealing with child injury or death, 3-13

disaster exercises and drills, 1-13–1-14

Emergency System for Advance Registration of Volunteer Health Professionals, 4-4

family concerns of, during nuclear and radiologic disasters, 7-39

legal issues for volunteer responders, 4-11–4-13

licensure issues, 4-11–4-12

mental health for emergency responders, 3-34–3-35

professional credentials and equipment (pre-disaster readiness), 4-9

professional liability, 4-11–4-12

professionalism and ethics, 5-25–5-26

protection following nuclear and radiologic disasters, 7-14–7-19

protection in chemical disasters, 8-7–8-8

readiness and disaster deployment, 4-1–4-27

reemployment after disasters, 4-11

self-deployment problems, 4-4

shortages following nuclear or radiologic events, 7-13

shortages in nuclear and radiologic disasters, 7-38

situational awareness and detection, 1-14–1-16

surge capacity and management, 1-21–1-23

volunteers, 4-4

Health system surge capacity, *See* Surge capacity

Hearing impairment, 3-20–3-21, 6-17

shelter information, 3-22–3-23

Heat emergencies, 10-18–10-21

types and causes of deaths, injuries, *10-7*

Heat exposure, 4-14

Heat-related injuries

cramps, edema, syncope, exhaustion, stroke, 10-19–10-20

from wildfires, 10-37

Heat waves, 1-16

Hematopoietic colony-stimulating factors, 7-31–7-32

Hematopoietic syndrome (radiation sickness), 7-28, *7-29*

Hemorrhagic fevers, viral, 9-28–9-30

HHS, *See* US Health and Human Services Department

History of medicine, notable epidemics and pandemics, 9-6

Homebush (triage system), 5-6

Hospitals, *See* Health facilities

Host, *See* Communicable diseases

Hot zones, 4-17–4-18

Housing

children and families, 3-11

disaster responders and volunteers, 4-13–4-14

evacuation vs shelter in place following nuclear and radiologic disasters, 7-11

Haiti earthquake, 10-13

Hurricane Katrina, 10-24

special needs populations, 3-22–3-23

women and children, 3-14, 3-15

Houston Astrodome, 10-24

Human systems failures, 1-2

classification of disasters, 1-4

Hurricane Ike (2008), 2-13, 10-21–10-22

Hurricane Katrina, 1-2, 1-24, 3-18, 4-10, 10-23–10-25

alternate care facilities, 10-5, 10-24

levee failures in New Orleans, 10-15

Hurricanes, 10-21–10-26

immediate and long-term aftermath, 10-23

types and causes of deaths, injuries, *10-7*, 10-23

Hydration, radioisotope decorporation therapies, countermeasures, *7-36*

Hydrogen cyanide, 8-19–8-21, 8-23, *8-25*, *8-26*

Hydrogen gases, hazardous (from volcanic eruptions), *10-34*

Hygiene, *See* Sanitation

Hyperkalemia, crush syndrome and, 6-16

Hypersomnia, depression symptoms, 3-29

Hypothermia, 4-14

child susceptibility, 3-4, 3-5

natural disasters and, 10-25, 10-40

Hypoxemia, 6-12

I

Ice-jam floods, 10-15

IDLH (immediately dangerous to life or health), *See* Hazard assessment

ID ME, glossary term, G-2

ID-MED, *See* Triage and treatment

IEDs, 6-2, 6-5–6-6

"Immediately dangerous to life or health" areas (IDLH), *See* Hazard assessment

Immunizations, disaster responders, 4-8

Impalement, 6-8, 6-20

Improvised explosive devices, 6-2, 6-5–6-6

Incident command system, 1-7, 1-17–1-18

public health emergencies, 2-15

Incident commander, 1-17

Incident management (DISASTER Paradigm™)

all-hazards disaster casualty management (discussion points), 1-31

biologic disasters, 9-36

chemical disaster discussion points, 8-38

chemical disaster reporting, 8-7

chemical disasters, 8-7–8-8

elements of DISASTER Paradigm™ described, A-A3

explosion disasters (discussion points), 6-23

glossary term, G-2

health-related considerations, 1-17–1-20

integration of public health and clinical services in disasters, 2-15–2-16

key elements of DISASTER Paradigm™, 1-6–1-7, 1-31

multiagency coordination in large-scale disasters, 2-16–2-17

natural disasters (discussion points), 10-43

public health aspects, 2-15–2-17

public health response (discussion points), 2-28

radiologic and nuclear disaster discussion points, 7-44

three C's (command, coordination, communication), 1-6–1-7

Incident management competencies (BDLS® course), *See* Competencies

Independence in personal activities, *See* Vulnerable populations

Indian Ocean, 10-21

Indonesia, tsunami (2004), 10-13

Infants, *See* Children

Infection control, 9-12–9-13

Infectious diseases, *See* Communicable diseases

Influenza epidemics and pandemics, 9-6

Inhalation injuries, 6-8

Injuries, *See* Ballistic injuries; Blast injuries; Burns; Crush injuries; Explosion disasters; Trauma management; names of particular body parts or organ systems, *eg*, Extremity injuries; Respiratory system

Insect bites and stings, 4-14

Insomnia, depression symptoms, 3-29

International health, 2-7–2-8

   Web sites for global health agencies and organizations, 2-7–2-8

International Red Cross and Red Crescent Movement, 2-8

Iodine isotopes, radioisotope decorporation therapies, countermeasures, *7-36*

Ionizing radiation, *See* Radiation

Iridium 192, radioisotope decorporation therapies, countermeasures, *7-36*

Isolation, 2-10–2-11, G-2

J-K

Japan, earthquake and tsunami (2011), 10-9, 10-10, 10-14

JumpSTART (triage system), 5-6

KI (Potassium iodide) 7-35

   radioisotope decorporation therapies, countermeasures, *7-36*

Kidney, *See* Renal injuries

L

Laboratory Response Network, *See* Laboratory services

Laboratory services, 2-23–2-24

Landslides, 10-15

Law

   disaster planning framework, 1-13

   Good Samaritan doctrine, 4-12

   issues for volunteer health responders, 4-11–4-13

   living wills, 4-6

   power of attorney for finance, 4-6

   power of attorney for health care, 4-6

Legal issues, *See* Law

Legs, *See* Extremity injuries

Levee failures, 10-15

Lewisite, 8-13

   diagnostic, clinical and treatment aspects, *8-15*

   pediatric management of chemical agents, *8-34*

Liability, professional, 4-11–4-12

Liaison officer, 1-17

Licensure and scope of practice, 4-11–4-14

Living wills, 4-6

Lodging, *See* Housing

Logistics, *See* Support

Lung, blast injuries, 6-7

M

Malaria, 10-25–10-26

Mass care, *See* Emergency Support Functions; Mass casualty incidents

Mass casualty incidents, 1-21, 1-22, 5-1–5-29

   all-hazards disaster management, 1-1–1-34

   casualty assessment, 5-15–5-19

   casualty transport and evacuation, 5-19–5-20

   chemical disasters, 8-8–8-12

   decontamination, 4-22–4-26

   documentation and recordkeeping, 5-12, 5-28

   history-taking (SAMPLE), 5-18

   mass fatality event, glossary term, G-2

   mass fatality management, 5-20–5-23, 5-27

   morgue operations, 5-22–5-23

   natural disasters, 10-5–10-8

   nuclear and radiologic disasters, 7-11–7-14

   nuclear and radiologic, casualty decontamination, 7-18–7-19

   nuclear and radiologic, casualty management, 7-19–7-36

   nuclear detonation, 7-2, 7-3

   physical examination, 5-19

   predeployment education and training of disaster responders, 4-9–4-11

   recovery of human remains, 5-22

   reporting, identification, tracking, 5-24–5-25

   triage principles, 5-3–5-5

   triage systems described, 5-5–5-14

visual assessment (exposure and environment), 5-17

Mass fatalities, *See* Mass casualty incidents

Mechanical explosions, 6-3–6-4

Medecins Sans Frontieres, 2-8

Media, *See* Communication

Medical records, 3-16–3-17

Medical Reserve Corps, description, Web site, 2-21

Medications, *See also* Triage and treatment (DISASTER Paradigm™);

   cutaneous radiation syndrome, 7-33

   cytokine therapy (nuclear and radiation casualties), 7-31–7-32

   disaster responders, 4-8

   emesis and diarrhea following nuclear and radiation disasters, 7-30

   hematopoietic colony-stimulating factors, 7-31–7-32

   infection control, neutropenia following nuclear and radiation disasters, 7-31

   pediatric, 3-9

   psychiatric symptom management, 3-34

Men, separation of sexes, 5-26

Mental health, 3-1, 3-2, 3-25–3-40

   adults in disasters, 3-31–3-35

   brief psychotic disorder, 3-29

   children and adolescents, 3-35–3-36

   crisis intervention, 3-34

   demobilization and deployment-related symptoms in responders, 4-25–4-26, 4-27

   disaster responders, 3-34–3-35

   earthquake aftermath, 10-13–10-14

   explosion disasters, 6-20

   generalized anxiety disorder, 3-30

   hurricane aftermath, 10-25

   medications, 3-34

   nuclear and radiologic disasters, 7-38

   planning and priorities, 3-26–3-27

   psychological first aid, 3-32–3-33

psychological impact of disasters on women, 3-15–3-16

psychological triage, 3-31–3-32

psychosocial effects of disasters, 3-26–3-27

psychosocial emergencies, 6-8

"SAD-A-FACES" depression symptom screening tool, 3-29

stress and psychological trauma, 3-27–3-28

"worried well," 3-36

Methemoglobin, 8-24, *8-26*

Methyl isocyanate, 8-35

Military triage, 5-6

Mitigation, glossary term, G-2

Mobilization, *See* Disaster responders

MODIS (Moderate Resolution Imaging Spectroradiometer), 10-38

Moment magnitude scale, 10-9

Morgues, 5-22–5-23

Mortality, *See* Deaths

MRC, *See* Medical Reserve Corps

Mudflows, 10-32

Mustards, *See* Distilled mustard; Sulfur mustard

Myocardial infarction, 6-8

N

NAC, radioisotope decorporation therapies, countermeasures, *7-36*

National Disaster Life Support program, definition of disasters, 1-4

National Disaster Medical System, 1-19

description, Web site, 2-21

National Health Security Strategy, goals and objectives of, *1-3*

National Hurricane Center, 10-22, 10-26

National Incident Management System, 1-6

glossary term, G-2

Implementation Plan for Hospitals and Healthcare, 4-10–4-11

incident command system, 1-17–1-18

public health emergencies, 2-15

National Oceanic and Atmospheric Administration, 10-26

National Response Framework, 1-20

special needs populations, 3-19–3-20

National Voluntary Organizations Active in Disaster, 2-6

National Weather Service

hurricane warnings, 10-22

NOAA flood warnings, 10-16

winter storm warnings, 10-39–10-40

Natural disasters, 1-2, 1-4, 10-1–10-48, G-2; *See also* Disasters; Earthquakes and tsunamis; Floods; Heat emergencies; Hurricanes; Tornadoes; Volcanic Eruptions; Wildfires; Winter storms;

aftermath, 10-41–10-42

casualty types, by type of disaster, *10-7–10-8*

deaths from, 1-2

disruption of supplies, resources and utilities, 10-4

economic damage from, 10-3

global statistics, 10-3

glossary term, G-2

mass casualty management, 10-5–10-8

medical needs timeline, *10-6*

risks of, on the rise, 10-1

specific considerations in, 10-3–10-5

warnings (early, limited, and none), *10-4*

Negative phase impulse, *See* Explosion disasters

Neonatal care, *See* Children

Nerve agents, 8-26–8-33

diagnostic, clinical and treatment aspects, *8-29*

mnemonics for symptoms of exposure, 8-28

therapy by age groups, *8-31*

Nervous system

chemical nerve agents, 8-26–8-33

explosion-related injuries, 6-11

identification of chemical agent exposures, *8-11*

Neutropenia, nuclear and radiation disaster infection control, 7-31

New Orleans, *See* Hurricane Katrina

New York City, West Nile virus cluster, 1-16

NGOs, *See* Nongovernmental organizations

NHSS, *See* National Health Security Strategy

9-11 attacks, *See* September 11, 2001, attacks

Nitrogen mustard, 8-13

Nitroglycerine, 6-4

NOAA, *See* National Oceanic and Atmospheric Administration

Nongovernmental organizations, 2-6

Nongovernmental organizations, international organizations, 2-7–2-8

NRF, *See* National Response Framework

Nuclear disasters, *See also* Radiologic disasters;

casualty management, 7-18–7-36

characteristic injuries, 7-6–7-8

evacuation vs shelter in place, 7-11

explosions, 6-3

fallout zone, 7-11

fallout, 7-7–7-8, 7-10

hazard assessment, 7-9–7-11

incident management, 7-11–7-14

neutrons in proximity to ground zero, 7-4

nuclear detonations, 7-2, 7-3

panic, 7-15

public health measures, 7-37–7-41

radiation exposure, 7-3–7-6, 7-10

radiologic disasters compared to, 7-3

reactor materials, 7-14

situational awareness and detection, 7-8–7-9

thermal burns, 7-6–7-7

weapons proliferation, 7-2

workforce protection, 7-14–7-19

workforce shortages, 7-38

Nutrition, disaster responders, 4-8

O

Occupational injuries, See Disaster responders

Ocular blast injuries, *See* Eye injuries

Oil spill (BP, Gulf of Mexico), 8-36–8-37

Oklahoma City bombing, 6-5
secondary blast injuries, 6-7

Online listings, *See* under specific topics, *eg*, State government

Orbital injuries, explosion-related injuries, 6-11

Organizations, nongovernmental and private, *See* Nongovernmental organizations

Overpopulation, *See* Population

Oxidative phosphorylation, 8-22

P

Pacific Ocean
"Ring of Fire," 10-30
typhoons, 10-21

Pain, compartment syndrome symptom, 6-16

Pandemic, glossary term, G-2

Pandemics, *See* Communicable diseases

Panic attacks, 3-30

Parents, communicating with, 3-8

Peak overpressure, *See* Explosions

Pediatric care, *See* Children

Pediatric Triage Tape (triage system), 5-6

Penetrating trauma, *See* Trauma management

Personal protective equipment, 4-18–4-22, 4-26–4-27
difficulties and challenges when wearing, 4-21–4-22, 5-19
infection control precautions, 9-12, 9-13
levels (A, B, C, D), 4-20–4-21
nuclear and radiologic disasters 7-15, 7-16–7-17
required in casualty examination and assessment, 5-15, 5-19

Personnel, *See* Disaster responders; Health personnel

Petroleum disasters (BP oil spill), 8-36–8-37

PGOs, *See* Private governmental organizations

Phosgene
choking/pulmonary chemical agent, 8-17, 8-18–8-19
pediatric management of chemical agents, *8-34*

Phosgene oxime, diagnostic, clinical and treatment aspects, *8-16*

Phosphorus, nonradioactive, radioisotope decorporation therapies, countermeasures, *7-36*

Phosphorus 32, radioisotope decorporation therapies, countermeasures, *7-36*

Physical assault, *See* Violence

Physical examination, explosion injuries, 6-10, *6-11*

PIOs, *See* Public information officers

Plague, 9-6
bubonic, 9-6
pneumonic, 9-20–9-22
potential bioterrorism agents (symptoms, differential diagnoses), *9-11*
speedy therapy necessary, 9-14
therapy and prophylaxis in children, *9-32*

Planning, *See* DISASTER Paradigm™; Disaster response; PRE-DISASTER Paradigm™; Emergency operations plans; Planning and practice (PRE-DISASTER Paradigm™)

Planning and practice
all-hazards disaster casualty management (discussion points), 1-30
biologic disasters, 9-35
chemical disaster discussion points, 8-38
elements of PRE-DISASTER Paradigm™ described, A-A3
explosion disasters (discussion points), 6-22

natural disasters (discussion points), 10-42
predeployment preparation, 4-3–4-13
public health response (discussion points), 2-27
radiologic and nuclear disaster discussion points, 7-43
volunteers' "go-kits," 4-8–4-9

Plutonium, radioisotope decorporation therapies, countermeasures, *7-36*

Pneumonic plague, *See* Plague

Population, *See also* Vulnerable populations;
health needs in disasters, 3-1–3-25
mental health needs, 3-1, 3-2, 3-25–3-40
overpopulation and disasters, 1-2, 10-41
surge management, 2-19–2-22

Portal of entry, infectious agents, 9-4–9-5

Portal of exit, infectious agents, 9-3

Positive phase impulse, *See* Explosions

Post-traumatic stress disorder, *See* Stress

Potassium, *See* Hyperkalemia

Potassium iodide, 7-35, *7-36*

Potassium salt, 8-21

Power of Attorney for Finance, 4-6

Power of Attorney for Health Care, 4-6

PPE, *See* Personal protective equipment

Pralidoxime, *8-32*

Pralidoxime chloride, 8-30–8-31

PRE-DISASTER Paradigm™, 1-1, 1-2, 1-5–1-6, 1-30
biologic disasters, 9-35
chemical disaster discussion points, 8-38
description of elements of, A-A3
explosion disaster discussion points, 6-22–6-23
glossary term, G-2
public health response (discussion points), 2-27–2-29

radiologic and nuclear disaster discussion points, 7-43

workforce readiness and disaster deployment, 4-1–4-27

Pregnancy, 3-14–3-15

risks in nuclear and radiologic disasters, 7-39–7-40

Preparation and planning, *See* Competencies

Preparedness, *See* DISASTER Paradigm™

Preparedness planning, glossary term, G-2

Privacy, casualty reporting and, 5-24, 5-26

Private governmental organizations, 2-6

Professional liability, *See* Liability, professional

Prussian blue, radioisotope decorporation therapies, countermeasures, *7-36*

Psychological first aid, 10-14, 10-25

Psychosocial effects of disasters, *See* Mental health

Psychosocial emergencies, 6-8

Psychotic disorder, *See* Mental health

PTSD (post-traumatic stress disorder), *See* Stress

Public health, *See also* Communicable diseases, Disaster response;

agencies, organizations 2-4–2-8

balancing rights of privacy and needs to know, 2-14

bioterror attacks, 9-32–9-35

core functions, 2-3

crisis and emergency risk communication, 2-17–2-18

description of public health system, infrastructure, 2-2–2-4

disaster response, 2-1–2-30

disease outbreak monitoring, recognition, 9-9–9-10

emergencies (definition and description of), 1-4

emergency aftermath, recovery and beyond, 2-25–2-26

emergency declaration and powers, 2-9–2-11

epidemiologic surveillance and investigation, 2-11–2-14

equipment and supplies (Strategic National Stockpile), 2-22

essential services, 2-3–2-4

evacuations, 2-18–2-19

explosion disasters (pre-existing conditions and other risks), 6-20

federal agencies listed, 2-5–2-6

flood aftermath, 10-17

glossary term, G-2

heat emergencies, 10-20

hurricane aftermath, 10-25–10-26

incident management, 2-15–2-17

international health agencies and organizations, 2-7–2-8

isolation and quarantine, 2-10–2-11

local government agencies, 2-4–2-5

mission, 2-3

National Voluntary Organizations Active in Disaster, 2-6

nongovernmental organizations, 2-6

notable epidemics and pandemics, 9-6

notification of serious biologic outbreak, 9-11

nuclear and radiologic disasters, 7-37–7-41

online directory of local agencies, 2-5

online listing of state health departments, 2-5

population-based surge management, 2-19–2-22

population monitoring after nuclear and radiologic disasters, 7-40–7-41

priorities in disasters, 2-8–2-9

private governmental organizations, 2-6

rapid needs assessment (RNA), 2-13

reporting, 2-14–2-15

restrictions on individual liberty and public trust, 1-13

situational awareness and detection, 1-14–1-16

state government agencies, 2-5

volcanic eruptions, 10-35

wildfires, 10-37–10-38

winter storms, 10-41

Public health competencies, *See* Competencies

Public health law and ethics, *See* Competencies

Public information officers, 1-17

Pulmonary agents, *See* Respiratory system

Pulmonary blast injuries, *See* Respiratory system

Pulmonary disease, chronic obstructive, 6-8

Pyroclastic flows, 10-32

Q-R

Quarantine, glossary term, G-2

Radiation, 7-3–7-6, *See also* Nuclear disasters; Radiologic disasters;

acute radiation sickness (ARS), 7-22–7-23, 7-27, 7-28–7-32

acute radiation sickness phases, 7-30

acute radiation sickness subsyndromes, 7-28, *7-29–7-30*

cutaneous radiation syndrome, 7-27, 7-32–7-33

decorporation and countermeasures for radioisotope contamination, 7-34–7-35

dosage determination for casualties, 7-26

exposure and contamination, 7-5–7-6, 7-21–7-36

exposure monitoring and limits, 7-17–7-18

exposure of pregnant women and fetuses, 7-39–7-40

exposure risks, 7-10

exposure, skin effects, *7-24*

fallout zone, 7-11

field determination, 7-11–7-12

gray (Gy) absorbed dose, 7-4

internal radioisotope contamination, 7-33–7-36

levels and workforce protection, 7-15–7-16

measurement terms and units, 7-4–7-5

nuclear fallout, 7-7–7-8, 7-10, 7-11

radioactive decay products (alpha, beta, gamma), 7-4

radioactive iodine in food chain, 7-8

radioactive materials half-life, 7-4–7-5

sievert (Sv) effective dose, 7-4

toxicity, 7-7–7-8

Radioactive decay products, *See* Radiation

Radioisotope contamination, *See* Radiation

Radiologic disasters, 7-1–7-47; *See also* Nuclear disasters;

casualty management, 7-18–7-36

characteristic injuries, 7-6–7-8

evacuation vs shelter in place, 7-11

hazard assessment, 7-9–7-11

incident management, 7-11–7-14

nuclear disasters compared to, 7-3

nuclear reactor materials, 7-14

nuclear weapons proliferation, 7-2

panic, 7-15

public health measures, 7-37–7-41

radiation exposure, 7-3–7-6, 7-10

situational awareness and detection, 7-8–7-9

workforce protection, 7-14–7-19

workforce shortages, 7-38

Radium 226, radioisotope decorporation therapies, countermeasures, *7-36*

Rape, 3-15

Rapid needs assessment, 2-13

Recovery (DISASTER Paradigm™)

all-hazards disaster casualty management (discussion points), 1-32

benefits of communal events, 3-33

biologic disasters, 9-37

chemical disaster discussion points, 8-39

elements of DISASTER Paradigm™ described, A-A3

explosion disasters (discussion points), 6-23

health-care related considerations, 1-25–1-28

key elements of DISASTER Paradigm™, 1-6, 1-8, 1-32

natural disasters (discussion points), 10-44

planning, glossary term, G-2

public health emergencies, 2-25–2-26

public health response (discussion points), 2-29

radiologic and nuclear disaster discussion points, 7-45

Recovery competencies (BDLS® course), *See* Competencies

Red Cross, *See* American Red Cross; International Red Cross and Red Crescent Movement

Religious issues, 5-26

Remains (mass fatalities), *See* Mass casualty incidents

Remote sensing, 1-11

Renal failure, crush injuries, 6-15

Renal injuries, explosion-related injuries, 6-11

Reservoir, description of, 9-3

Resilience (PRE-DISASTER Paradigm™), 1-28, 1-30, 2-25–2-26

all-hazards disaster casualty management (discussion points), 1-30

biologic disasters, 9-35

chemical disaster discussion points, 8-38

elements of PRE-DISASTER Paradigm™ described, A-A3

explosion disasters (discussion points), 6-22

natural disasters (discussion points), 10-42

PRE-DISASTER Paradigm™, 1-5–1-6, 1-30

public health response (discussion points), 2-27

radiologic and nuclear disaster discussion points, 7-43

Resource allocation, 1-13

Respirators

air-purifying, 4-19

infection control precautions, 9-12, 9-13

levels A, B and C, 4-20–4-21, 7-17

nuclear and radiologic disasters, 7-16–7-17

Respiratory distress, 6-8

Respiratory system

arterial gas embolism, 6-12–6-13

asthma and, 6-8

common explosion-related injuries, 6-11–6-12

COPD and, 6-8

explosion-related injuries, 6-11

identification of chemical agent exposures, 8-11

inhalation injuries, 6-8

inhalational anthrax, 9-16

mechanical ventilation, 6-12

pulmonary agents (chemicals), 8-16–8-19, *8-20*

respiratory distress, 6-8

traumatic asphyxiation, 6-13–6-14

volcanic eruption injuries, 10-7, 10-33, 10-34

wildfires, 10-8, 10-37

Responders, *See* Disaster responders

Retinal burns, 7-7

Richter scale, 10-9

Risk, differentiation between and hazard and, 1-10

Risk awareness, *See* Safety and security

Risk communication

notification of serious biologic outbreak, 9-11

nuclear and radiologic disasters, 7-37–7-41

principles, rules, 2-17–2-18

Risks, *See* Hazard assessment

S

Safety and security (DISASTER Paradigm™)

all-hazards disaster casualty management (discussion points), 1-31

biologic disasters, 9-36

chemical disaster discussion points, 8-39

dangers to disaster responders ("second hit"), 6-10

disaster responders' risk awareness and mitigation, 4-13–4-15

disaster workforce protection, 4-16–4-22

elements of DISASTER Paradigm™ described, A-A3

explosion disasters (discussion points), 6-23

explosion disasters, 6-9–6-10

key elements of DISASTER Paradigm™, 1-6, 1-7, 1-31

natural disasters (discussion points), 10-43

public health response (discussion points), 2-28

radiologic and nuclear disaster discussion points, 7-44

related BDLS® course chapters and objectives, A-B-5

workforce protection following nuclear and radiologic disasters, 7-14–7-19

Safety officer, 1-17

SALT (triage system), 5-6, 5-12–5-14

glossary term, G-2

SAMPLE, See Mass casualty incidents

Sanitation

drinking water, 2-23

human waste, 2-25

responders' personal hygiene, 4-13

women's needs, 3-14

Sarin

pediatric management of chemical agents, 8-34

subway attack, 8-35–8-36

SARS, See Severe acute respiratory syndrome

Scope of practice, See Licensure and scope of practice

Sea-level rises, 10-15

SEIRV triage model, 9-13, G-2

Self-esteem, depression symptoms, 3-29

Semtex, 6-4

September 11, 2001 attacks, fatalities and injuries, 6-3

Severe acute respiratory syndrome, 9-22–9-23

Sexual assault, 3-15

Shelter, See Housing

Shigellosis, potential bioterrorism agents (symptoms, differential diagnoses), 9-11

Shock, children, 3-4, 3-5

Sichuan earthquake (2008), 10-9

SIEVE (triage system), 5-6

Sievert (Sv; effective radiation dose), See Radiation

Simple Triage and Rapid Treatment (START) (triage system), 5-6

Situational awareness, See Detection

Skin

blistering agents, 8-13–8-16

cutaneous anthrax, 9-15–9-16

cutaneous radiation syndrome, 7-27, 7-32–7-33

identification of chemical agent exposures, 8-11

radiation exposure effects, 7-24, 7-24–7-25, 7-27, 7-32–7-33

Sleep problems

depression symptoms, 3-29

disaster responders, 4-7

SLUDGEM (nerve agent mnemonic), 8-28

Smallpox, 9-23–9-26

potential bioterrorism agents (symptoms, differential diagnoses), 9-11

therapy and prophylaxis in children, 9-31

SNS, See Strategic National Stockpile

Social distancing, glossary term, G-2

Sodium cyanide, 8-21–8-22

Soman, pediatric management of chemical agents, 8-34

Special needs, See Children; Vulnerable populations

Stafford Act, 2-20

START (Simple Triage and Rapid Treatment) (triage system), 5-6

State government

online listing of health departments, 2-5

public health emergency powers, 2-10

public health reporting, 2-14–2-15

Stem cell transplantation, radiation casualties, 7-32

Storm surges, 10-21

Strategic National Stockpile, 1-19, 1-21, 2-22

Stress, 3-27–3-28

acute stress disorder, 3-28–3-29

critical incident debriefing (not recommended), 3-34

demobilization and deployment-related, 4-25–4-26, 4-27

disaster responders, 4-2

PTSD (post-traumatic stress disorder), 3-30, 3-36

PTSD and earthquakes, 10-13–10-14

PTSD and explosion disasters, 6-20

Strontium 90, radioisotope decorporation therapies, countermeasures, 7-36

Structural collapse, See Building collapses

Substance abuse, 3-30-3-31

Suicide, 3-29, 3-31

Sulfur dioxide, 10-34

Sulfur mustard, 8-13

diagnostic, clinical, treatment aspects, 8-15

pediatric management of chemical agents, 8-34

Supervision, See Vulnerable populations

Supplies

pediatric, 3-9

Strategic National Stockpile, 2-22

"Supply and demand," See Surge capacity

Support (DISASTER Paradigm™), See also Emergency Support Functions;

all-hazards disaster casualty management (discussion points), 1-31

biologic disasters, 9-36

chemical disaster discussion points, 8-39

elements of DISASTER Paradigm™ described, A-A3

explosion disasters (discussion points), 6-23

health-related considerations, 1-19–1-20

key elements of DISASTER Paradigm™, 1-6, 1-7, 1-31

natural disasters (discussion points), 10-43

nuclear and radiologic disasters, 7-12

public health response (discussion points), 2-28

radiologic and nuclear disaster discussion points, 7-44

Support competencies (BDLS® course), *See* Competencies

Surge capacity, 1-12–1-13

alternative care environment, 1-23, 1-24

assessment, 1-10

capacity assessment (glossary term), G-1

continuum, 1-23

conventional, contingency and crisis capacity, 1-23

definition, 1-12

glossary term, G-2

health-related considerations, 1-20–1-24

inadequacy of US health facilities, 1-22

natural disasters, 10-5

population-based surge management, 2-19–2-22

surge capability and, 1-12

Surveillance, epidemiologic, *See* Communicable diseases; Public health

Susceptible host, *See* Communicable diseases

Sv (effective radiation dose), *See* Radiation

T

Tabun, pediatric management of chemical agents, *8-34*

TATP, *See* Triacetone triphosphate (TATP)

Teamwork, 4-4

Teenagers, *See* Adolescents

Terminology, *See* Definitions

Terrorism, *See also* Bioterrorism;

explosive devices, 6-2

glossary term, G-2

targeting of explosion disaster responders, 6-9

Tokyo sarin subway attack, 8-35–8-36

Thermal burns, *See* Burns

Thyroid gland, internal radioisotope contamination and, 7-33–7-36

TNT, 6-4

Tokyo sarin subway attack, 8-35–8-36

Tornadoes, 10-26–10-30

key facts about, 10-27

personal safety measures, protective actions, *10-30*

severe outbreaks in 2011, 10-26–10-27

types and causes of deaths, injuries, *10-7*

Tourniquets, 6-14

avoidance in penetrating ballistic injuries, 6-19

Toxic agents, particular dangers to children, 3-3, 3-4, 3-5

Toxidrome, glossary term, G-2

Toxidromes, *See* Chemical disasters

Training, *See* Education and training

Transportation, *See also* Evacuation (DISASTER Paradigm™);

casualties, 5-19–5-20

nuclear and radiologic casualties, 7-20–7-21

vulnerable and special needs populations, 3-19

Trauma management, 6-1–6-27, *See also* Triage and treatment;

blast injuries, 6-10–6-20

blunt ballistic injuries, 6-18

blunt trauma, 6-7, 6-8

compartment syndrome, 6-16–6-17

crush injuries and crush syndrome, 6-15–6-16

earthquakes and tsunamis, 10-7, 10-11–10-12

floods, 10-16–10-17

heat emergencies, 10-19–10-20

hurricanes, 10-7, 10-23–10-25

injuries following nuclear and radiologic disasters, 7-6

natural disasters, 10-5–10-8

nuclear and radiation disasters, 7-25–7-26

penetrating ballistic injuries, 6-19

penetrating stabs or impalement, 6-20

penetrating trauma, 6-7

tornadoes, 10-7, 10-29

tourniquets, 6-14

types of injuries by type of natural disaster, *10-7–10-8*

volcanic eruptions, 10-32–10-34

wound management, 10-6, 10-8

Triacetone triphosphate (TATP), 6-4

Triage and treatment (DISASTER Paradigm™), *See also* Trauma management;

A, B, C casualty assessment (airway, breathing, circulation), 5-15-5-17

acute radiation syndrome, cutaneous radiation syndrome, 7-28–7-33

all-hazards disaster casualty management (discussion points), 1-31–1-32

biologic disasters, 9-36–9-37

chemical disaster discussion points, 8-39

chemical disasters, 8-8–8-33

children in chemical disasters, 8-33–8-34

disease outbreaks, 9-13–9-14

elements of DISASTER Paradigm™ described, A-A3

emesis and diarrhea following nuclear and radiation disasters, 7-30

examples of symptoms and injuries correlated with triage categories, 5-8–5-10

explosion disasters (discussion points), 6-23

explosion injuries, 6-10–6-20

ID-MED triage categories (immediate, delayed, minimal, expectant, dead), 5-7–5-11

internal radioisotope contamination, 7-33–7-36

internal radioisotope contamination, 7-33–7-36

key elements of DISASTER Paradigm™, 1-6, 1-7–1-8, 1-31–1-32

mass casualty incidents, 5-3–5-14

natural disasters (discussion points), 10-43

nuclear and radiologic casualties, 7-19–7-36

primary triage, 5-5

psychological, 3-31–3-32, 3-34

public health response (discussion points), 2-28

radiation dose effect, 7-24

radiologic and nuclear disaster discussion points, 7-44–7-45

SALT methodology, 5-12–5-14

secondary triage, 5-5

SEIRV triage model for infectious diseases, 9-13

self-evacuation of casualties, 5-4–5-5

SIEVE triage system, 5-6

specific chemical agents, 8-12–8-33

tertiary triage, 5-5

triage as dynamic and continuous process, 5-5

triage color codes and tags (red, yellow, green, gray, black), 5-7–5-11

triage (glossary term), G-2

use of same, common terminology and methodology, 5-6

2,4,6-trinitrotoluene (TNT), 6-4

Tritium, radioisotope decorporation therapies, countermeasures, *7-36*

Trust, 1-13

Tsunamis, *See* Earthquakes and tsunamis

Tularemia, 9-26–9-28

Tympanic membrane, 6-17

Typhoons, *See* Hurricanes

U

Union Carbide Bhopal India chemical disaster, 8-35

United Nations, 2-7

Universal precautions, *See* Communicable diseases

Uranium, radioisotope decorporation therapies, countermeasures, *7-36*

Urbanization, 10-41

US agencies beginning with "National," *See headings at* National

US Agency for International Development, 2-7

US Centers for Disease Control and Prevention, *See also* Strategic National Stockpile;

crisis and emergency risk communication, 2-17–2-18

Epidemic Intelligence Service, 2-21–2-22

US Forest Service, 10-38

US Geological Survey, 10-11

US government

federal public health agencies, 2-5–2-6

population-based surge management, 2-20–2-22

Web sites for federal agencies, 2-5–2-6

US Health and Human Services Department

crisis and emergency risk communication, 2-17–2-18

emergency powers, 2-10

public health activities, 2-5–2-6

US Medical Reserve Corps, *See* Medical Reserve Corps

US National…*See headings beginning with* National

US Public Health Service, Commissioned Corps, description, Web site, 2-21

V

V-agents, *See* Nerve agents

Variola major, *See* Smallpox

Vector-mediated disease transmission, 9-4

Ventilation, mechanical, 6-12

Vesicants, 8-13–8-16

Violence, physical assault of women, 3-15

Viral hemorrhagic fevers, 9-28–9-30

Viruses, *See* Communicable diseases

Visual impairment, 3-20–3-21

Volcanic eruptions, 10-30–10-35

ash, 10-32, 10-33

notable historic eruptions showing major causes of deaths, injuries, 10-31

types and causes of deaths, injuries, *10-7*

types of, 10-30–10-31

Voluntary organizations, *See* Nongovernmental organizations

Volunteers, 4-4; *See also* Disaster responders; Health personnel;

activation and mobilization, 4-15–4-16

legal issues for health personnel, 4-11–4-13

personal equipment and packing ("go kits"), 4-8–4-9

personal health and wellness, 4-7–4-8

pre-approvals for work leave, 4-5

predeployment education and training, 4-9–4-11

professional credentials and equipment, 4-9

Vulnerable populations, *See also* Children; Chronic diseases; Disabilities; Mental health; Women;

assessment, 1-10–1-12

child and adolescent mental problems, 3-35–3-36

children, 3-2–3-13

chronic disease, 3-16–3-18

communication challenges, 3-20–3-21

community registries, 3-24

decontamination, 4-22–4-26

definitions for special needs populations, 3-19–3-20

description of groups in, 1-11–1-12

disaster-prone regions, 1-2

evacuation, 2-19, 3-21–3-22

explosions, 6-2

functional disabilities, 3-18–3-19

health care access, 3-24

health needs in disasters, 3-1–3-25

heat emergencies, 10-7

hurricanes and, 10-23

issues regarding independence, communication, transportation, supervision, medical care, 3-19–3-20

mental health needs, 3-1, 3-2, 3-25–3-40

nuclear and radiologic disasters, 7-38–7-40

psychological distress, 3-24

risk analysis, 1-10

sheltering needs, 3-22–3-23

surge management, 2-19–2-22

winter storms, 10-41

women, 3-13–3-16

VX (nerve agent), 8-26-8-27, 8-29

pediatric management of chemical agents, *8-34*

W-Z

War

conflict-based disaster, glossary term, G-1

disaster classification, 1-4

Warm zones, 4-18

Warning systems, *See* Detection (DISASTER Paradigm™)

Waste management, 2-25

Water solubility, choking/pulmonary chemical agents, 8-17–8-18

Water supply, 2-23

Web sites, *See* under specific topics, *eg*, US government

Weight change, depression symptoms, 3-29

West Nile virus, 1-16

Wildfires, 10-35–10-38

controlled burns, 10-38

environmental effects, 10-36

firebreaks, 10-38

floods in aftermath of, 10-36

types and causes of deaths, injuries, *10-8*

Wills (estate disposition), 4-6

Winter storms, 10-38–10-41

types and causes of deaths, injuries, *10-8*

Women, 3-13–3-16

Women

physical and sexual assault, 3-15

pregnant, 3-14–3-15, 7-39–7-40

psychological impact of disasters, 3-15–3-16

sanitation and hygiene, 3-14

separation of sexes, 5-26

Workforce, *See* Disaster responders; Health personnel

World health, *See* International health

World Health Organization, 2-7, 10-3

World War I, 9-7

chemical agents in, 8-13, 8-17

influenza/Spanish flu, 9-6

World War II

nerve agents, 8-26–8-27

Wounds, *See* Trauma management

Yellowstone fire (1988), 10-37

Yersinia pestis, *See* Plague, pneumonic

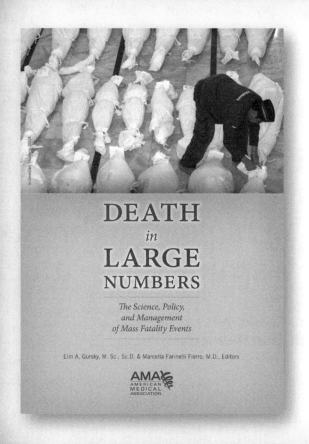

Comprehensive one-stop guide in dealing with mass fatality events

DEATH IN LARGE NUMBERS:
The Science, Policy, and Management of Mass Fatality Events

Written by respected leaders and experts in their fields who have made mass fatality policy and planning a priority in their careers, *Death in Large Numbers* provides the most current information on diagnostics and technologies. It offers epidemiological and outbreak scenarios as context, and pertains to current thought in national policy and strategy considerations.

- **Scientific information**—offers a valuable resource to practitioners of body identification, and response and recovery activities following a mass fatality incident

- **Relevant and unique issues**—address the science, policy implications, and management strategies

- **Tables and figures**—serve as quick resources with information ranging from historical timelines to radiological images for identification

- Forward by The Honorable Michael Chertoff, the nation's second United States Secretary of Homeland Security and co-author of the USA PATRIOT Act.

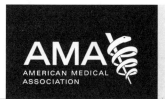

Visit amabookstore.com
or call (800) 621-8335 to order.

"Written and assembled by the leading experts in the field—this book does the essential work of updating our knowledge about biological weapons and documenting the lessons learned from the anthrax attacks of October 2001. It's a must-read for any health professional whom may be called upon to respond to a future bioterrorist attack."

Senator Bill Frist, MD, Author of "When Every Moment Counts"

Prompt recognition of biological threats can provide an early warning to an attack

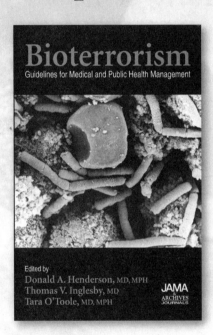

Bioterrorism: Guidelines for Medical and Public Health Management

Edited by leading experts in their field, this peer-reviewed clinical resource provides guidelines and recommendations for the medical and public health community following a bioterrorist attack. *Bioterrorism* guides health care personnel through diagnosis and management of infections caused by Category A agents used in bioterror weapons. The idea of early recognition of organisms or toxins that cause such uncommon illnesses as anthrax, smallpox, plague, and viral hemorrhagic fevers can provide a community with an early warning of an attack and allow health care personnel to take steps to protect the public from further spread of infection.

Bioterrorism presents:

- Each disease/syndrome in logical and practically grounded order
- History and potential for each disease/syndrome as a biological weapon
- Epidemiology and microbiology
- Pathogenesis and clinical presentation
- Diagnosis, treatment, prevention and prophylaxis
- Infection control and decontamination
- Specific diseases covered include Category A agents: anthrax, smallpox, plague, botulinum toxin and tularemia
- Seminal articles describing the first bioterrorist attack with anthrax in the United States and an article on the principles of quarantine and isolation

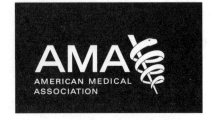

Visit **amabookstore.com**
or call **(800) 621-8335** to order.